Understand Cancer

Research and Treatment

Understand Cancer – Research and Treatment

Publisher: iConcept Press Ltd.

ISBN: 978-1-922227-386

Printed in the United States of America

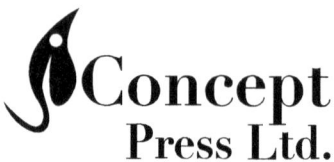

𝄐Concept
Press Ltd.

www.iconceptpress.com

Contents

Preface

Cancer is a broad group of diseases involving unregulated cell growth, in which cells divide and grow uncontrollably, forming malignant tumors, and invade nearby parts of the body. Cancer may also spread to different parts of the body through the lymphatic system or the bloodstream. *Understand Cancer – Research and Treatment* discusses some recent advances in cancer research and treatment methods.

There are totally 14 chapters in this book. In Chapter 1, the biological significance of a duplicated GGAA motif in the human gene promoter is discussed. The imbalance in the GGAA motif dependent transcription may lead to dysregulation of mitochondrial function, which subsequently could cause cancer generation. Chapter 2 reviewed the redefined mutational landscape of acute lymphoblastic leukemia as drawn by next generation sequencing technology in the last decade. It also discussed how the massively parallel sequencing works, and the currently available platforms, underlying their strengths and their applications to cancer genomics. Chapter 3 is dedicated to tumor vascularization aiming to show its complexity and explaining the central role of VEGF and its receptors in this phenomenon. This complexity is corrobrated by the failure of anti-angiogenic therapy, showing once again that the dynamic network of vessels formation into and within a malignant neoplasia is far from being completely known. Chapter 4 focuses on the presentation and discussion of existing literature in the field of Bcl2 and tumor angiogenesis, and especially provide an overview of the field of tumor angiogenesis research assisted with LCM. In addition, it presents a brief protocol of cDNA synthesis following immune-LCM from paraffin-embedded tissue sections.

Chapter 5 proposes a stem cell therapy for malignant tumors. The co-transplantation of thymus and stem cells are discussed, which is better than stem cell transplantation only as therapy for malignant tumors. Chapter 6 reviews the anti-cancer effect of Coptidis Rhizoma and berberine. They can be summarized as preventing carcinogenesis, inhibiting proliferation, inducing apoptosis, preventing angiogenesis, and suppressing migration and invasion. In addition, their preventive and therapeutic effects in hepatocellular carcinoma will be highlighted as well. Chapter 7 focuses on the altered status of heme and iron metabolism, transport, uptake, and metabolism in cancer, and thus how heme and iron manipulation is a plausible target of cancer prevention and treatment. Chapter 8 discusses the critical activity of p53 (the DNA damage monitor gene) and the DNA repair system – with a focus on the nucleotide excision repair (NER) pathway – in acquired chemo-resistance in cancer treatment. One improved clinical outcome might be achieved by targeting the key regulators/controllers in the development of resistance during chemotherapy.

Chapter 9 attempts to identify indications for tomosynthesis technique for chest imaging. Moreover, the author performed experiments to measure the pulmonary nodules detection (clinical and phantom study) capabilities of the tomosynthesis imaging system for use as an effective screening method and compared the results with those of radiography and computed tomography imaging. Chapter 10 reviews the current standard treatments and future research directions of gallbladder cancer. Specifically, molecular genetics of gallbladder carcinomas and precursor lesions including abnormalities of adenosine triphosphate-binding cassette transporter ABCG8, membrane-bound enzyme ADAM-17 of multi-functional gene family, and other genes including p53, COX2, XPC, and RASSF1A are covered. Chapter 11 discusses oncofetal GPC-3 as a specific biomarker for HCC diagnosis and a valuable target for HCC gene therapy through the Wnt/beta-catenin and hedgehog singling pathways. Chapter 12 gives a comprehensive review in the current thinking Oral Cavity Tumors. It discusses generalities of the disease process, diagnostic workup and current management options available for oral squamous cell carcinomas.

In Chapter 13, the morbidity of inguinofemoral lympadenectomy through the triple incision technique with the possible predictors of its development and the technique modifications aiming at a lower morbidity rate are highlighted and discussed. Moreover, the advantages and disadvantages of the sentinel lymph node over the triple incision technique are covered. Chapter 14 reviews the literature on the various cervical tumors/ growths. Around ten high resolution clinical and histological pictures from the author's collection would be included.

Editing and publishing a book is never an easy task. Each chapter in this book has gone through a peer review, a selection and an editing process so as to guarantee its quality. Without the supports and contributions of the authors and reviewers, this book can never be able to complete. We would like to thank all of the authors in this book and all of the reviewers who participated in the reviewing process: Shahla Alalaf, Frank Arfuso, Manjit Singh Bal, Giovanni Blandino, Dr. Koushik Chattopadhyay, Lee-Young Chau, Xiaohong Chen, Jean E. Crabtree, Fabrizio Dal Piaz, Françoise Debierre-Grockiego, Dr. Prasanna R. Deshpande, Muzeyyen Duran, Diana English, Heng-Yu Fan, Giovanna Giordano, Salvatore Gizzo, Naoki Hashimoto, ATSUSHI IMAI, Tavan Janvilisri, Vijay K. Kalra, Koji Kawakami, Benjamin Kefas, Katsumasa Kuroi, Bin Li, Lishu Li, XIAOMING LI, Fabio Luciani, Maria Lyra, Thumuluru Kavitha Madhuri, Giovanni Marfia, Atsuko Masumi, Masaaki Miyazawa, Anthony Oyekunle, Kajsa Paulsson, Maria Marjorette O. Peña, Paola Perego, Roman Pfister, James R. Reed, Bernhard Schaller, Jörg D. Seebach, Prachi Sharma, Cornelis F. M. Sier, Daniel Sinnett, Luís Ricardo Martinhão Souto, Yutaka Suzuki, Gaurav Tomar, Aruna V Vanikar, Eric Vela, Vaclav Vetvicka, Hao Wen, Erxi Wu, Wei-Zhong Wu, Xifeng Wu, Samantha M. Yeligar, Ae-Kyung Yi, Yoshihito Yokoyama, Linquan Zang, Zong-De Zhang and Quan Zhao. We hope that you, the reader, will find this book interesting and useful. Any advices please feel free and are always welcome to tell us.

iConcept Press Editorial Office

January 2016

Possible Roles of a Duplicated GGAA Motif as a Driver *Cis*-element for Cancer-associated Genes

Fumiaki Uchiumi[*], Steven D. Larsen[†] and Sei-ichi Tanuma[‡]

1   Introduction

Transcription is a fundamental biological process in all living cells to synthesize mRNAs that are translated into proteins. In eukaryotic cells, formation of pre-initiation complex, including RNA polymerase II (RNA pol II), has been acknowledged as a consensus first step of transcription reaction from TATA-box (Carey *et al.*, 2009). Recent studies in yeast genomics indicated that TATA-like elements are frequently found near transcription start site (TSS) of yeast genes (Rhee & Pugh, 2012). However, obvious TATA boxes or TATA like sequences are not always found in close proximity of TSSs of human genes. It has been estimated that 76% of upstream regions of human genes could be classified as TATA-less promoters (Yang *et al.*, 2007). From a bioinformatic analysis, we have reported that 81% of the promoters having at least one duplicated 14-bp, in a 2.0-kbp upstream region contain overlapped GGAA (TTCC) motifs within 500-bp upstream but have no authentic TATA-boxes (Uchiumi *et al.*, 2011b). The GGAA motif containing sequences are recognized and bound by ETS family proteins (Oikawa & Yamada, 2003), (Hsu *et al.*, 2004). Moreover, genome wide ChIP analysis estimated that promoter regions of human genes are very frequently occupied with ETS family or GGAA-binding proteins (Hollenhorst *et al.*, 2007). This transcription system enables competitive binding of different GGAA-binding proteins to the same duplicated or overlapped GGAA sequences in the 5′-flanking region of a specific gene. Duplication of the GGAA-motif might be advantageous to organisms to control gene expression just dependent on the expression profile of the GGAA-binding proteins in the cells. Further surveillance of the 5′-upstream regions of DNA repair-, interferon response-, and mitochondrial function-associated genes revealed that their expression regulatory regions contain duplicated GGAA motifs near the TSSs (Uchiumi *et al.*, 2013b), (Uchiumi *et al.*, 2013c), (Uchiumi *et al.*, 2015). The observations imply that some of the characteristics of cancer, including DNA damage and mutations, inflammation, and failure in mitochondrial respiratory system, could be caused by changes in the profile of the GGAA (TTCC)-binding factors. In this chapter, we will focus on the duplicated GGAA-motifs near TSSs of various human genes and propose possible mechanisms for transcription regulatory systems that cause cancer and malignant tumors, providing an insight into a novel treatment for cancer by transcription targeted gene-therapy.

[*] Department of Gene Regulation, Faculty of Pharmaceutical Sciences and Research Center for RNA Science, RIST, Tokyo University of Science, Japan

[†] Research Center for RNA Science, RIST, Tokyo University of Science, Japan

[‡] Department of Biochemistry, Faculty of Pharmaceutical Sciences and Research Center for RNA Science, RIST, Tokyo University of Science, Japan

2   Identification of GGAA-motifs Adjacent to TSSs of Various Genes

The GGAA-motifs are the ETS-targets that are very frequently found within a variety of regulatory region of human genes (Xie *et al.*, 2005), (Sementchenko & Watson, 2000). We found the duplicated GGAA-motifs in the promoter regions of the *PARG*, *IGHMBP2*, and *RB1* that are up-regulated during TPA-induced HL-60 cell differentiation into macrophage like cells (Uchiumi *et al.*, 2011b). The *RB1* gene belongs to a group of TPA-inducible late genes (Zheng *et al.*, 2002), and its encoding protein RB1 is involved in the regulation of cell fate by inducing differentiation (Goodrich, 2006). Also, the 5′-upstream regions of the *IL1R1*, *IL1R2*, *IL1RAPL2*, *S100A3*, *eIF3A*, *ECM1*, and the macrophage marker *CD68* (O'Reilly *et al.*, 2003) genes have tandem repeated GGAA (TTCC)-motifs. These observations suggest that duplicated GGAA motifs regulate genes that are up-regulated during TPA-induced differentiation of HL-60 into macrophage like cells. Comparison of the sequence in the 5′-upstream regions of the *PARG*, *IGHMBP2*, *ATR*, *XPB*, *RTEL*, and *RB1* genes determined a tentative consensus 14-bp as 5′-(A/G/C)N(A/G/C)(C/G)(C/G)**GGAA**(A/G)(C/T)(G/C/T)(A/G/C)(A/G/C)-3′ (Uchiumi *et al.*, 2010). Surveillance of this 14-bp sequence within 500-bp from TSSs of human genes retrieved nearly two hundred genes, including *TRAF1*, *TNFSF12*, and *TNFSF13* (Uchiumi *et al.*, 2011b). Notably, the human *TNF* gene promoter contains a duplication of the GGAA-motif (Steer *et al.*, 2000), implying that the motif plays a role in response to TNF. Several of these retrieved gene-encoding proteins are classified into groups such that are involved in DNA-repair, interferon (IFN)-response, glucose metabolism, mitochondrial functions, and apoptosis. Other features of the upstream regions of these genes are that some of them have bidirectional partner genes, linked in a head-head configuration, and that most of them have no obvious TATA-box or TATA-like elements near TSSs (Table 1).

3   Duplicated GGAA-motifs in the DNA Repair Factor Encoding Gene Promoters

The duplicated GGAA-motif is present in the promoter region of the human *PARP1* gene, encoding poly(ADP-ribose) polymerase (Yokoyama *et al.*, 1990), (Uchiumi *et al.*, 2013a). Moreover, the GGAA duplication is contained in the 5′-regulatory region of the human *XRCC1* gene, which encodes a single strand break repair factor accumulating at poly(ADP-ribose)s that are synthesized by the PARP enzyme (Wei *et al.*, 2013). Furthermore, the duplicated GGAA-motifs are located near the TSS of the *ADPRHL2* (*ARH3*) gene, encoding poly(ADP-ribose) degrading enzyme that localizes mainly in mitochondria (Niere *et al.*, 2012). GGAA-duplication is found near the TSS of the *ZC3HAV1* gene that encodes PARP13, an anti-viral RNA binding protein (Leung *et al.*, 2012), (Gibson & Kraus, 2012). Taken together, these findings suggested that expression of genes encoding poly(ADP-ribose)-mediated DNA repair factors are commonly regulated by the duplicated GGAA-motifs.

    The human *WRN* and *TERT* promoters positively respond to 2-deoxy-D-glucose (2DG), which is a caloric restriction (CR) mimetic drug having the effect of elongating life span in several organisms (Zhou *et al.*, 2009). Similar results were obtained with *trans*-resveratrol (Rsv), which is a natural polyphenolic compound having effects on various organisms to elongate life spans (Uchiumi *et al.*, 2011a). These 5′-flanking regions of the telomere maintenance factor-encoding genes harbor duplicated GGAA-motifs (Zhou *et al.*, 2009). Hence, we tentatively concluded that expression of these genes are up-regulated by CR or CR mimetic drugs, and hypothesized that telomere maintenance- and DNA repair-factor encoding genes are regulated by the duplicated GGAA-motifs in their promoter regions. Next, we further checked the 5′-regulatory regions of the *XPB, RB1, RTEL1, ATR, TP53,* and *CDKN1A (p21)* genes to confirm that they contain the GGAA duplications near TSSs (Table 1).

Functions	Gene
Apoptosis	*ABL1, AEN, APC, BARD1, BCL2, CASP1, DFFA, DAPK, FAS (TNFRSF6), FASLG (TNFSF6), HMGB2, PDCD1, PIM3, SUMO1, TP53, XIAP …*
ATP synthase	*ATP5A1, ATP5C1, ATP5F1, ATP5H, ATP5J*
Cell adhesion	*CDH5, CTGF (CCN2), ICAM2, UTRN*
Cytochrome c oxidase	*COX10, COX15, COX17, SCO1*
DNA repair (BER)	*APC, APEX1, BRCA1, CDKN1A, CHEK1, ERCC1, ERCC2, FEN1, LIG1, NBN …*
DNA repair (NER)	*ATR, CDKN1A, PARP1, ERCC1-4, GTF2H1-3, PARP1, POLD1, POLD3, POLD4 …*
DNA repair (TCR)	*APEX1, BRCA1, CDK1/2, CDKN1A, CDKN2A, ERCC1-4, GTF2H1-3, LIG1, MRE11*
DNA (DSB) repair	*APC, APEX1, ATM, ATR, BLM, BRCA1, BRCA2, CHEK1, DCLRE1A-C, DDX1 …*
Endocrine system	*GIP, INSIG2, LXRB (NR1H2)*
FA core complex	Genes encoding protein components of the Fanconi anemia (FA) core complex
Glucose metabolism	*G6PD, GYS1, SLC2A13*
IFN response	*CD40 (TNFSF5), IRF2BP2, OAS1, OASL, IL18, RUNX1, STAT3, TREX1 …*
Interleukin signal	*IL1B, IL1R1, IL1R2, IL1RAPL2, IL2, IL2RB, IL7R*
Macrophage marker	*CD68*
Megakaryocyte marker	*ITGA2B (CD41)*
NAD⁺ synthesis	*NAMPT*
NADH dehydrogenase	*NDUFA1-3, NDUFB3, NDUFB9, NDUFC1, NDUFS1*
Sirtuins	*SIRT1, SIRT3*
Sumoylation	*SUMO1, UBA1*
TCA cycle	*ACLY, ACO2, CS, FH, IDH1, IDH3A, IDH3B, SUCLG1, SDHAF2, SDHB, SDHD*
TGF-beta signal	*TGFBR2*
TNF signal	*TNF, TRAF1, TNFSF12, TNFSF13*
Tumor suppressor	*CDKN1A, RB1, TP53*
Tumor invasion	*MMP3, MMP7*
Transcription	*BTAF1, GTF2A1, GTF2B, IGHMBP2, MYBBP1A, RUNX1, SP1, SPI1 (PU.1), TAF1, TAF12, TBP*
Ubiquitination	*BTRC, FANCD2, OTUB1, UBB, UBC, UBXN1, USP19, USP28, USP32, USP47 …*

Table 1: Human genes that contain duplicated GGAA motifs in their 5′-flanking regions.

Several of them are linked with both the telomere maintenance and mitochondrial functions. We also confirmed that duplicated GGAA-motifs are contained near TSSs of the *ATM, BRCA1,* and *FANCD2* genes, which have bidirectional partner genes (Table 1). For instance, *ATM/NPAT, BRCA1/NBR2, FANCD2/CIDECP,* and *TP53/WRAP53* are found in head-

head configured gene pairs. These DNA-repair factor-encoding genes are hypothesized to be simultaneously regulated by duplicated GGAA-motifs.

4   Duplicated GGAA-motifs in the Interferon Stimulated Gene (ISG) Promoters

Innate immune system ligands are up-regulated by DNA damage signaling pathway (Gasser *et al.*, 2005). Moreover, TTCC-duplication is found adjacent to the TSS of the human *TP53* gene (Sementchenko & Watson, 2000), which expression is regulated by IFN-α and β (Takaoka *et al.*, 2003). IRF1 was reported to be a negative regulator for the human *TERT* promoter in response to IFN-γ (Lee *et al.*, 2003). In addition, IRF-5 has been shown to up-regulate expression of DNA-repair and apoptosis-associated genes (Barnes *et al.*, 2003). DNA damage initiates an immune response to regulate DNA repair genes (Xiong & Gasser, 2011). Therefore, we hypothesized that immune responses and DNA damage responses might be depending on each other, and that the overlapped GGAA-motifs may provoke expression of genes encoding DNA repair-associated factors in response to IFN-induced signals. Previous studies revealed that the duplication of GGAA-motifs are present in the 5′-upstream of the ISGs, such as *ISG15* (Perry *et al.*, 1999), *TAP1* (Rouyez *et al.*, 2005), and *CD40 (TNFRSF5)* (Nguyen & Benveniste, 2000). We previously confirmed the GGAA-motifs in the promoter regions of cytokine signal associated genes, such as *TNF, TRAF1, TNFSF12 (TWEAK), TNFSF13 (APRIL), IL-1β, IL1R1, IL1R2, IL1RAPL2, IL-2, IL-2Rβ,* and *IL7R* (Table 1). Moreover, overlapped GGAA-motifs are found in the interferon (IFN)-stimulated response element (ISRE)-like sequences in the promoter regions of the mouse *Itga2b* (Masumi *et al.*, 2009), and *Pdcd1* (Cho *et al.*, 2008) genes. These lines of evidences suggest that the location of the duplicated GGAA-motifs near TSSs is one of the features of ISG promoters.

Over 300 ISGs have been known to encode proteins that are signaling factors, transcription factors (TFs), immune modulators, or apoptosis mediators (De Veer *et al.*, 2001). The duplicated GGAA-motifs are found in ISGs whose anti-viral functions have been analyzed (Schoggins *et al.*, 2011). We thus further surveyed the upstream regions of ISGs, whose expression responds against hepatitis C virus (Brodsky *et al.*, 2007), Classical Swine Fever virus (Renson *et al.*, 2010) and West Nile virus infections (Scherbik *et al.*, 2007), and that of other ISGs (De Veer *et al.*, 2001), (Hilkens *et al.*, 2003), (Indraccolo *et al.*, 2007), (Sandhya Rani *et al.*, 2007). The surveillance revealed that the redundant GGAA-motifs are found within 500-bp upstream from the TSS of numbers of the ISGs (Uchiumi *et al.*, 2013b).

Collectively, the majority of the promoter regions from ISGs contain the duplicated GGAA motifs but rarely with TATA-element, suggesting that the transcription initiation mechanism is different from that of the house-keeping genes or essentially required genes such that encode cell structure components. IFNs play important roles in response to viral infection and cancer generation by inducing expression of ISGs that should be elevated only when they are required, but suppressed under normal conditions. The duplicated GGAA motifs might have some advantages for the gene expression controlling system by a total net contribution of many GGAA-binding factors, including the ETS family proteins. Furthermore, GGAA-binding factors may associate with other TFs around TSSs to facilitate the expression of each ISG with subtle changes responding to IFN-induced signals.

5   Transcription Factors that Recognize and Bind to the GGAA-Motifs

Comparing the GGAA-motifs that are present in the 5'-upstream regions of 168 ISGs, the consensus sequence was tentatively determined as 5'-RVVVRGGAARNNVR-3' (Uchiumi *et al.*, 2013b) that matches the binding motif of the ETS family Type III, including SPI1 (PU.1), SPIB, and SPIC (Wei *et al.*, 2010). Some of the duplicated GGAA motifs could be classified as ISRE, whose consensus sequence is 5'-GGAAANNGAAACT-3' (Kerr & Stark, 1991), implying that ISG expression is competitively regulated by Type III of the ETS family and ISRE-binding proteins. The GGAA containing motifs have been ranked within the top 50 discovered motifs in human promoters (Xie *et al.*, 2005). The IRF1 binding motif AACTTT could be generated when CT was inserted between GGAA and TTCC. Deficiency of IRF1, which is a negative regulator of *IL23A* gene, causes prolonged RELA occupancy on the NF-κB site (Sheikh *et al.*, 2011). The c-REL binds to the *CXCL10*, *GIP2*, *GRB2*, *IFIT1*, *IFIT3*, and *IFI203* promoters to regulate expression of those genes (Wei *et al.*, 2008). Moreover, NF-κB p65 (RELA) homodimer binds to two symmetric sequences, 5'-**GGAA**TTTCC-3' and 5'-**GGAA**TTCCC-3', which are contained in the *IL8* and *COL7A1* enhancers, respectively (Chen *et al.*, 2000). ETS family proteins are known to regulate gene expression of the *OAS1* (Rutherford *et al.*, 1997) , (Larsen *et al.*, 2015) and *IL7R* (*CD127*) (Grenningloh *et al.*, 2011). STAT4 complex binds to (T/A)TTCC (C/G)GGAA(T/A) that contains duplication of the GGAA (TTCC) motif (Yamamoto *et al.*, 1997). IRF8 (ICSBP) is a negative transcriptional regulator for ISGs through binding to ISRE (Nelson *et al.*, 1993), but positively regulates the *IL-12B* gene (Wang *et al.*, 2000). Moreover, STAT1 and ETS family proteins regulate *CD40* and *FCGR1A* promoters (Nguyen & Benveniste, 2000), (Aittomäki *et al.*, 2004). HSF1 and HSF2 are also candidates to recognize the GGAA-motif (Kroeger & Morimoto, 1994), (Manuel *et al.*, 2002). In summary, a variety of TFs, including ETS family, IRFs, STATs, c-Rel/NF-κB, and HSF proteins are involved in the regulation of ISG transcription.

Promoter regions of the *TGFBR2*, *CCND1*, *ID2*, *MYC*, *IGFBP3*, *PTPN13*, *HERC5*, *STYXL1*, and *CAV1* genes, in which multiple GGAA motifs are contained, respond to the aberrant protein EWS/FLI fusion oncoprotein, which is generated by chromosomal translocation of Ewing's sarcoma (Delattre *et al.*, 1992), (Guillon *et al.*, 2009). It has been suggested that IRF and IFN down-regulate *MYC* (Pathak *et al.*, 2011) and *CAV1* (Navarro-Lérida *et al.*, 2004) gene expression, respectively, but IFN up-regulates the *CCND1* (Mannonen *et al.*, 2007), *IGFBP3* (Kitaya *et al.*, 2007), *PTPN13* (Huang *et al.*, 2008), and *HERC5* (Wong *et al.*, 2006) genes. HERC plays a role in antiviral responses to activate IRF3 *via* ISGylation (Shi *et al.*, 2010). The GGAA-containing microsatellites, which are contained in the promoter regions of the *NR0B1*, *FCGRT*, *CACNB2*, *FEZF1*, *KIAA1797*, and *GSTM4* genes (Garcia-Aragoncillo *et al.*, 2008), (Guillon *et al.*, 2009), (Luo *et al.*, 2009), may be regulated by a total net of weak interactions with GGAA binding factors. The recent report of the crystal structure of murine Elf3 interacting with the *Tgfbr2* promoter (Agarkar *et al.*, 2010) offers a model of how ETS family protein can associate with duplicated GGAA motifs. Competitive or cooperative binding of multiple GGAA binding proteins would control transcription initiation efficiency, with a subtle change dependent on the signals that are induced by various stresses. Thus the duplicated GGAA motifs may present a platform for TFs. Transcriptional initiation will be thus determined by competition of such TFs for occupation around the TSSs.

ETS family and other TFs could dependently or independently control transcription of human genes. For example, SPI1 (PU.1) and IRF proteins synergistically cause IFN-inducible transcription (Marecki *et al.*, 2001), (Meraro *et al.*, 2002). Sp1, SPI1 (PU.1), and OCT1 binding sites independently co-regulate basal transcription of the human *PTGIR* gene (Turner & Kinsella, 2009). Sp1 and Ets1 interact with each other to regulate mouse *Npr1* gene expression (Kumar *et al.*, 2010). The ETS-binding consensus sequence is frequently found with a second ETS-binding sequence and with Sp1-binding sequence, but not with a TATA-element (FitzGerald *et al.*, 2004), implying the exclusive role of GGAA- and TATA-elements. SPI1 (PU.1) and STAT1 bind independently to the TATA-less *FCGR1A* promoter, where SPI1 (PU.1) associates with TBP and RNA polymerase II to initiate transcription (Aittomäki *et al.*, 2004). Recently, ANP32A was shown to interact with STAT1 and STAT2 to regulate transcription initiation of ISGs (Kadota & Nagata, 2010). The human *VEGFR1* promoter region contains overlapping GGAA motifs and it is also regulated by CREB, and EGR-binding elements (Jin *et al.*, 2009). Furthermore, Creb, Ets1, Ap2, and Sp1bind to the mouse *Ppp2r1a* gene promoter carrying duplicated TTCC motifs (Chen *et al.*, 2009). The promoter region of the *IFNB* gene represents transcriptional regulation by an enhanceosome (Merika & Thanos, 2001). Multiple elements around the duplicated GGAA motifs may recruit various TFs, including OCT, Sp1, and CREB, to form a pre-initiation complex near TSSs. Association of multiple TFs or enhanceosome assembly will make transcription start easier, and it might be advantageous for a rapid response to stresses in a TATA-independent manner.

6 Duplicated GGAA-Motifs in the Promoter Regions of the TCA Cycle Associated Genes

Our survey of human genomic promoters to find putative TPA-responsive elements with GGAA-duplication retrieved the *MRPL32*, *NDUFB3*, *NDUFS3*, *SDHB*, and *SDHAF2* genes, encoding mitochondrial ribosomal proteins, components that are involved in TCA cycle, and oxidative phosphorylation (OXPHOS) (Vafai & Mootha, 2012). The surveillance also retrieved mitochondrial function-associated genes such as *CFL1* (*Cofilin1*), *COX17*, *ELAC2*, *ERO1L*, *FASN*, *HSPA5*, and *SUMO1*. Interestingly, 13% of the retrieved genes have bidirectional partners (Uchiumi *et al.*, 2011b). At least 30% of these bidirectional gene pairs are associated with mitochondrial function (Uchiumi *et al.*, 2013c). In addition, duplicated GGAA-motifs are very frequently found in the upstream regions of the mitochondrial function-associated genes that encode ATP synthase, cytochrome c oxidase, NADH dehydrogenase, and TCA cycle enzymes (Table 1).

The duplicated GGAA-motifs are present in the upstream regions of the *SDHAF2*, *SDHD*, *ACO2*, and *IDH1* genes, encoding enzymes that work for TCA cycle progression. Dysfunction of mitochondria is thought to cause either cellular senescence or cancer generation (Seyfried & Shelton, 2010), (Schulze & Harris, 2012), (López-Otín *et al.*, 2013), (Gomes *et al.*, 2013). Remarkably, TCA-cycle enzymes, FH (Fumarate hydratase) and SDH (succinate dehydrogenase) have been suggested as tumor suppressors (Pollard *et al.*, 2005). Hence, mutations of the TCA cycle factor-encoding genes give rise to an abnormal mitochondrial respiration that is one of the characteristics of tumor or cancer (Hoekstra & Bayley, 2013), (Desideri *et al.*, 2014). Mutations on *IDH1* and *IDH2* genes have been identified in human brain cancer cells

(Dang *et al.*, 2009), (Yan *et al.*, 2009), (Vogelstein *et al.*, 2013). A recent study demonstrated that mutation-introduced IDH2 could generate sarcomas (Lu *et al.*, 2013). Moreover, we confirmed the existence of duplicated GGAA-motifs in the upstream region of the *NAMPT*, encoding a nicotinamide phosphoribosyltransferase that catalyzes the first rate-limiting step of NAD$^+$ synthesis from nicotinamide (Tan *et al.*, 2012). NAMPT may modulate biologically important reactions, such as the TCA (Citrate/Krebs) cycle, poly(ADP-ribosyl)ation, and sirtuin-mediated de-acetylation all that depend on NAD$^+$.

   Aberrant pyruvate metabolism is thought to play a prominent role in cancer (Gray *et al.*, 2013). Duplicated GGAA-motif is present in the bidirectional promoter of the *PDHX* (Uchiumi *et al.*, 2013c), encoding one of the components of the PDH enzyme to metabolize pyruvate to acetyl-CoA (Barnerias *et al.*, 2009). The *IDH3G*, encoding NAD$^+$ dependent iso-citrate dehydrogenase (IDH) gamma subunit, has a bidirectional partner *SSR4*, but has no obvious GGAA-motif duplications near the TSS. However, 5'-upstreams of the *IDH3A* and *IDH3B*, encoding α and β subunits of the IDH3 complex, contain sequences 5'-GGGGA**GGAA**GAAGCT**TTCC**CG GAG-3' and 5'-GTCAC**TTCC**CACGCGAC**TTCC**TGCG **GGAA**ACATG-3', respectively. The duplicated GGAA-motifs are present near the TSSs of the human *FH*, *SUCLG1*, *CS*, and *ACLY*, encoding fumarate hydratase, succinate-CoA ligase alpha subunit, citrate synthase, and ATP citrate lyase, respectively. The *CS* and *ACLY* genes have bidirectional partners, *LOC102724133* and *TTC25*, respectively.

7   Various Stresses that Modulate Gene Expression

Expression of the ISGs, DNA repair- and mitochondrial function-associated genes, is hypothesized to be regulated by duplicated GGAA-motifs, implying that the profile of the TFs may affect expression of these genes to various stresses (Figure 1). IFN-induced signals have been well studied as JAK/STAT and NF-κB systems. Similar to the response to IFNs, DNA-damage would alter the transcriptional state (Wolters & Schumacher, 2013). The cellular responses against DNA damage are thought to be relevant to the oxidative stress that is mediated by mitochondria (Pohjoismäki *et al.*, 2012), (Kazak *et al.*, 2012). Transcription mediated by NF-κB and p53 could be modulated by oxidative stresses (Rehmani *et al.*, 2013). Moreover, metabolites that are mainly generated from mitochondria play roles in the regulation of transcription (Gut & Verdin, 2013), (Liu *et al.*, 2013). The concept of coordination between metabolism and gene expression has been postulated as REM (RNA/enzyme/metabolite) networks (Hentze & Preiss, 2010). Metabolites, such as NAD$^+$, acetyl-CoA, S-adenosylmethionine, epigenetically affect transcription of various genes by poly (ADP-ribosyl)ation, acetylation, and methylation of chromosomal proteins and TFs (Gut & Verdin, 2013). Among these, the NAD$^+$ molecule, which are the substrate for PARP enzyme to synthesize poly(ADP-ribose), has been considered to play a key role in linking nuclear DNAs with mitochondria (Gomes *et al.*, 2013). PARP is activated in tumor and cancer cells (Gibson & Kraus, 2012). The first step in cancer development would be the imbalances in the GGAA-binding factors. When NAD$^+$ molecules are accumulated in accordance with the insufficient TCA cycle progression, they would be used for both glycolysis and poly(ADP-ribosyl)ation. If then DNA-damage occurred persistently, activation of PARP enzyme that leads to consumption of the NAD$^+$ molecules will down-regulate NAD$^+$-dependent enzymes, including SIRT1, IDH2, malate dehydrogenase (MDHB),

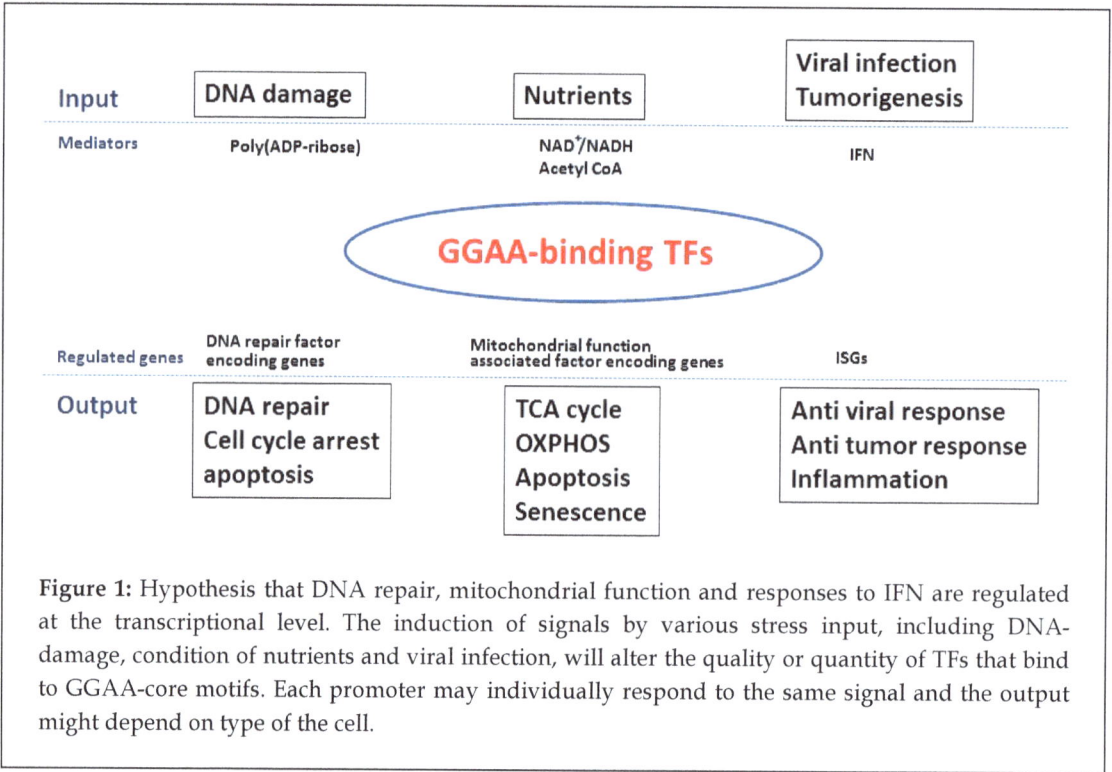

Figure 1: Hypothesis that DNA repair, mitochondrial function and responses to IFN are regulated at the transcriptional level. The induction of signals by various stress input, including DNA-damage, condition of nutrients and viral infection, will alter the quality or quantity of TFs that bind to GGAA-core motifs. Each promoter may individually respond to the same signal and the output might depend on type of the cell.

pyruvate dehydrogenase complex (PDH), and lactate dehydrogenase (LDHB). Despite the decrease in the amount of the NAD^+, cells need to produce ATP to survive. In this situation, the metabolic state of the cells could be referred to as the "Warburg effect" (Seyfried, 2012). This is a possible scenario explaining the reason why lactic acid fermentation is up-regulated, but in contrast, TCA cycle and OXPHOS is down-regulated in cancerous cells. Mitochondria may utilize L-glutamate, which is metabolized to 2-oxo-glutarate. Thus, the elevated metabolism of L-glutamate, which is frequently observed in tumor cells (Prickett & Samuels, 2012), would be accompanied with an insufficient NAD^+ level. This hypothesis could be drawn if we figure out consequences from the gradual alteration in the profile of the multiple GGAA-binding TFs that simultaneously disturbs the expression of the TCA cycle enzyme- and DNA repair factor-encoding genes.

8   IFN Responses and Mitochondrial Functions

In regards to the immunological system, lymphocyte functions are thought to be dependent on nutrients and changes in metabolic state (Pearce & Pearce, 2013), (Pearce *et al.*, 2013). Conversely, the metabolic state could be regulated by actions of the immune system (Odegaard & Chawla, 2013). Metabolic changes in macrophages, Th_{17} and T_{reg} cells have been reviewed and it was suggested that they are under the control of the AMPK signaling system (O'Neill & Graham Hardie, 2013). Mitochondrial OXPHOS, and generation of reactive oxygen species (ROS) are demonstrated to regulate T-cell activation (Chang *et al.*, 2013), (Sena *et al.*, 2013). In addition, activation of Ca^{2+}-dependent dehydrogenases of TCA cycle has been shown to regulate production of NADH and ATP to activate T-cells (Krauss *et al.*, 2001). Glucose metabolism does not only influence the activation, but also differentiation of T-cells (Michalek *et al.*, 2011). Taken together, these observations imply that metabolic state and integrity of the mitochondria plays a key role in the communication between the metabolism and the immune system.

The JAK-STAT signaling pathway has been widely believed as a main system to respond to IFNs (Berry *et al.*, 2010), (Stark & Darnell Jr., 2012). The duplicated GGAA-motif is present near the TSS of the *SUMO1* gene (Uchiumi *et al.*, 2011b). SUMOylation is associated with not only mitochondrial function (Harder *et al.*, 2004), but also DNA-damage response through modification of PARP1 (Martin *et al.*, 2009), (Ryu *et al.*, 2010). Interestingly, transcriptional activity of the GGAA binding factor STAT1 is suppressed by SUMOylation that is catalyzed by PIAS1 (Ungureanu *et al.*, 2005), (Shuai, 2006), (Tahk *et al.*, 2007). Hence, GGAA-motif dependent transcription could be negatively regulated by SUMOylation. The STAT3 protein acts in mitochondria to control respiration and energy management in a transcription independent manner (Tammineni *et al.*, 2014). Importantly, NDUFA13 (GRIM-19) is a component of the mitochondrial respiratory chain complex I (Chen *et al.*, 2012) that acts as a chaperone recruiting STAT3 to mitochondria. In addition, mitochondrial antiviral signaling (MAVS) is an antiviral innate immune signaling protein that localizes in mitochondrial outer membranes (Koshiba, 2013). The MAVS protein regulates anti-viral or inflammatory responses, and cell-death and metabolic functions, which is suggested to be under the control of IFN and NF-κB pathways (West *et al.*, 2011), (Belgnaoui *et al.*, 2011). The MAVS signalosome contains TNF receptor-associated factors (TRAFs), TNF receptor-associated death domain (TRADD) proteins, and Tom70, HSP90, IFIT3, and STING (Jacobs & Coyne, 2013). As expected, the duplicated GGAA-motifs are present in the 5′-upstream regions of the *ATG12, DDX3X, IFIT3, IRF7, MAVS*, and *TRADD* genes (Uchiumi *et al.*, 2013c).

IFN-γ and IL-4 commonly induce eighty four mitochondrial function-associated mouse genes, including *Ndufc1, Ndufs1, Ndufs3, Sdha, Sdhd, Aco2, Atp5a1, Atp5h, Atp5j, Atp5c1, Hadhb,* and *Usmg5,* in ERRα knock out macrophages (Sonoda *et al.*, 2007). Induction of expression for these genes, which may lead to mitochondrial ROS generation and host defense, is mediated by the induction of the *Pgc-1β* gene. Because expression patterns of the ISGs in monocytes from IFN-β non responders resembles to that of the mitochondrial function-associated genes (Bustamante *et al.*, 2013), mitochondria might be up-regulated by type I IFN-induced signals that induce antiviral activities. Moreover, IFN-γ-induced signaling affects poly(ADP-ribosyl)ation of DNA-PKcs that in turn regulates p53 (Sajish *et al.*, 2013). Interestingly, this process is mediated by Trp-tRNA synthetase, implying that amino acid metabolism links the IFN-induced signal with DNA damage response. The finding suggests that poly (ADP-ribose) metabolism, which is closely associated with mitochondrial function, cross-talks with the IFN-induced signals.

Cytokines have therapeutic potential for enhancing antitumor immunity (Margolin *et al.*, 2013). Two cytokines, IFN-α and IL-2 have been approved for the treatment of cancer. Given that IFN-induced signals are mainly mediated by cell-membrane receptors and the JAK-STAT system, the outcome would be up-regulation of genes whose promoters contain GGAA (TTCC)-motifs, the target sequence of the STATs. Therefore, not only ISGs, but also several mitochondrial function-associated genes could be simultaneously induced by IFNs.

9   Implicative Link between DNA-Repair and Mitochondria

Several nuclear DNA-repair factors are suggested to play roles in the maintenance of mitochondrial DNAs (mtDNAs), and damaged mtDNAs in turn exert signals to regulate nuclear transcription (Kazak *et al.*, 2012). Duplicated GGAA-motifs are present in the bidirectional promoter of the human *PARG* and *TIM23B* genes, encoding poly(ADP-ribose) glycohydralase and mitochondrial inner membrane translocase 23B, respectively (Meyer *et al.*, 2003), (Uchiumi *et al.*, 2015). The motif is also contained in the human *PARP1* promoter region (Yokoyama *et al.*, 1990), (Uchiumi *et al.*, 2013a). Importantly, isoforms of the PARG protein localize in the mitochondria (Whatcott *et al.*, 2009). PARP enzymes synthesize poly(ADP-ribose)s, and the poly(ADP-ribosyl)ation of target proteins, including p53 (Mendoza-Alvarez & Alvarez-Gonzalez, 2001), (Lee *et al.*, 2012) and PARP1 itself, regulate DNA-repair synthesis (Gibson & Kraus, 2012). Moreover, PARP1 and PARP2 influence mitochondrial function and oxidative metabolism (Bai & Cantó, 2012). Localization of the PARP1protein in mitochondria and its role to maintain mitochondrial DNA integrity has been revealed (Rossi *et al.*, 2009).

As described, the human *TP53* and *RB1* promoters harbor tandem repeated GGAA (TTCC) motifs (Uchiumi *et al.*, 2010), (Uchiumi *et al.*, 2016). It is widely known that damage on DNAs activates p53, which is transcribed from the *TP53* gene, and let it bind to the responsive elements and activate genes encoding cell cycle regulators, apoptosis- and autophagy-inducers (Menendez *et al.*, 2009), (Green & Kroemer, 2009). Recent studies indicated that the p53 protein does not only act as a "guardian of the genome", but also serves as a metabolism regulator (Vousden & Lane, 2007), (Vousden & Ryan, 2009). Moreover, p53 has been reported to accumulate in mitochondria in response to stress (Green & Kroemer, 2009). One recent study revealed that mitochondrial disulfide relay causes translocation of p53 into mitochondria to facilitate its function for repairing oxidative damage to mitochondrial DNA (Zhuang *et al.*, 2013). However, overexpression of p53 in mitochondria would lead to depleted mitochondrial DNA abundance and a reduction in oxidative stress (Koczor *et al.*, 2012). Oncogenic *RAS*-induced mitochondrial dysfunction, which causes oncogene induced senescence, is dependent on either p53 or RB (Moiseeva *et al.*, 2009). The tumor suppressor protein RB plays a role in linking cell cycle exit with mitochondrial biogenesis (Sankaran *et al.*, 2008). RB is widely known to control cell cycle progression, maintenance of genome stability and apoptosis by interacting with the E2F family proteins (Dick & Rubin, 2013). Recently, it was reported that mutation of E2F1 leads to mitochondrial defects in human cells (Ambrus *et al.*, 2013). Notablly, DNA sequence, 5′-CAATA**GGAA**CCGCCGCCGTTG**TTCC**CGTC-3′ is present near the TSS of the human *E2F1* gene. These lines of evidences imply that tumors could be generated from mitochondrial dysfunctions when p53 and RB proteins lose their intrinsic biological functions as tumor suppressors, and that expression of their encoding genes are under the control of GGAA-motif binding TFs.

Besides, p53 and RB, other DNA repair factors localize in mitochondria or regulate their biological functions. For example, mutations of the *BRCA1* gene have become one of the hallmarks for diagnosis of breast cancer (Miki *et al.*, 1994) (King, 2014). BRCA1 protein, which plays a part in the repair synthesis of double-strand DNA breaks (Huen *et al.*, 2010), is also involved in the mitochondrial genome maintenance to be trans-located into mitochondria especially when it is phosphorylated (Coene *et al.*, 2005). Deficiency of BRCA1, which interacts with FANCD2 protein, leads to phenotypes that resemble to Fanconi anemia (FA) (Garcia-

Higuera *et al.*, 2001). A number of additional DNA repair factors associate with FA proteins (Banerjee *et al.*, 2013). Recent study of transcripts from bone marrow cells revealed that FA patients have deficiencies in mitochondrial, redox and DNA repair pathways (Pagano *et al.*, 2013), (Cappelli *et al.*, 2013). Another DNA-repair deficient disease is Ataxia Telangiectasia that is caused by mutations on the *ATM* gene (Negrini *et al.*, 2010). The lack of ATM reduces mitochondrial DNA integrity and mitochondrial dysfunction (Sharma *et al.*, 2014). Moreover, mitochondria are suggested to be required for the oxidative activation of ATM (Morita *et al.*, 2014). The duplicated GGAA-motifs are present in the 5'-upstream regions of the *BRCA1*, *FANCD2*, and *ATM*, which have bidirectional partner *NBR2*, *CIDECP*, and *NPAT*, respectively (Uchiumi *et al.*, 2015). Although *BRCA2*, encoding a tumor suppressor to repair double-strand DNA breaks (Yuan *et al.*, 1999), (Venkitaraman, 2014), has no bidirectional partner gene, the duplication of the GGAA-motif is also present near its TSS.

GGAA-motif duplications are found in the bidirectional *APEX1/OSGEP* promoter region. The *APEX1* encodes apurinic/apyrimidinic endonuclease 1 (APE1) that regulates both base excision repair (BER) and mitochondrial DNA-repair systems (Mohan & Madhusuden, 2013), (Kazak *et al.*, 2012). APE1does not only regulate a redox system in a cell (Tell *et al.*, 2009), but also interacts with XRCC1, which is recruited to the poly(ADP-ribosyl)ated site (Fishel *et al.*, 2013). The GGAA-duplication is contained in the regulatory region of the head-head configured *ACO2/PHF5A* genes (Uchiumi *et al.*, 2013c). The *ACO2* gene encodes aconitase that plays an important role in the TCA cycle to produce citrate and isocitrate and also serves as a mitochondrial redox-sensor (Liu & Kamp, 2011). More importantly, aconitase and mitochondrial BER enzyme OGG1 (8-oxoguanine DNA glycosylase) cooperatively preserve mitochondrial DNA integrity (Kim *et al.*, 2014). Additionally, Cockayne syndrome proteins CSA and CSB, which play roles in nucleotide excision repair (NER), accumulate in mitochondria upon oxidative stress (Kamenisch *et al.*, 2010). Although no obvious duplication of the GGAA-motif is found, putative ETS1 binding motif is present in the *ERCC8* (*CSA*)/*NDUFAF2* bidirectional promoter region.

Apoptosis is mediated by mitochondria in response to various stresses including DNA-damage and immunological stress signals (Estaquier *et al.*, 2012), (Galluzzi *et al.*, 2012). It has been reviewed that ETS family proteins regulate apoptosis (Oikawa & Yamada, 2003). As expected, the GGAA-duplications are contained in the 5'-regulatory regions of the human *PDCD1*, *DFFA*, *BCL2*, and *FAS* genes (Table 1), implying that expression of the apoptosis regulating factor-encoding genes is under the control of the duplicated GGAA-motifs. Previous studies revealed that mitochondrial functions closely associate with the execution of apoptosis (Kroemer, 1997), (Tait & Green, 2010), (Estaquier *et al.*, 2012). For instance, cytochrome c is released from mitochondria during induction of DNA-damage signals, and that apoptosis regulator BAX and BCL2 localize in mitochondria (Estaquier *et al.*, 2012). Interestingly, *ATG12/AP3S1*, *APOPT1/BAG5*, *COX10/COX10AS1*, *COX15/CUTC* and *HTRA2/AUP1* gene pairs have duplicated GGAA-motifs in the bidirectional promoter regions (Uchiumi *et al.*, 2013c). The *ATG12* and *HTRA2* genes encode an autophagy protein that takes a part in the quality control after mitochondrial damage (Rubinstein *et al.*, 2011), (Mai *et al.*, 2012) and a serine protease that is localized in mitochondria (Goo *et al.*, 2013), respectively. Collectively, it was suggested that transcription of a large numbers of the DNA repair/apoptosis/mitochondrial function associated genes are regulated by bidirectional and duplicated GGAA-motif-containing promoters.

10   Modulation of Transcription Status May Reprogram Cancer Cells

A fertilized Egg usually proliferates without cell cycle arrest, and does not need to increase either the number or the amount of mitochondria because it is preset or embedded before fertilization. The mtDNA is known to be inherited in a maternal manner, and paternal mtDNA is actively degraded after fertilization of an egg of *C. elegans* (Friedman & Nunnari, 2014), (Rawi *et al.*, 2011), (Sato & Sato, 2011). When cell-division has to proceed to generate several cells, they will grow and enlarge their sizes and to differentiate. Under certain circumstances in which cells are proliferating rapidly without increasing their sizes, the energy for survival should be supplied from glycolysis or from existing mitochondria. However, when cells are increasing in size, keeping the differentiated state, they need more energy from TCA-cycle and OXPHOS. Most (99%) of the mitochondrial proteins are encoded in nuclear genomes (Vafai & Mootha, 2012). Therefore, especially when cells differentiate, transcription of mitochondrial function associated genes should be efficiently controlled by some biological mechanisms. Duplicated GGAA motifs are commonly contained near TSSs of large numbers of the mitochondrial function-associated genes that have bidirectional partners and a lot of the DNA repair- and IFN signal-associated genes, implying that mitochondrial functions and responses to IFNs and DNA-damage need to be coordinately regulated at transcriptional level.

Introduction of several TFs (OSKM factors or Yamanaka factors) into somatic cells could reprogram and convert them with pluripotency (Takahashi & Yamanaka, 2006), (Apostolou & Hochedlinger, 2013). It was demonstrated that three TFs, *Blimp1*, *Prdm14*, and *Tfap2c*, could direct epiblast-like cells into primordial germ cells (Nakaki *et al.*, 2013). Moreover, C/EBPα enhances effects of the OSKM factors to reprogram B cells (Di Stefano *et al.*, 2014). These lines of evidences imply that the transcriptional state or the profile could determine cell behaviors towards proliferation, cell cycle arrest, differentiation, senescence or even to undergo programmed cell death. Furthermore, it has been postulated that nutrient or metabolite state affect the balance between quiescence and proliferation of stem cells (Ito & Suda, 2014). Hence, we tentatively hypothesize that mitochondrial functions are regulated by the same or similar signals that affect IFN- and DNA damage-responses. We propose a scenario that transcriptional dysregulation occurred before cancerous cells are generated. In other words, pre-cancerous state could be reprogrammed to be benign by altering TF profile.

11   Mitochondrial Dysfunction and Cancer

Mitochondria have specific features that resemble bacteria, namely, being surrounded by double membrane and having a circular genome (Vafai & Mootha, 2012). Comparison of amino acid sequences of small subunit rRNA and HSP-90 proteins suggested that mitochondria are evolved from endosymbiosis of prokaryotic cells that might have been similar to the alpha-proteobacteria (Yang *et al.*, 1985), (Viale & Arakaki, 1994). Mitochondrial functions, including TCA-cycle, OXPHOS, and stress responses, are essentially required for cells to survive. In cases where cells were overexposed to damaging stress, mitochondria will exert signals to the host cell to undergo programmed death or apoptosis. If the damage on nuclear DNAs, including telomeres, could be manageable to repair, mitochondria will evoke the

DNA-repair system to protect their own function-associated genes. This overview would be supported by the deep insight that mitochondrial dysfunction is associated with cancer generation (Scatena, 2012). Cancer is widely acknowledged as aberrant state of cells that are forced to proliferate in accordance with an abnormally respiration system (Seyfried, 2012). Recently, it was shown that mitochondria and nuclear DNAs are communicating each other (Houtkooper *et al.*, 2013). Almost all (99%) of the mitochondrial proteins are encoded in nuclear genomes, and mitochondria in turn exert damage responding signals to nuclei. In this chapter, we proposed a possible mechanism that expression of genes encoding three major TCA-cycle-enzymes or the components, SDHAF2/SDHB/SDHD (complex II), ACO2, and IDH1, could be simultaneously regulated at the transcriptional level. Similarly, the duplicated GGAA-motifs are present near TSSs of other TCA-cycle enzyme-encoding genes, including *IDH3A, IDH3B, FH, SUCLG1, CS,* and *ACLY*. Moreover, the *NAMPT* gene expression could be regulated by a similar system mediated by the duplicated GGAA-motifs. However, no obvious GGAA duplications are identified near TSSs of the *IDH2, IDH3GL, MDH1B (malate dehydrogenase)* and *OGDH (oxoglutarate dehydrogenase)* genes. It is implicative that expression of these genes might not be affected if multiple GGAA-driven transcriptions were not working well. Competitive binding of multiple TFs to these GGAA-motifs might have enabled cells to control expression of various genes in a comparatively stable manner, and the system would have worked as a buffer against subtle changes in the profile of GGAA-binding TFs. However, repeated cell division and damage on the DNAs may gradually disturb the balance of those TFs, and finally attenuate mitochondrial functions, DNA-repair system, and IFN-response simultaneously. Prior to the fatal mutations on the genomes, extra damage on DNAs may eventually activate PARP enzyme that synthesizes poly(ADP-ribose) consuming NAD^+ as a substrate. Under the circumstance that both TCA cycle and NAD^+ synthesis by NAMPT would not function efficiently, cells may produce ATP mainly by glycolysis and lactic acid fermentation. As a consequence, cells might develop ultimate aberrances in mitochondrial respiration system that is one of the hallmarks of cancer.

Cancer incidence in humans increase exponentially with age, suggesting that aging is a risk factor for most human malignancies (Benz & Yan, 2008). Aging is accompanied with epigenetic change and alteration of gene expression profile (Geigl *et al.*, 2004), (Cencioni *et al.*, 2013). It should be noted that GGAA microsatellites are the sites of epigenetic regulation (Gangwal *et al.*, 2008), (Monument *et al.*, 2012). Here we tentatively draw a hypothesis that DNA-repair, IFN-response and mitochondrial function-related genes are coordinately regulated by multiple GGAA-binding TFs. Altered expression of the TCA-cycle enzyme-encoding genes might take place before causing dysfunction of mitochondria in developing cancer cells. Transcriptional state in the cells would be gradually or very slowly altered by repeated cell-divisions and by ROS generation that is believed to cause senescence. This subtle alteration in the profile of GGAA-binding TFs would be the very first step in the cancer generation (Figure 2). A recent study showed that decrease in $NAD^+/NADH$ ratio, which is thought to be occurred by an aberrances in mitochondria, does not only enhance cancer progression but also metastasis (Santidrian *et al.*, 2013). IFNs have been successfully utilized for therapy of a variety of cancers (Margolin *et al.*, 2013). IFN therapy might be also effective for specific type of cancer by up-regulating DNA-repair- and mitochondrial function-associated genes.

It is paradoxical and controversial that depletion of NAD^+ molecules from cytoplasm and mitochondria could be caused by the DNA-damage dependent activation of the PARP,

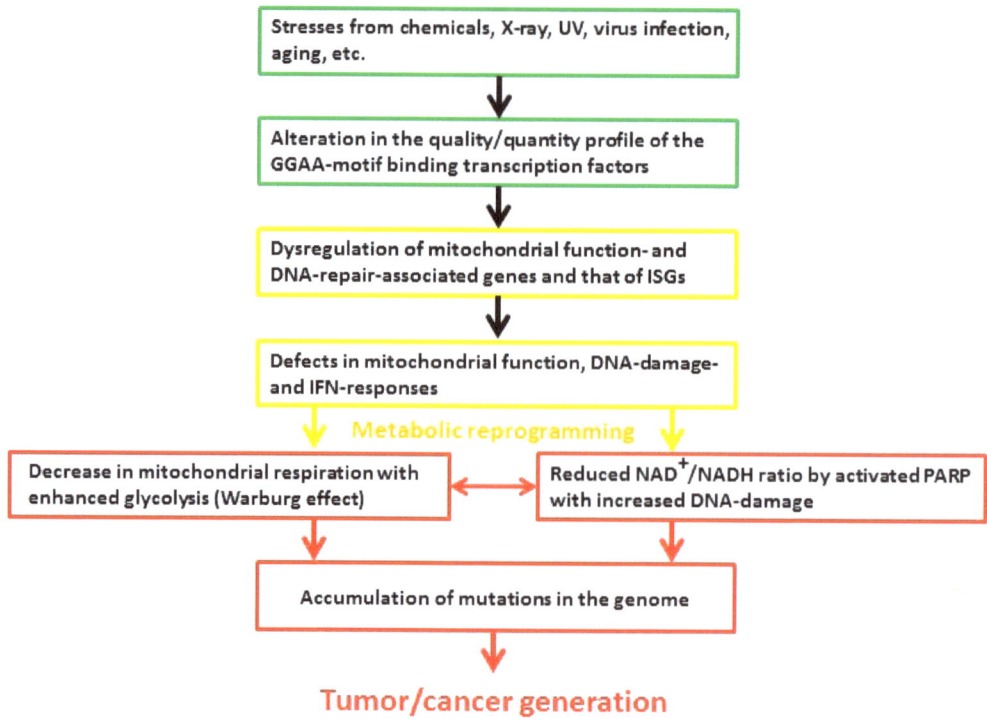

Figure 2: Hypothesis of cancer generation. Chemicals, X-ray and UV irradiation, virus infection, and aging, may alter the quality and/or quantity profile of the GGAA-binding factors to lead to disruption of the mitochondrial function-associated gene expression. DNA-damage will up-regulate PARP that consumes NAD$^+$ molecule as a substrate. The outcome would be a metabolic reprogramming decreasing NAD$^+$/NADH ratio to cause dysfunction of the TCA-cycle, and more glucose will be required to synthesize ATP. This hypothesis implies that cancer could be prevented if NAD$^+$/NADH ratio were ameliorated at an early stage.

which play important roles in the DNA-repair synthesis. Nevertheless, several PARP inhibitor drugs have been already developed and are now clinical trials were undertaken successfully (Gibson & Kraus, 2012), (Curtin *et al.*, 2012). One of the possible explanations for various PARP inhibitors to suppress cancer development might be the resulting increase in the NAD$^+$/NADH ratio, which would occur by preventing the incorporation of the NAD$^+$ molecule into poly(ADP-ribose). However, because poly(ADP-ribosyl)ation is an essential response to DNA damage, complete inhibition of the PARP might be rather deleterious for cells. Therefore, advantages and disadvantages of the PARP inhibitors on treatment of tumors might have been observed in different clinical setting (Venkitaraman, 2014). Inhibitors of the poly(ADP-ribose) degrading enzyme PARG could be also utilized as anticancer drugs to induce cell death or apoptosis. Knockdown of *PARG* by siRNAs in HeLa S3 cells enhanced the staurosporine-induced cell-death (Uchiumi *et al.*, 2013a). Moreover, it was demonstrated that individual inhibition of either PARP1 or PARG is effective for cancer treatment, whereas combined inhibition of the both enzymes does not affect cancer cell-death (Feng & Kho, 2013). These observations might be partly explained by a homeostasis of the cellular abundance of the NAD$^+$ that has to be biologically maintained in an appropriate level. Maintaining concentration of NAD[+] at an appropriate level might be required to avoid a pseudohypoxic state that disrupts nuclear-mitochondrial communication (Gomes *et al.*, 2013). Thus, it is valuable to develop new drugs that ameliorate the NAD[+] level. Low dose of Rsv stimulates NADH dehydrogenases and mitochondrial complex I activity to increase the NAD[+]/NADH ratio (Desquiret-Dumas *et al.*, 2013). Rapamycin, which inhibits mTor, rescues the mitochondrial defects in a Leigh syndrome-model *Ndufs4* knockout mouse (Johnson *et al.*, 2013). An anti-diabetic agent, metformin could serve as an anti-cancer agent by decreasing glucose oxidation and increasing dependency on reductive glutamine metabolism in generation of prostate cancer cells (Fendt *et al.*, 2013). In addition to these drugs, we propose introduction of genes encoding specific GGAA-binding TFs into cancerous cells may be a new therapy to integrate mitochondrial functions, DNA-repair, and IFN-responses.

12   Conclusions and Future Prospects

Mitochondria do not only control respiration to produce energy, but also serve as stress-sensors to determine cell fate toward differentiation, proliferation, senescence, or death. Most of the biological stresses such that are induced by IFNs, DNA-damage, and metabolic state should be properly managed in mitochondria. That is consistent with the observation that common sequence motif is contained in the 5'-regulatory region of the ISGs and DNA repair/mitochondrial-function associated genes.

In cancerous cells, mutations are selectively integrated in specific genes encoding tumor suppressors, p53, RB, CDKN2A, BRCA1 (Vogelstein *et al.*, 2013), (Kandoth *et al.*, 2013), (Rahman, 2014). Such accumulating information will greatly help to establish a genomic prediction, prognosis or diagnosis of cancer. However, the observations that *TP53* and *RB1* genes are so frequently mutated to generate loss-of-function protein products in cancer cells raises questions how and why specific genes are highly mutated in cancer cells. In other words, by what mechanisms, the *TP53* and the *RB1* genes are more frequently damaged than other genes? These tumor suppressor proteins are not only localize in nuclei but also in mitochondria, suggesting that cancer cells carry aberrance in mitochondrial functions, such as respiration system. Mitochondria are serving as a damage-sensor of nuclear DNAs, including telomeres (Sahin *et al.*, 2011), (Kazak *et al.*, 2012), (Galluzzi *et al.*, 2012). It seems as if certain mechanisms have worked to cause mutations on tumor suppressor genes before tumorigenesis.

In this article, we tentatively tethered a hypothesis that explains the gradual or age-dependent generation of cancer (Figure 2). This hypothesis does not only denote the reason why usually it takes a long time to generate cancer, but also explains why the up-regulated glycolysis is very frequently observed in cancer. Prior to the reduction in the NAD[+]/NADH ratio that is caused by PARP activation, subtle alterations in the quality/quantity profile of the GGAA-binding TFs might have occurred. Cancer has been already considerably developed when genetic changes, such as the *TP53* mutation, were diagnosed. Moreover, this hypothesis supports the medical use of drugs that ameliorate the NAD[+]/NADH ratio as one of the appropriate remedies for cancer patient. In order to develop a new gene therapy for treatment of patient with malignant tumor and cancer, the precise mechanisms how mitochondrial function-associated genes are controlled, and why specific genes are frequently mutated in cancer cells should be elucidated.

Acknowledgement

This work was supported in part by JSPS KAKENHI Grant Number 24510270 and a Research Fellowship from the Research Center for RNA Science, RIST, Tokyo University of Science.

Abbreviations

BER: base excision repair; CR: calorie restriction; DSB: double strand break; FA: Fanconi anemia; IFN: interferon; ISG: interferon stimulated gene; ISRE: interferon-stimulated response element; NAD: nicotine amide dinucleotide; NER: nucleotide excision repair; OXPHOS: oxidative phosphorylation; PARG: poly(ADP-ribose) glycohydrolase; PARP: poly(ADP-ribose) polymerase; ROS: reactive oxygen species; Rsv: resveratrol; TCR: transcription coupled repair; TF: transcription factor; TSS: transcription start site.

References

Agarkar V.B., Babayeva N.D., Wilder P.J., Rizzino A., & Tahirov T.H. (2010). *Crystal structure of mouse Elf3 C-terminal DNA-binding domain in complex with type II TGF-β receptor promoter DNA.* J. Mol. Biol., 397, 278-289.

Aittomäki S., Yang J., Scott E.W., & Simon M.C. (2004). *Silvennoinen, O. Molecular basis of Stat1 and PU.1 cooperation in cytokine-induced Fcg receptor 1 promoter activation.* Int. Immunol., 16, 265-274.

Ambrus A.M., Islam A.B.M.M.K., Holmes K.B., Moon N.S., Lopez-Bigas N., Benevolenskaya E.V., & Frolov M.V. (2013). *Loss of dE2F compromises mitochondrial function.* Dev. Cell, 27, 438-451.

Apostolou E. & Hochedlinger K. (2013). *Chromatin dynamics during cellular reprogramming.* Nature, 502, 462-471.

Bai P. & Cantó C. (2012). *The role of PARP-1 and PARP-2 enzymes in metabolic regulation and disease.* Cell Metab., 16, 290-295.

Banerjee T., Bharti S.K., & Brosh Jr. R.M. (2013). *Fanconi anemia, interstrand cross-link repair, and cancer. In DNA Repair and Cancer-From Bench to Clinic,* (S. Madhusudan, D.M. Wilson III eds.), CRC Press, Taylor & Francis Group, Boca Raton, FL. (pp. 310-324).

Barnerias C., Saudubray J.M., Touati G., De Lonlay P., Dulac O., Ponsot G., Marsac C., Brivet M., & Desguerre I. (2009). *Pyruvate dehydrogenase complex deficiency: four neurological phenotypes with differing pathogenesis.* Dev. Med. Child Neurol., 52, e1-e9.

Barnes B.J., Kellum M.J., Pinder K.E., Frisancho J.A., & Pitha P.M. (2003). *Interferon regulatory factor 5, a novel mediator of cell cycle arrest and cell death.* Cancer Res., 63, 6424-6431.

Belgnaoui S.M., Paz S., & Hiscott J. (2011). *Orchestrating the interferon antiviral response through the mitochondrial antiviral signaling (MAVS) adapter.* Curr. Opin. Immunol., 23, 564-572.

Benz C.C. &Yau C. (2008). *Aging, oxidative stress and cancer: paradigms in parallax.* Nat. Rev. Cancer, 8, 875-879.

Berry M.P.R., Graham C.M., McNab F.W., Xu Z., Bloch S.A.A., Oni T., Wilkinson K.A., Banchereau R., Skinner J., Wilkinson R.J., Quinn C., Blankenship D., Dhawan R., Cush J.J., Mejias A., Ramilo O., Kon O.M., Pascual V., Banchereau J., Chaussabel D., & O'Garra A. (2010). *An interferon-inducible neutrophil-driven blood transcriptional signature in human tuberculosis.* Nature, 466, 973-977.

Brodsky L.I., Wahed A.S., Li J., Tavis J.E., Tsukahara T., & Taylor M.W. (2007). *A novel unsupervised method to identify genes important in the anti-viral response: application to Interferon/Ribavirin in Hepatitis C patients.* PLoS ONE, 7, e584.

Bustamante M.F., Nurtdinov R.N., Río J., Montalban X., & Comabella M. (2013). *Baseline gene expression signatures in monocytes from multiple sclerosis patients treated with Interferon-beta.* PLoS ONE, 8, e60994.

Cappelli E., Ravera S., Vaccaro D., Cuccarolo P., Bartolucci M., Panfoli I., Dufour C., & Degan P. (2013). Mitochondrial respiratory complex I defects in Fanconi anemia. Trends Mol. Med., 19, 513-514.

Carey M.F., Peterson C.L., & Smale S.T. (2009). Transcription and preinitiation complex assembly in vitro. In Transcriptional Regulation in Eukaryotes. 2nd ed. Cold Spring Harbor Laboratory Press. (pp. 439-538).

Cencioni C., Spallotta F., Martelli F., Valente S., Mai A., Zeiher A.M., & Gaetano C. (2013). Oxidative stress and epigenetic regulation in ageing and age-related diseases. Int. J. Mol. Sci., 14, 17643-17663.

Chang C.H., Curtis J.D., Maggi L.B., Faubert B., Villarino A.V., O'Sullivan D., Huang S.C.-C., van der Windt G.J.W., Blagih J., Qiu J., Weber J.D., Pearce E.J., Jones R.G., & Pearce E.L. (2013). Posttranscriptional control of T cell effector function by aerobic glycolysis. Cell, 153, 1239-1251.

Chen H.G., Han W.J., Deng M., Qin J., Yuan D., Liu J.P., Xiao L., Gong L., Liang S., Zhang J., Liu Y., & Li D.W. (2009). Transcriptional regulation of PP2A-A alpha is mediated by multiple factors including AP-2alpha, CREB, ETS-1, and SP-1. PLoS One, 4, e7019.

Chen Y., Lu H., Liu Q., Huang G., Lim C.P., Zhang L., Hao A., & Cao X. (2012). Function of GRIM-19, a mitochondrial respiratory chain complex I protein, in innate immunity. J. Biol. Chem., 287, 27227-27235.

Chen Y.Q., Sengchanthalangsy L.L., Hackett A., & Ghosh G. (2000). NF-kappaB p65 (RelA) homodimer uses distinct mechanisms to recognize DNA targets. Structure, 8, 419-428.

Cho H.Y., Lee S.W., Seo S.K., Choi I.W., Choi I., & Lee S.W. (2008). Interferon-sensitive response element (ISRE) is mainly responsible for IFN-α-induced upregulation of programmed death-1 (PD-1) in macrophages. Biochim. Biophys. Acta, 1779, 811-819.

Coene E.D., Hollinshead M.S., Waeytens A.A.T., Schelfhout V.R.J., Eechaute W.P., Shaw M.K., Van Oostveldt P.M.V., & Vaux D.J. (2005). Phosphorylated BRCA1 is predominantly located in the nucleus and mitochondria. Mol. Biol. Cell, 16, 997-1010.

Curtin N.J., Mukhopadhyay A., Drew Y., & Plummer R. (2012). The role of PARP in DNA repair and its therapeutic exploitation. InDNA repair in cancer therapy-Molecular targets and clinical applications, (M.R. Kelley ed.), Academic Press, Elsevier Inc., London, UK. (pp. 55-73).

Dang L., White D.W., Gross S., Bennett B.D., Bittinger M.A., Driggers E.M., Fantin V.R., Jang H.G., Jin S., Keenan M.C., Marks K.M., Prins R.M., Ward P.S., Yen K.E., Liau L.M., Rabinowitz J.D., Cantley L.C., Thompson C.B., Vander Heiden M.G., & Su S.M. (2009). Cancer-associated IDH1 mutations produce 2-hydroxyglutarate. Nature, 462, 739-744.

Delattre O., Zucman J., Plougastel B., Desmaze C., Melot T., Peter M., Kovar H., Joubert I., de Jong P., Rouleau G., Aurias A., & Thomas G. (1992). Gene function with an ETS DNA-binding domain caused by chromosome translocation in human tumors. Nature, 359, 162-165.

Desideri E., Vegliante R., & Ciriolo M.R. (2015). Mitochondrial dysfunctions in cancer: genetic defects and oncogenic signaling impinging on TCA cycle activity. Cancer Lett., 356, 217-223.

Desquiret-Dumas V., Gueguen N., Leman G., Baron S., Nivet-Antoine V., Chupin S., Chevrollier A., Vessières E., Ayer A., Ferré M., Bonneau D., Henrion D., Reynier P., & Procaccio V. (2013). Resveratrol induces a mitochondrial complex I-dependent increase in NADH oxidation responsible for sirtuin activation in liver cells. J. Biol. Chem., 288, 36662-36675.

De Veer M.J., Holko M., Frevel M., Walker E., Der S., Paranjape J.M., Silverman R.H., & Williams B.R.G. (2001). Functional classification of interferon-stimulated genes identified using microarrays. J. Leukoc. Biol., 69, 912-920.

Dick F.A. & Rubin S.M. (2013). Molecular mechanisms underlying RB protein function. Nat. Rev. Mol. Cell Biol., 14, 297-306.

Di Stefano B., Sardina J.L., van Oevelen C., Collombet S., Kallin E.M., Vincent G.P., Lu J., Thieffry D., Beato M., & Graf T. (2014). C/EBPα poises B cells for rapid reprogramming into induced pluripotent stem cells. Nature, 506, 235-239.

Estaquier J., Vallette F., Vayssiere J.L., & Mignotte B. (2012). The mitochondrial pathways of apoptosis. In Advances in Mitochondrial Medicine, (R. Scatena, P. Bottoni, B. Giardina eds.), Springer Science+Business Media B.V., Dordrecht, Germany. (pp. 157-183).

Fendt S.M., Bell E.L., Keibler M.A., Davidson S.M., Wirth G.J., Fiske B., Mayers J.R., Schwab M., Bellinger G., Csibi A., Patnaik A., Blouin M.J., Cantley L.C., Guarente L., Blenis J., Pollak M.N., Olumi A.F., Vander Heiden M.G., & Stephanopoulos G. (2013). Metformin decreases glucose oxidation and increases the dependency of prostate cancer cells on reductive glutamine metabolism. Cancer Res., 73, 4429-4438.

Feng X. & Kho D. (2013). *Inhibition of poly(ADP-ribose) polymerase-1 or poly(ADP-ribose) glycohydrolase individually, but not in combination, leads to improved chemotherapeutic efficacy in HeLa cells. Int. J. Oncol., 42, 749-756.*

Fishel M.L., Vascotto C., & Kelley M.R. (2013). *DNA base excision repair therapeutics: Summary of targets with a focus on APE1. In DNA Repair and Cancer-From Bench to Clinic, (S. Madhusudan, D.M. Wilson III eds.), CRC Press, Taylor & Francis Group, Boca Raton, FL. (pp. 233-287).*

FitzGerald P.C., Shlyakhtenko A., Mir A.A., & Vinson C. (2004). *Clustering of DNA sequences in human promoters. Genome Res., 14, 1562-1574.*

Friedman J.R. & Nunnari J. (2014). *Mitochondrial form and function. Nature, 505, 335-343.*

Galluzzi L., Kepp O., & Kroemer G. (2012). *Mitochondria: master regulators of danger signalling. Nat. Rev. Mol. Cell Biol., 13, 780-788.*

Gangwal K., Sankar S., Hollenhorst P.C., Kinsey M., Haroldsen S.C., Shah A.A., Boucher K.M., Watkins W.S., Jorde L.B., Graves B.J., & Lessnick S.L. (2008). *Microsatellites as EWS/FLI response elements in Ewing's sarcoma. Proc. Natl. Acad. Sci. USA, 105, 10149-10154.*

Garcia-Aragoncillo E., Carrillo J., Lalli E., Agra N., Gomez-Lopez G., Pestana A., & Alonso J. (2008). *DAX1, a direct target of EWS/FLI1 oncoprotein, is a principal regulator of cell-cycle progression in Ewing's tumor cells. Oncogene, 27, 6034-6043.*

Garcia-Higuera I., Taniguchi T., Ganesan S., Meyn M.S., Timmers C., Hejna J., Grompe M., & D'Andrea A.D. (2001). *Interaction of the Fanconi anemia proteins and BRCA1 in a common pathway. Mol. Cell, 7, 249-262.*

Gasser S., Orsulic S., Brown E.J., & Raulet D.H. (2005). *The DNA damage pathway regulates innate immune system ligands of the NKG2D receptor. Nature, 436, 1186-1190.*

Geigl J.B., Langer S., Barwisch S., Pfleghaar K., Lederer G., & Speicher M.R. (2004). *Analysis of gene expression patterns and chromosomal changes associated with aging. Cancer Res., 64, 8550-8557.*

Gibson B.A. & Kraus W.L. (2012). *New insights into the molecular and cellular functions of poly(ADP-ribose) and PARPs. Nat. Rev. Mol. Cell Biol., 13, 411-424.*

Gomes A.P., Price N.L., Ling A.J.Y., Mosiehi J.J., Montgomery M.K., Rajman L., White J.P., Teodoro J.S., Wrann C.D., Hubbard B.P., Mercken E.M., Palmeira C.M., de Cabo R., Rolo A.P., Turner N., Bell E.L., & Sinclair D.A. (2013). *Declining NAD$^+$ induces a pseudohypoxic state disrupting nuclear-mitochondrial communication during aging. Cell, 155, 1624-1638.*

Goo H.-G., Jung M.K., Han S.S., Rhim H., & Kang S. (2013). *HtrA2/Omi deficiency causes damage and mutation of mitochondrial DNA. Biophim. Biophys. Acta, 1833, 1866-1875.*

Goodrich D.W. (2006). *The retinoblastoma tumor-suppressor gene, the exception that proves the rule. Oncogene, 25, 5233-5243.*

Gray L.R., Tompkins S.C., & Taylor E.B. (2014). *Regulation of pyruvate metabolism and human disease. Cell. Mol. Life Sci., 71, 2577-2604.*

Green D.R. & Kroemer G. (2009). *Cytoplasmic functions of the tumor suppressor p53. Nature, 458, 1127-1130.*

Grenningloh R., Tai T.-S. Frahm N., Hongo T.C., Chicoine A.T., Brander C., Kaufmann D.E., & Ho I.-C. (2011). *Ets-1 maintains IL-7 receptor expression in peripheral T cells. J. Immunol., 286, 969-976.*

Guillon N., Tirode F., Boeva V., Zynovyev A., Barillot E., & Delattre O. (2009). *The oncogenic EWS-FLI1 protein binds in vivo GGAA microsatellite sequences with potential transcriptional activation function. PLoS One, 4, e4932.*

Gut P. & Verdin E. (2013). *The nexus of chromatin regulation and intermediary metabolism. Nature, 502, 489-498.*

Harder Z., Zunino R., & McBride H. (2004). *Sumo1 conjugates mitochondrial substrates and participates in mitochondrial fission. Curr. Biol., 14, 340-345.*

Hentze M.W. & Preiss T. (2010). *The REM phase of gene regulation. Trends Biochem. Sci., 35, 423-426.*

Hilkens C.M.U., Schlaak J.F., & Kerr I.M. (2003). *Differential responses to IFN-α subtypes in human T cells and dendritic cells. J. Immunol., 171, 5255-5263.*

Hoekstra A.S. & Bayley J.-P. (2013). *The role of complex II in disease. Biochim. Biophys. Acta, 1827, 543-551.*

Hollenhorst P.C., Shah A.A., Hopkins C., & Graves B.J. (2007). Genome-wide analyses reveal properties of redundant and specific promoter occupancy within the ETS gene family. Genes Dev., 21, 1882-1894.

Houtkooper R.H., Mouchiroud L., Ryu D., Moullan N., Katsyuba E., Knott G., Williams R.W., & Auwerx J. (2013). Mitonuclear protein imbalance as a conserved longevity mechanism. Nature, 497, 451-457.

Hsu T., Trojanowska M., & Watson D.K. (2004). Ets proteins in biological control and cancer. J. Cell. Biochem., 91, 896-903.

Huang W., Zhu C., Wang H., Horvath E., & Eklund E.A. (2008). The interferon consensus sequence-binding protein (ICSBP/IRF8) represses PTPN13 gene transcription in differentiating myeloid cells. J. Biol. Chem., 283, 7921-7935.

Huen M.S., Sy S.M., & Chen J. (2010). BRCA1 and its toolbox for the maintenance of genome integrity. Nat. Rev. Mol. Cell Biol., 11, 138-148.

Indraccolo S., Pfeffer U., Minuzzo S., Esposito G., Roni V., Mandruzzato S., Ferrari N., Anfosso L., Dell'Eva R., Noonan D.M., Chieco-Bianchi L., Albini A., & Amadori A. (2007). Identification of genes selectively regulated by IFNs in endothelial cells. J. Immunol., 178, 1122-1135.

Ito K & Suda T. (2014). Metabolic requirements for the maintenance of self-renewing stem cells. Nat. Rev. Mol. Cell Biol., 15, 243-256.

Jacobs J.L. & Coyne C.B. (2013). Mechanisms of MAVS regulation at the mitochondrial membrane. J. Mol. Biol., 425, 5009-5019.

Jin E., Liu J., Suehiro J., Yuan L., Okada Y., Nikolova-Krstevski V., Yano K., Janes L., Beeler D., Spokes K.C., Li D., Regan E., Shih S.C., Oettgen P., Minami T., & Aird W.C. (2009). Differential roles for ETS, CREB, and EGR binding sites in mediating VEGF receptor 1 expression in vivo. Blood, 114, 5557-5566.

Johnson S.C., Yanos M.E., Kayser E.-B., Quintana A., Sangesland M., Castanza A., Uhde L., Hui J., Wall V.Z., Gagnidze A., Oh K., Wasco B.M., Ramos F.J., Palmiter R.D., Rabinovitch P.S., Morgan P.G., Sedensky M.M., & Kaeberlein M. (2013). mTOR inhibition alleviates mitochondrial disease in a mouse model of Leigh syndrome. Science, 342, 1524-1528.

Kadota S. & Nagata K. (2010). pp32, an INHAT component, is a transcription machinery recruiter for maximal induction of IFN-stimulated genes. J. Cell Sci., 124, 892-899.

Kamenisch Y., Fousteri M., Knoch J., von Thaler A.-K., Fehrenbacher B., Kato H., Becker T., Dollé M.E.T., Kuiper R., Majora M., Schaller M., van der Horst G.T.J., van Steeg H., Röcken M., Rapaport D., Krutmann J., Mullenders L.H., & Berneburg M. (2010). Proteins of nucleotide and base excision repair pathways interact in mitochondria to protect from loss of subcutaneous fat, a hallmark of aging. J. Exp. Med., 207, 379-390.

Kandoth C., McLellan M.D., Vandin F., Ye K., Niu B., Lu C., Xie M., Zhang Q., McMichael J.F., Wyczalkowski M.A., Leiserson M.D.M., Miller C.A., Welch J.S., Walter M.J., Wendl M.C., Ley T.J., Wilson R.K., Raphael B.J., & Ding L. (2013). Mutational landscape and significance across 12 major cancer types. Nature, 502, 333-339.

Kazak L., Reyes A., & Holt I.J. (2012). Minimizing the damage: repair pathways keep mitochondrial DNA intact. Nat. Rev. Mol. Cell Biol., 13, 659-671.

Kerr I.M. & Stark G.R. (1991). The control of interferon-inducible gene expression. FEBS Lett., 285, 194-198.

Kim S.J., Cheresh P., Williams D., Cheng Y., Ridge K., Schumacker P.T., Weitzman S., Bohr V.A., & Kamp D.W. (2014). Mitochondria-targeted Ogg1 and aconitase-2 prevent oxidant-induced mitochondrial DNA damage in Alveolar Epithelial cells. J. Biol. Chem., 289, 6165-6176.

King M.-C. (2014). "The race" to clone BRCA1. Science, 343, 1462-1465.

Kitaya K., Yasuo T., Yamaguchi T., Fushiki S., & Honjo H. (2007). Genes regulated by interferon-gamma in human uterine microvascular endothelial cells. Int. J. Mol. Med., 20, 689-697.

Koczor C.A., White R.C., Zhao P., Zhu L., Fields E., & Lewis W. (2012). p53 and mitochondrial DNA. Am. J. Pathol., 180, 2276-2283.

Koshiba T. (2013). Mitochondrial-mediated antiviral immunity. Biochim. Biophys. Acta, 1833, 225-232.

Krauss S., Brand M.D., & Buttgereit, F. (2001). Signaling takes a breath – new quantitative perspectives on bioenergetics and signal transduction. Immunity, 15, 497-502.

Kroeger P.E. & Morimoto R.I. (1994). Selection of new HSF1 and HSF2 DNA-binding sites reveals differences in tumor cooperativity. Mol. Cell. Biol., 14, 7592-7603.

Kroemer G. (1997). *Mitochondrial implication in apoptosis. Towards an endosymbiont hypothesis of apoptosis evolution. Cell Death Differ., 4, 443-546.*

Kumar P., Garg R., Bolden G., & Pandey K.N. (2010). *Interactive roles of Ets-1, Sp1, and acetylated histones in the retinoic acid-dependent activation of guanylyl cyclase/atrial natriuretic peptide receptor-A gene transcription. J. Biol. Chem., 285, 37521-37530.*

Larsen S., Kawamoto S., Tanuma S., & Uchiumi F. (2015). *The hematopoietic regulator, ELF-1, enhances the transcriptional response to interferon-β of the OAS1 anti-viral gene. Sci. Rep., 5, 17497.*

Lee M.-H., Na H., Kim E.-J., Lee H.-W., & Lee M.-O. (2012). *Poly(ADP-ribosyl)ation of p53 induces gene-specific transcriptional repression of MTA1. Oncogene, 31, 5099-5107.*

Lee S.H., Kim J.W., Lee H.W., Cho Y.S., Oh S.H., Kim Y.J., Jung C.H., Zhang W., & Lee J.H. (2003). *Interferon regulatory factor-1 (IRF-1) is a mediator for interferon-gamma induced attenuation of telomerase activity and human telomerase reverse transcriptase (hTERT) expression. Oncogene, 22, 381-391.*

Leung A., Todorova T., Ando Y., & Chang P. (2012). *Poly(ADP-ribose) regulate post-transcriptional gene regulation in the cytoplasm. RNA Biol., 9, 542-548.*

Liu G. & Kamp D.W. (2011). *Mitochondrial DNA damage: role of Ogg1 and aconitase. In DNA Repair, (I. Kruman ed.), InTech-Open Access Publisher, Inc., Rijeka, Croatia. (pp. 85-102).*

Liu J., Kim J., & Oberdoerffer P. (2013). *Metabolic modulation of chromatin: implications for DNA repair and genomic integrity. Front. Genet., 4, 182.*

López-Otín C., Serrano M., Partridge L., Blasco M.A., & Kroemer G. (2013). *The hallmarks of aging. Cell, 153, 1194-1217.*

Lu C., Ward P.S., Kapoor G.S., Rohle D., Turcan S., et al. (2012). *IDH mutation impairs histonedemethylation and results in a block to cell differentiation. Nature, 483, 474-478.*

Luo W., Gangwal K., Sankar S., Boucher K.M., Thomas D., & Lessnick S.L. (2009). *GSTM4 is a microsatellite-containing EWS/FLI target involved in Ewing's sarcoma oncogenesis and therapeutic resistance. Oncogene, 28, 4126-4132.*

Mai S., Muster B., Bereiter-Hahn J., & Jendrach M. (2012). *Autophagy proteins LC3B, ATG5 and ATG12 participate in quality control after mitochondrial damage and influence life span. Autophagy, 8, 47-62.*

Mannonen L., Nikula T., Haveri A., Reinikainen A., Vuola J.M., Lahesmaa R., & Puolakkainen M. (2007). *Up-regulation of host cell genes during interferon-gamma-induced persistent Chlamydia pneumonia infection in HL cells. J. Infect. Dis., 195, 212-219.*

Manuel M., Rallu M., Loones M.-T., Zimarino V., Mezger V., & Morange M. (2002). *Determination of the consensus sequence for the purified embryonic heat shock factor 2. Eur. J. Biochem., 269, 2527-2537.*

Marecki S., Riendeau C.J., Liang M.D., & Fenton M.J. (2001). *PU.1 and multiple IFN regulatory factor proteins synergize to mediate transcriptional activation of the human IL-1β gene. J. Immunol., 166, 6829-6838.*

Margolin K., Lazarus M., & Kaufman H.L. (2013). *Cytokines in the treatment of cancer. In Cancer Immunotherapy. Paradigms, Practice and Promise. (T.J. Curiel ed.), Springer Science +Business Media, New York, NY (pp. 173-210).*

Martin N., Schwamborn K., Schreiber V., Werner A., Guillier C., Zhang X.-D., Bischof O., Seeler J.-S., & Dejean A. (2009). *PARP-1 transcriptional activity is regulated by sumoylation upon heat shock. EMBO J., 28, 3534-3548.*

Masumi A., Hamaguchi I., Kuramitsu M., Mizukami T., Takizawa K., Momose H., Nuito S., & Yamaguchi K. (2009). *Interferon regulatory factor-2 induces megakaryopoiesis in mouse bone marrow hematopoietic cells. FEBS Lett., 583, 3493-3500.*

Mendoza-Alvarez H. & Alvarez-Gonzalez R. (2001). *Regulation of p53 sequence-specific DNA-binding by covalent poly(ADP-ribosyl)ation. J. Biol. Chem., 276, 36425-36430.*

Menendez D., Inga A., & Resnick M.A. (2009). *The expanding universe of p53 targets. Nat. Rev. Cancer, 9, 724-737.*

Meraro D., Gleit-Kielmanowicz M., Hauser H., & Levi B.-Z. (2002). *IFN-stimulated gene 15 is synergistically activated through interactions between the myelocyte/lymphocyte-specific transcription factors, PU.1, IFN regulatory factor-8/IFN consensus sequence binding protein, and IFN regulatory factor-4: characterization of a new subtype of IFN-stimulated response element. J. Immunol., 168, 6224-6231.*

Merika M. & Thanos D. (2001). *Enhanceosomes. Curr. Opin. Genet. Dev., 11, 205-208.*

Meyer R.G., Meyer-Ficca M.L., Jacobson E.L., & Jacobson, M.K. (2003). Human poly(ADP-ribose) glycohydrolase (PARG) gene and the common promoter sequence it shares with inner mitochondrial membrane translocase 23 (TIM23). Gene, 314, 181-190.

Michalek R.D., Gerriets V.A., Jacobs S.R., Macintyre A.N., MacIver N.J., Mason E.F., Sullivan S.A., Nichols A.G., & Rathmell J.C. (2011). Cutting edge: Distinct glycolytic and lipid oxidative metabolic programs are essential for effector and regulatory CD4+ T cell subsets. J. Immunol., 186, 3299-3303.

Miki Y., Swensen J., Shattuck-Eidens D., Futreal P.A., Harshman K., Tavtigian S., Liu Q., Cochran C., Bennett L.M., Ding W., Bell R., Rosenthal J., Hussey C., Tran T., McClure M., Frye C., Hattier T., Phelps R., Haugen-Strano A., Katcher H., Yakumo K., Gholami Z., Shaffer D., Stone S., Bayer S., Wray C., Bogden R., Dayananth P., Ward J., Tonin P., Narod S., Bristow P.K., Norris F.H., Helvering L., Morrison P., Rosteck P., Lai M., Barrett J.C., Lewis C., Neuhausen S., Cannon-Albright L., Goldgar D., Wiseman R., Kamb A. & Skolnick M.H. (1994). A strong candidate for the breast and ovarian cancer susceptibility gene BRCA1. Science, 266, 66-71.

Mohan V. & Madhusuden S. (2013). DNA base excision repair: evolving biomarkers for personalized therapies in cancer. In New Research Directions in DNA Repair, (C. Chen ed.), InTech-Open Access Publisher, Inc., Rijeka, Croatia. (pp. 529-557).

Moiseeva O., Bourdeau V., Roux A., Deschênes-Simard X., & Ferbeyre G. (2009). Mitochondrial dysfunction contributes to oncogene-induced senescence. Mol. Cell. Biol., 29, 4495-4507.

Monument M.J., Johnson K.M., Grossmann A.H., Schiffman J.D., Randall R.L., & Lessnick S.L. (2012). Microsatellites with macro-influence in ewing sarcoma. Genes, 3, 444-460.

Morita A., Tanimoto K., Murakami T., Morinaga T., & Hosoi Y. (2014). Mitochondria are required for ATM activation by extranuclear oxidative stress in cultured human hepatoblastoma cell line Hep G2 cells. Biochem. Biophys. Res. Commun., 443, 1286-1290.

Nakaki F., Hayashi K., Ohta H., Kurimoto K., Yabuta Y., & Saitou M. (2013). Induction of mouse germ-cell fate by transcription factors in vitro. Nature, 501, 222-226.

Navarro-Lérida I., Portolés M.T., Barrientos A.A., Gavilanes F., Boscá L., & Rodríguez-Crespo I. (2004). Induction of nitric oxide synthase-2 proceeds with the concomitant downregulation of the endogenous caveolin levels. J. Cell Sci., 117, 1687-1697.

Negrini S., Gorgoulis V.G., & Halazonetis T.D. (2010). Genomic instability – an evolving hallmark of cancer. Nat. Rev. Mol. Cell Biol., 11, 220-228.

Nelson N., Marks M.S., Driggers P.H., & Ozato K. (1993). Interferon consensus sequence-binding protein, a member of the interferon regulatory factor family, suppresses interferon-induced gene transcription. Mol. Cell. Biol., 13, 588-599.

Nguyen V.T. & Benveniste E.N. (2000). Involvement of STAT-1 and Ets family members in interferon-γ induction of CD40 transcription in microglia/macrophages. J. Biol. Chem., 275, 23674-23684.

Niere M., Mashimo M., Agledal L., Dölle C., Kasamatsu A., Kato J., Moss J., & Ziegler M. (2012). ADP-ribosylhydrolase 3 (ARH3), not poly(ADP-ribose) glycohydrolase (PARG) isoforms, is responsible for degradation of mitochondrial matrix-associated poly(ADP-ribose). J. Biol. Chem., 287, 16088-16102.

Odegaard J.I. & Chawla A. (2013). The immune system as a sensor of the metabolic state. Immunity, 38, 644-654.

Oikawa T. & Yamada T. (2003). Molecular biology of the Ets family of transcription factors. Gene, 303, 11-34.

O'Neill L.A.J. & Grahame Hardie D. (2013). Metabolism of inflammation limited by AMPK and pseudo-starvation. Nature, 493, 346-355.

O'Reilly D., Quinn C.M., El-Shanawany T., Gordon S., & Greaves D.R. (2003). Multiple Ets factors and interferon regulatory factor-4 modulate CD68 expression in a cell type-specific manner. J. Biol. Chem., 278, 21909-21919.

Pagano G., Talamanca A.A., Castello G., d'ischia M., Pallardó F.V., Petrovi□ S., Porto B., Tiano L., & Zatterale A. (2013). Bone marrow cell transcripts from Fanconi anaemia patients reveal in vivo alterations in mitochondrial, redox and DNA repair pathaways. Eur. J. Haematol., 91, 141-151.

Pathak S., Ma S., Trinh L., Eudy J., Wagner K.-U., Joshi S.S., & Lu R. (2011). IRF4 is a suppressor of c-Myc induced B cell leukemia. PLoS One, 6, e22628.

Pearce E.L., & Pearce E.J. (2013). Metabolic pathways in immune cell activation and quiescence. Immunity, 38, 633-643.

Pearce E.L., Poffenberger M.C., Chang C.-H., & Jones R.G. (2013). *Fueling immunity: insights into metabolism and lymphocyte function. Science, 342, 1242454.*

Perry D.J., Austin K.J., & Hansen T.R. (1999). *Cloning of interferon-stimulated gene 17: the promoter and nuclear proteins that regulate transcription. Mol. Endocrinol., 13, 1197-1206.*

Pohjoismäki J.L.O., Boettger T., Liu Z., Goffart S., Szibor M., & Braun T. (2012). *Oxidative stress during mitochondrial biogenesis compromises mtDNA integrity in growing hearts and induces a global DNA repair response. Nucleic Acids Res., 40, 6595-6607.*

Pollard P.J., Brière J.J., Alam N.A., Barwell J., Barclay E., Wortham N.C., Hunt T., Mitchell M., Olpin S., Moat S.J., Hargreaves I.P., Heales S.J., Chung Y.L., Griffiths J.R., Dalgleish A., McGrath J.A., Gleeson M.J., Hodgson S.V., Poulsom R., Rustin P., & Tomlinson I.P. (2005). *Accumulation of Krebs cycle intermediates and over-expression of HIFalpha in tumors which result from germline FH and SDH mutations. Hum. Mol. Genet., 14, 2231-2239.*

Prickett T.D. & Samuels Y. (2012). *Molecular pathways: dysregulated glutamatergic signaling pathways in cancer. Clin. Cancer Res., 18, 4240-4246.*

Rahman N. (2014). *Realizing the promise of cancer predisposition genes. Nature, 505, 302-308.*

Rawi S.A., Louvet-Vallée S., Djeddi A., Sachse M., Culetto E., Hajjar C., Boyd L., Legouis R., & Galy V. (2011). *Postfertilization autophagy of sperm organelles prevents paternal mitochondrial DNA transmission. Science, 334, 1144-1147.*

Rehmani I., Liu F., & Liu A. (2013). *Cell signaling and transcription. InMolecular Basis of Oxidative Stress: Chemistry, Mechanisms, and Disease Pathogenesis, (F.A. Villamena ed.), John Wiley & Sons, Inc., Hoboken, NJ. (pp. 179-201).*

Renson P., Blanchard Y., Le Dimna M., Felix H., Cariolet R., Jestin A., & Le Potier M.-F. (2010). *Acute induction of cell death-related IFN stimulated genes (ISG) differentiates highly from moderately virulent CSFV strains. Vet. Res., 41, 07.*

Rhee H.S., & Pugh B.F. (2012). *Genome-wide structure and organization of eukaryotic pre-initiation complexes. Nature, 483, 295-301.*

Rossi M.N., Carbone M., Mostocotto C., Mancone C., Tripodi M., Maione R., & Amati P. (2009). *Mitochondrial localization of PARP-1 requires interaction with mitofilin and is involved in the maintenance of mitochondrial DNA integrity. J. Biol. Chem., 284, 31616-31624.*

Rouyez M.C., Lestingi M., Charon M., Fichelson S., Buzyn A., & Dusanter-Fourt I. (2005). *IFN regulatory factor-2 cooperates with STAT1 to regulate transporter associated with antigen processing-1 promoter activity. J. Immunol., 174, 3948-3958.*

Rubinstein A.D., Eisenstein M., Ber Y., Bialik S., & Kimchi A. (2011). *The autophagy protein Atg12 associates with antiapoptotic Bcl-2 family members to promote mitochondrial apoptosis. Mol. Cell, 44, 698-709.*

Rutherford M.N., Kumar A., Haque S.J., Ghysdeal J., & Williams B.R. (1997). *Specific binding of the ETS-domain protein to the interferon-stimulated response element. J. Interferon Cytokine Res., 17, 1-10.*

Ryu H., Al-Ani G., Deckert K., Kirkpatrick D., Gygi S.P., & Dasso M. (2010). *PIASy mediates SUMO-2/3 conjugation of poly(ADP-ribose) polymerase 1 (PARP1) on mitotic chromosomes. J. Biol. Chem., 285, 14415-14423.*

Sahin E., Colla S., Liesa M., Moslehi J., Müller F.L., Guo M., CooperM., Kotton D., Fabian A.J., Walkey C., Maser R.S., Tonon G., Foerster F., Xiong R., Wang Y.A., Shukla S.A., Jaskelioff M., Martin E.S., Heffernan T.P., Protopopov A., Ivanova E., Mahoney J.E., Kost-Alimova M., Perry S.R., Bronson R., Liao R., Mulligan R., Shirihai O.S., Chin L., & DePinho R.A. (2011). *Telomere dysfunction induces metabolic and mitochondrial compromise, Nature, 470, 359-365.*

Sajish M., Zhou Q., Kishi S., Valdez Jr. D.M., Kapoor M., Guo M., Lee S., Kim S., Yang X.-L., & Schimmel P. (2013). *TrptRNA synthetase bridges DNA-PKcs to PARP-1 to link IFN-γ and p53 signaling. Nat. Chem. Biol., 8, 547-554.*

Sandhya Rani M.R., Shrock J., Appachi S., Rudick R.A., Williams B.R.G., & Ransohoff R.M. (2007). *Novel interferon-b-induced gene expression in peripheral blood cells. J. Leukoc. Biol., 82, 1353-1360.*

Sankaran V.G., Orkin S.H., & Walkley C.R. (2008). *Rb intrinsically promotes erythropoiesis by coupling cell cycle exit with mitochondrial biogenesis. Genes Dev., 22, 463-475.*

Santidrian A.F., Matsuno-Yagi A., Ritland M., Seo B.B., LeBoeuf S.E., Gay L.J., Yagi T., & Felding-Habermann B. (2013). *Mitochondrial complex I activity and NAD+/NADH balance regulate breast cancer progression. J. Clin. Invest., 123, 1068-1081.*

Sato M. & Sato K. (2011). *Degradation of paternal mitochondria by fertilization-triggerd autophagy in C. elegans embryos. Science, 334, 1141-1147.*

Scatena R. (2012). *Mitochondria and cancer: A growing role in apoptosis, cancer cell metabolism and differentiation. In Advances in Mitochondrial Medicine*, (R. Scatena, P. Bottoni, B. Giardina eds.), Springer Science+Business Media B.V., Dordrecht, Germany. (pp. 287-308).

Scherbik S.V., Stockman B.M., & Brinton M.A. (2007). *Differential expression of Interferon (IFN) regulatory factors and IFN-stimulated genes at early times after West Nile virus infection of mouse embryo fibroblasts.* J. Virol., 81, 12005-12018.

Schoggins J.W., Wilson S.J., Panis M., Murphy M.Y., Jones C.T., Bieniasz P., & Rice C.M. (2011). *A diverse range of gene products are effectors of the type I interferon antiviral response.* Nature, 472, 481-485.

Sementchenko V.I. & Watson D.K. (2000). *Ets target genes: past, present and future.* Oncogene, 19, 6533-6548.

Sena L.A., Li S., Jairaman A., Prakriya M., Ezponda T., Hildeman D.A., Wang C.-R., Schumacker P.T., Licht J.D., Perlman H., Bryce P.J., & Chandel N.S. (2013). *Mitochondria are required for antigen-specific T cell activation through reactive oxygen species signaling.* Immunity, 38, 225-236.

Seyfried T.N. & Shelton L.M. (2010). *Cancer as a metabolic disease.* Nutr. Metabol., 7, 7.

Seyfried T.N. (2012). *Confusion surrounds the origin of cancer. In Cancer as a metabolic disease*, A John Wiley & Sons, Inc., Publication, Hoboken, NJ. (pp. 15-29).

Sharma N.K., Lebedeva M., Thomas T., Kovalenko O.A., Stumpf J.D., Shadel G.S., & Santos J.H. (2014). *Intrinsic mitochondrial DNA repair defects in Ataxia Telangiectasia.* DNA Repair (Amst), 13, 22-31.

Sheikh S.Z., Kobayashi T., Matsuoka K., Onyiah J.C., & Plevy S.E. (2011). *Characterization of an interferon-stimulated response element (ISRE) in the Il23a promoter.* J. Biol. Chem., 286, 1174-1180.

Shi H.X., Yang K., Liu X.Y., Wei B., Shan Y.F., Zhu L.H., & Wang C. (2010). *Positive regulation of interferon regulatory factor 3 activation by HERC5 via ISG15 modification.* Mol. Cell. Biol., 30, 2424-2436.

Shuai K. (2006). *Regulation of cytokine signaling pathways by PIAS proteins.* Cell Res., 16, 196-202.

Shultze A. & Harris A.L. (2012). *How cancer metabolism is tuned for proliferation and vulnerable to disruption.* Nature, 491, 364-373.

Sonoda J., Laganière J., Mehl I.R., Barish G.D., Chong L.-W., Li X., Scheffler I.E., Mock D.C., Bataille A.R., Robert F., Lee C.-H., Giguère V., & Evans R.M. (2007). *Nuclear receptor ERRα and coactivator PGC-1β are effectors of IFN-γ-induced host defense.* Genes Dev., 21, 1909-1920.

Stark G.R. & Darnel Jr. J.E. (2012). *The JAK-STAT pathway at twenty*, Immunity, 36, 503-514.

Steer J.H., Kroeger K.M., Abraham L.J., & Joyce D.A. (2000). *Glucocorticoids suppress tumor necrosis factor-α expression by human monocytic THP-1 cells by suppressing transactivation through adjacent NF-κB and c-Jun-activating transcription factor-2 binding sites in the promoter.* J. Biol. Chem., 275, 18432-18440.

Tahk S., Liu B., Chernishf V., Wong K.A., Wu H., & Shuai K. (2007). *Control of speficicity and magnitude of NF-kappa B and STAT1-mediated gene activation through PIASy and PIAS1 cooperation.* Proc. Natl. Acad. Sci. USA, 104, 11643-11648.

Tait S.W. & Green D.R. (2010). *Mitochondria and cell death: outer membrane permeabilization and beyond.* Nat. Rev. Mol. Cell Biol., 11, 621-632.

Takahashi K. & Yamanaka S. (2006). *Induction of pluripotent stem cells from mouse embryonic and adult fibroblast cultures by defined factors.* Cell, 126, 663-676.

Takaoka A., Hayakawa S., Yanai H., Stoiber D., Negishi H., Kikuchi H., Sasaki S., Imai K., Shibue T., Honda K., & Taniguchi T. (2003). *Integration of interferon-α/β signaling to p53 responses in tumor suppression and antiviral defense.* Nature, 424, 516-523.

Tammineni P., Anugula C., Mohammed F., Anjaneyulu M., Larner A.C., & Sepuri N.B.V. (2013). *The import of the transcription factor STAT3 into mitochondria depends on GRIM-19, a component of the electron transport chain.* J. Biol. Chem., 288, 4723-4732.

Tan B., Young D.A., Lu Z.-H., Meier T.I., Shepard R.L., Roth K., Zhai Y., Huss K., Kuo M.-S., Gillig J., Parthasarathy S., Burkholder T.P., Smith M.C., Geeganage S., & Zhao G. (2012). *Pharmacological inhibition of nicotinamide phosphoribosyltransferase (NAMPT), an enzyme essential for NAD+ biosynthesis, in human cancer cells.* J. Biol. Chem., 288, 3500-3511.

Tell G., Quadrifoglio F., Tiribelli C., & Kelley M.R. (2009). *The many functions of APE1/Ref-1: Not only a DNA repair enzyme. Antioxid Redox Signal*, 11, 601-620.

Turner E.C. & Kinsella B.T. (2009). *Transcriptional regulation of the human prostacyclin receptor gene is dependent on Sp1, PU.1 and Oct-1 in megakaryocytes and endothelial cells. J. Mol. Biol.*, 386, 579-597.

Uchiumi F., Watanabe T., & Tanuma S. (2010). *Characterization of various promoter regions of human DNA helicase-encoding genes and identification of duplicated ets (GGAA) motifs as an essential transcription regulatory element. Exp. Cell Res.*, 316, 1523-1534.

Uchiumi F., Watanabe T., Hasegawa S., Hoshi T., Higami Y., & Tanuma S. (2011a). *The effect of Resveratrol on the Werner Syndrome RecQ helicase gene and telomerase activity. Curr. Aging Sci.*, 4, 1-7.

Uchiumi F., Miyazaki S., & Tanuma S. (2011b). *The possible functions of duplicated ets (GGAA) motifs located near transcription start sites of various human genes. Cell. Mol. Life Sci.*, 68, 2039-2051.

Uchiumi F., Watanabe T., Ohta R., Abe H., & Tanuma S. (2013a). *PARP1 gene expression is downregulated by knockdown of PARG gene. Oncol. Rep.*, 29, 1683-1688.

Uchiumi F., Larsen S., Masumi A., & Tanuma S. (2013b). *The putative implications of duplicated GGAA-motifs located in the human interferon regulated genes (ISGs). In Genomics I-Humans, Animals and Plants, (iConcept ed.), iConcept Press Ltd., Hong Kong. (pp. 87-105).*

Uchiumi F., Fujikawa M., Miyazaki S., & Tanuma S. (2013c). *Implication of bidirectional promoters containing duplicated GGAA motifs of mitochondrial function-associated genes. AIMS Mol. Sci.*, 1, 1-26.

Uchiumi F., Larsen S., & Tanuma S. (2015).*Transcriptional regulation of the human genes that encode DNA repair- and mitochondrial function-associated proteins. In Advances in DNA Repair, (C. Chen ed.), InTech-Open Access Publisher, Inc., Rijeka, Croatia. (pp. 129-167).*

Uchiumi F., Shoji K., Sasaki Y., Sasaki M., Sasaki Y., Oyama T., Sugisawa K., & Tanuma S. (2016). *Characterization of the 5'-flanking region of the human TP53 gene and its response to the natural compound, Resveratrol. J. Biochem.*, doi:10.1093/jb/mvv126, in press.

Ungureanu D., Vanhatupa S., Gronholm J., Palvimo J.J., & Silvennoinen O. (2005). *SUMO-1 conjugation selectively modulates STAT1-mediated gene responses. Blood*, 106, 224-226.

Vafai S.B. & Mootha V.K. (2012). *Mitochondrial disorders as windows into an ancient organelle. Nature*, 491, 374-383.

Venkitaraman A.R. (2014). *Cancer suppression by the chromosome custodians, BRCA1 and BRCA2. Science*, 343, 1470-1475.

Viale A.M. & Arakaki A.K. (1994).*The chaperone connection to the origins of the eukaryotic organelles. FEBS Lett.*, 341, 146-151.

Vogelstein B., Papadopoulos N., Velculescu V.E., Zhou S., Diaz Jr. L.A., & Kinzler K.W. (2013). *Cancer genome landscapes. Science*, 339, 1546-1558.

Vousden K.H. & Lane D.P. (2007). *p53 in health and disease. Nat. Rev. Mol. Cell Biol.*, 8, 275-283.

Vousden K.H. & Ryan K.M. (2009). *p53 and metabolism. Nat. Rev. Cancer*, 9, 691-700.

Wang I.-M., Contursi C., Masumi A., Ma X., Trinchieri G., & Ozato K. (2000). *An IFN-γ-inducible transcription factor, IFN consensus sequence binding protein (ICSBP), stimulates IL12 p40 expression in macrophages. J. Immunol.*, 165, 271-279.

Wei G.H., Badis G., Berger M.F., Kivioja T., Palin K., Enge M., Bonke M., Jolma A., Varjosalo M., Gehrke A.R., Yan J., Talukder S., Turunen M., Taipale M., Stunnenberg H.G., Ukkonen E., Hughes T.R., Bulyk M.L. & Taipale J. (2010). *Genome-wide analysis of ETS-family DNA-binding in vitro and in vivo. EMBO J.*, 29, 2147-2160.

Wei L., Fan M., Xu L., Heinrich K., Berry M.W., Homayouni R., & Pfeffer L.M. (2008). *Bioinformatic analysis reveals cRel as a regulator of a subset of interferon-stimurated genes. J. Interferon Cytokine Res.*, 28, 541-552.

Wei L., Nakajima S., Hsieh C.L., Kanno S., Masutani M., Levine A.S., Yasui A., & Lan L. (2013). *Damage response of XRCC1 at sites of DNA single strand breaks is regulated by phosphorylation and ubiquitylation after degradation of poly(ADP-ribose). J. Cell Sci.*, 126, 4414-4423.

West A.P., Shadel G.S., & Ghosh S. (2011). *Mitochondria in innate immune responses. Nat. Rev. Immunol.*, 11, 389-402.

Whatcott C.J., Meyer-Ficca M.L., Meyer R.G., & Jacobson M.K. (2009). *A specific isoform of poly(ADP-ribose) glycohydrolase is targeted to the mitochondrial matrix by a N-terminal mitochondrial targeting sequence. Exp. Cell Res.*, 315, 3477-3485.

Wolters S. & Schumacher B. (2013). Genome maintenance and transcription integrity in aging and disease. Front. Genet., 4, 19.

Wong J.J., Pung Y.F., Sze N.S., & Chin K.C. (2006). HERC5 is an IFN-induced HECT-type E3 protein ligase that mediates type I IFN-induced ISGylation of protein targets. Proc. Natl. Acad. Sci. USA, 103, 10735-10740.

Xie X., Lu J., Kulbokas E.J., Golub T.R., Mootha V., Lindblad-Toh K., Lander E.S., & Kellis M. (2005). Systematic discovery of regulatory motifs in human promoters and 3' UTRs by comparison of several mammals. Nature, 434, 338-345.

Xiong G.M. & Gasser S. (2011). Integration of the DNA damage response with innate immune pathways. In DNA Repair and Human Health, (Vengrova S. ed.), InTech-Open Access Publisher, Inc., Rijeka, Croatia. (pp. 715-742).

Yamamoto K., Miura O., Hirosawa S., & Miyasaka N. (1997). Binding sequence of STAT4: STAT4 complex recognizes the IFN-gamma activation site (GAS)-like sequence (T/A)TTCC(C/G)GGAA(T/A). Biochem. Biophys. Res. Commun., 233, 126-132.

Yan H., Parsons D.W., Jin G., McLendon R., Rasheed B.A., Yuan W., Kos I., Batinic-Harberle I., Jones S., Riggins G.J., Friedman H., Friedman A., Reardon D., Herndon J., Kinzler K.W., Velculescu V.E., Vogelstein B., & Bigner D.D. (2009). IDH1 and IDH2 mutations in gliomas. N. Engl. J. Med., 360, 765-773.

Yang C., Bolotin E., Jiang T., Sladek F.M., & Martinez E. (2007). Prevalence of the initiator over the TATA box in human and yeast genes and identification of DNA motifs enriched in human TATA-less core promoters. Gene, 389, 52-65.

Yang D., Oyaizu Y., Oyaizu H., Olsen G.J., & Woese C.R. (1985). Mitochondrial origins. Proc. Natl. Acad. Sci. USA, 82, 4443-4447.

Yokoyama Y., Kawamoto T., Mitsuuchi Y., Kurosaki T., Toda K., Ushiro H., Terashima M., Sumimoto H., Kuribayashi I., Yamamoto Y., Maeda T., Ikeda H., Sagara Y., & Shizuta Y. (1990). Human poly(ADP-ribose) polymerase gene. Cloning of the promoter region. Eur. J. Biochem., 194, 521-526.

Yuan S.S., Lee S.Y., Chen G., Song M., Tomlinson G.E., & Lee E.Y. (1999). BRCA2 is required for ionizing radiation-induced assembly of Rad51 complex in vivo. Cancer Res., 59, 3547-3551.

Zheng X., Ravatn R., Lin Y., Shih W.-C., Rabson A., Strair R., Huberman E., Conney A., & Chin K.V. (2002). Gene expression of TPA induced differentiation in HL-60 cells by DNA microarray analysis. Nucleic Acids Res., 30, 4489-4499.

Zhou B., Ikejima T., Watanabe T., Iwakoshi K., Idei Y., Tanuma S., & Uchiumi F. (2009). The effect of 2-deoxy-D-glucose on Werner syndrome RecQ helicase gene. FEBS Lett., 583, 1331-1336.

Zhuang J., Wang P.-Y., Huang X., Chen X., Kang, J.-G., & Hwang, P.M. (2013). Mitochondrial disulfide relay mediates translocation of p53 and partitions its subcellular activity. Proc. Natl. Acad. Sci. USA, 110, 17356-17361.

The Genetic Landscape of Acute Lymphoblastic Leukemia as drawn by Next Generation Sequencing Technology

Ilaria Iacobucci[*], Annalisa Lonetti[†], Anna Ferrari[*], Marco Togni[‡],
Margherita Perricone[*], and Giovanni Martinelli[*]

1   Acute lymphoblastic leukemia

Acute lymphoblastic leukemia (ALL) is a heterogeneous group of lymphoid disorders with different clinical and biological aspects, characterized by the aberrant proliferation and expansion of immature B or T lymphoid cells in the bone marrow, blood, and other organs. There are no specific symptoms of ALL, but the presentation encompasses different complaints which correlate to bone marrow failure and infiltration of the proliferating leukemic blasts, such as fatigue, fever, loss of weight, hemorrhagic manifestations, lymphadenopathy, hepatomegaly, and splenomegaly (Inaba *et al.*, 2013). Regarding the possible environmental causes, e.g. the exposure to radiations, their role remains controversial, also because the absence of *in vitro* or *in vivo* models.

ALL is the most common childhood acute leukemia, representing about 80% of acute leukemias, whereas it makes up only 20% of adult leukemias. Its incidence has a bimodal distribution with an early peak at approximately age 4 to 5 years, and a subsequent increase over 50 years (Sallan, 2006). Although the precise pathogenetic events leading to development of ALL are still unknown, different studies indicated that multiple mutations are required to induce leukemia as well as drug resistance in both pediatric and adult patients (Iacobucci *et al.*, 2009; Mullighan *et al.*, 2007). The use of intensive and multi-agent chemotherapy regimens allowed a 5-year event-free survival of > 80% in children, whereas adult ALL patients have a worse prognosis with cure rate estimated to be between 20% and 40% (Pui *et al.*, 2009; 2010; Sive *et al.*, 2012). Even now, the initial leukocyte count, age at diagnosis, T-cell immunophenotype and early treatment response, continue to be important indicators for risk assessment (Pui *et al.*, 2010). However, their influence is reduced by ameliorated risk-adapted therapeutic protocols (Pui *et al.*, 2009). Despite the remarkable progress achieved, the treatment of refractory or relapsed ALL remains a major challenge, strengthen the requirement to improve the knowledge about genetic alterations in order to better predict the risk of treatment failure, and develop novel targeted therapies.

Diagnosis of ALL relies on the assessment of morphology, flow cytometry, immunophenotyping, and on the identification of cytogenetic or molecular abnormalities as the major-

[*] Institute of Hematology "L. and A. Seràgnoli", Department of Experimental, Diagnostic and Specialty Medicine, University of Bologna, Italy

[†] Department of Biomedical and Neuromotor Sciences, University of Bologna, Italy

[‡] Paediatric Oncology and Haematology "Lalla Seragnoli", University of Bologna, Italy

ity of ALL carries genomic anomalies. Standard genetic analyses based on karyotyping, fluorescence in situ hybridization (FISH) or molecular approaches can detect some recurring abnormalities, which differ in frequencies between adult and children. In B-ALL the most common pediatric chromosomal alterations include rearrangements of *MLL* at 11q23, t(1;19) *TCF3-PBX1* and t(12;21) *ETV6-RUNX1* (Iacobucci, Papayannidis *et al.*, 2012). In adult B-ALL the presence of Philadelphia chromosome, due to t(9:22) and consequent *BCR-ABL1* fusion transcript, is the most common translocation and is associated with a poor prognosis. Hyperdiploid (more than 50 chromosomes) and hypodiploid (less than 44 chromosomes) ALL are associated with a good and poor prognosis, respectively (Iacobucci, Papayannidis *et al.*, 2012). In T-ALL, chromosomal rearrangements frequently involve *TCR* genes, and the main partners are the transcription factors *TAL1, TAL2, LYL1, LMO1, LMO2*. Other less common abnormalities involve rearrangements of *NUP214* and *ABL1* genes, whereas *NOTCH1* and *FBXW7* are the most common mutated genes (Iacobucci, Papayannidis *et al.*, 2012; Kraszewska *et al.*, 2012).

In more recent years, the development and application of microarray technologies have broadly extended the genetic landscape of ALL. Since 2007, SNP (single nucleotide polymorphism) microarray-based studies have uncovered the presence of submicroscopic copy number alterations (CNAs) especially in B-ALL not previously detected with conventional cytogenetic. These CNAs generally target one or few genes involved in crucial cellular pathways. Deletion of *IKZF1* gene is probably the most important alteration identified in B-ALL, due to its correlation to prognosis. *IKZF1* encodes a lymphoid transcription factor required for the development of all lymphoid lineages, and broad or focal *IKZF1* deletions frequently occur in pediatric and adult B-ALL patients (Iacobucci *et al.*, 2009; Mullighan *et al.*, 2008; Mullighan, Su *et al.*, 2009). Most importantly, deleted *IKZF1* is unable to regulate specific target genes, conferring a distinctive gene expression signature which define a unique and poor outcome B-ALL subgroup, irrespective to the presence of other genetic lesions (e.g. *BCR-ABL1*) (Iacobucci, Iraci *et al.*, 2012). Other frequently observed alterations affect the transcription factor *PAX5* (Mullighan *et al.*, 2007; Iacobucci *et al.*, 2010) and the tumor suppressor genes *CDKN2A/B* (Iacobucci *et al.*, 2011) and *CRLF2* (Mullighan, Collins-Underwood *et al.*, 2009). Of note, several alterations associate among them, for instance *IKZF1* deletions and *BCR-ABL1* fusion transcript (Iacobucci, Iraci *et al.*, 2012), or *CRLF2* rearrangements and *JAK1/2* activating mutations (Mullighan, Collins-Underwood *et al.*, 2009). These observations suggest their cooperative role in B-ALL pathogenesis.

In 2002, Ferrando *et al.* identified for the first time three molecular subtypes of T-ALL related to the activation of distinct oncogenes (*HOX11+, LYL1+* and *TAL1+*), and indicative of leukemic arrest at specific stages of normal thymocyte development (Ferrando *et al.*, 2002). Subsequent studies revealed the presence of mutations in genes involved in T-cell differentiation, including *BCL11B* (Gutierrez *et al.*, 2011), *PTPN2* which is specifically associated with *TLX1+* expression (Kleppe *et al.*, 2010), *IL7R* which is enriched in *TLX3* rearranged and *HOXA* deregulated cases (Zenatti *et al.*, 2011), and duplications of the *MYB* oncogene (Lahortiga *et al.*, 2007). Deregulation of both PTPN2 and IL7R converge on the JAK-STAT pathway, and the discovery of these alterations provided new insight for the development of targeted therapies. Another frequent aberration detected in T-ALL is the loss of PTEN function, due both by gene deletion or post-translational inactivation (Silva *et al.*, 2008). This lipid phosphatase plays a crucial role in regulating PI3K (Phosphoinositide 3-kinase)-AKT pathway and concurrently it is regulated by NOCTH1 (Palomero *et al.*, 2007). The complex interplay between PI3K-AKT upregulation, loss of PTEN function and NOTCH1 mutations is crucial for risk assessment, prediction of response and identification of effective targeted therapies (Larson Gedman *et al.*, 2009).

2   Next Generation Sequencing Technology

Over the past ten years, through the development of novel –omic approaches such as the Next-Generation Sequencing technologies (NGS) also named as second-generation sequencing or massively-parallel sequencing technologies, our ability to analyze the cancer genome has been prominently improved, ensuring a complete picture of all molecular alterations harbored by cancer cells. Actually, the complete sequence of the genome, exome and transcriptome of a cancer cell could be obtain in a relative short time and in a financially sustainable manner, paving the way to the improvement of diagnosis, stratification of the patients in the correct risk classes, and personalized therapy. The most radical improvements of NGS compared to Sanger sequencing consist in: i) *in vitro* generation and clonal amplification of the DNA fragments of interest, avoiding the bottleneck of the cloning in bacteria required for Sanger sequencing and ensuring the possibility to run a large number of sequencing reaction in parallel. ii) The sequences are generated through repeated cycles, avoiding the termination of the sequencing reaction ad each cycle. Based on the approach used for the DNA libraries preparation, immobilization and sequencing, several NGS platforms with specific output characteristics (e.g. reads length, numbers, and reliability of the sequences obtained) are currently available (Table 1) and the choice of a NGS system rather than one another depends on the specific aim of the study (Marguerat *et al.*, 2008).

The Roche 454 Genome Sequencer (GS) FLX (2005) (Droege & Hill, 2008), Illumina Genome Analyzer/Solexa (2006) (Fedurco *et al.*, 2006; Turcatti *et al.*, 2008), and Applied Biosystems (AB) Supported Oligonucleotide Ligation and Detection (SOLiD) (2007) (Shendure *et al.*, 2005) have represented the first tree next-generation sequencing platforms released on the market. The first one, as well as the SOLiD, takes advantage of emulsion PCR (emPCR) in order to amplify the DNA of interest. Briefly, the emPCR is based on the immobilization through adapters of each single DNA fragment of interest to beads in oil–aqueous droplets. Then, a PCR reaction is performed within these droplets to obtain beads containing several thousand copies of the same template sequence. The emPCR beads can then be chemically attached to a physic support and sequenced: 454 Genome Sequencer (GS) FLX adopts a synthesis-mediated sequencing technique that is based on pyrosequencing (Huse *et al.*, 2007); the SOLiD does not use DNA polymerase for sequencing but DNA ligase (ligation-sequencing) (Marguerat *et al.*, 2008; Niedringhaus *et al.*, 2011; Wong *et al.*, 2011). Different are both the approach of immobilization/amplification and sequencing of the DNA in the Illumina Genome Analyzer. In this platform the immobilization is mediated by oligo-adaptors that ensure the link of each DNA fragment to a flow cell. By the Solid-phase "bridge" amplification, each fragment is amplified creating a cluster of molecules of the same DNA fragment. Then, synthesis-mediated sequencing is made through the use of labeled reversible ddNTPs which, after the acquisition of the fluorophore signal by a camera, can be reactivated guaranteeing the continuation of the reaction (Turcatti *et al.*, 2008). Currently, the HiSeq Sequencing Systems series represent one of the most widely used NGS platforms in cancer discovery studies (Cancer Genome Atlas Research N, 2013; Corces-Zimmerman *et al.*, 2014; Roberts *et al.*, 2012; 2014). However, due to a constantly improvement of technologies, additional next-generation sequencers, and eventually third-generation sequencers, are now available (Illumina MiSeq, Pacific Bioscience PACBIO RS II, and Life Technology Ion Proton) (Table 1).

NGS platform	Company/ Former Company	Library Preparation	Sequencing Method	Applications
GS FLX+ System	Roche	Emulsion PCR	Pyrosequencing	WGS (small genome), targeted sequencing, Metagenomics
454 GS Junior System	Roche	Emulsion PCR	Pyrosequencing	WGS (small genome), targeted sequencing
SOLiD™ 4 System	Life Technologies / Applied Biosystems	Emulsion PCR	Sequencing by ligation	WGS, WES, WTS, Metagenomics
HiSeq Sequencing System	Illumina/Solexa	Bridge PCR	Sequencing by synthesis with fluorescent reversible ddNTP	WGS, WES, RNA-seq, RNA profiling, ChIP-seq, Metagenomics
MiSeq System	Illumina/Solexa	Bridge PCR	Sequencing by synthesis with fluorescent reversible ddNTP	WGS (small genome), WES, targeted sequencing, RNA profiling, ChIP-seq
Ion Torrent System	Life Technologies	Emulsion PCR	Pyrosequencing coupled with H^+ ion production detection	WGS (small genome), WES, RNA-seq, targeted sequencing, RNA profiling, ChIP-seq
PACBIO RS II	Pacific Biosciences / Nanofluidics	Not required	Single molecule real time sequencing	WGS (small genome), targeted sequencing

Table 1: Mostly used next-generation platforms in cancer mutation discovery studies. Abbreviations: WGS, whole-genome sequencing; WES, whole-exome sequencing.

With the advent of the NGS, our ability to interrogate the cancer genome has been completely changed. However, with great improvements come also challenges that we need to take in account especially referring to mutations discovery studies in cancer. The i) mutations calling error rate, the ii) discrimination between somatic or germ-line mutations, the iii) tumor clonality and heterogeneity, the iv) lineage tracing and the v) data collection/annotation represent crucial issues that need to be considered when a NGS study is designed. Specific strategies/tools need to be used in order to overtake these challenges. With the technological advance, the NGS sequencers have lower mutations calling error rate, although, so far, a validation for the novel mutations identified by NGS trough conventional sequencing (Sanger seq) or novel deep targeted sequencing techniques is usually required. To overcome the discrimination between somatic or germline mutations, a common strategy is to analyze by NGS not only the tumor sample, but also the paired germline wild-type sample in order to identify the mutations that are only present in the cancer cells and that could be the ones with a role in the tumorigenesis. The tumor heterogeneity is another important aspect to consider when studying cancer genome. By definition, the tumor is a genetic and heterogenic disease in which different cancer cells belonging to the same tumor could have different genetic alterations. The ability to identify and quantify the extension of each clone by next generation sequencing present in a tumor is crucial to make a correct lineage tracing of each clone during the treatment and for monitoring of the minimal residual disease during the follow-up, both of which may have clinical implications and may contribute to therapy resistance. Recently, a novel computational method, SciClone, which identifies the number and genetic composition of subclones by analyzing the variant allele frequencies of somatic mutations, has been developed. It was successfully used to detect subclones in acute myeloid leukemia (AML) and breast cancer samples that, though present at disease onset, were not evident from a single primary tumor sample (Miller *et al.*, 2014).

With specific focus on hematopoietic malignancies as well as acute lymphoblastic leukemia, NGS has been widely used in order to clarify the mutational scenario of specific subgroups of ALL with dismal outcome and/or lacking the most common alterations known to be associated with the disease. These studies will be discussed in details in the next session.

3   NGS and B-cell Acute Lymphoblastic Leukemia

B-cell acute lymphoblastic leukemia (B-ALL) is the most prevalent childhood hematological malignancy, as well as the leading cause of childhood cancer-related mortality. Novel exciting insights into the genetic basis of this disease have been identified using array-based technologies and next-generation sequencing techniques, opening the therapeutic way to individualized treatment plans for affected children.

Whole genome sequencing (WGS) studies have applied to understanding the genetic basis of t(4;11) (q21;q23)/*MLL-AFF1* (AF4)-positive ALL (Meyer *et al.*, 2006; 2009). The incidence of this translocation is influenced by age. In infants (<1 years) the t(4;11) has a 40 – 50% frequency, whereas in children older than 1 year, the incidence is very low (2 – 3%) but increases with age among adults (~10%; >20 years old) (Moorman, 2012). The very high incidence in infants, especially among those under 6 months of age, suggests that the latency period for this subtype of leukemia can be very short (Greaves, 2003). Studies have shown that in these cases the gene fusion arises in utero (Mullighan *et al.*, 2007). Patients with t(4;11) have been reported to have an aggressive disease with consequent high probability of treatment failure and poor outcome at all ages especially in infants who have a worst survival (<20 % 5-year DFS) (Bueno *et al.*, 2011) and are classified as high risk in the international infant treatment protocol (Pieters *et al.*, 2007). WGS showed few somatic alterations (single nucleotide variants, loss of heterozygosity or copy number abnormalities) with most of them affecting important pathways, such as the PI3K-RAS signaling (Dobbins *et al.*, 2013). *RAS* mutations have been already demonstrated to frequently occur in infant *MLL* rearranged ALL cases, especially in t(4;11) ones, and their presence represents an independent poor prognostic factor (Driessen *et al.*, 2013; Liang *et al.*, 2006). The comparison of these data with exome sequencing results from 13 *MLL* cases in older children (7 – 19 years of age; 8 ALLs and 5 AMLs) highlights the significant increase of non-silent mutations in the second group, speculating that the target cell of transformation differs between infants and older children, with the cells present during early development requiring fewer cooperating mutations to induce leukemia (A. Andersson *et al.*, 2012). Whole exome sequencing (WES) has been recently performed to analyze paired tumor-normal (diagnosis versus remission) DNA samples from two patients with congenital t(4;11) ALL. Only few somatic mutations were identified. Specifically, one patient had somatic single mutations in *FAM78B* and *SHH* (*G143S*, not previously reported in ALL), the other one harbored a single somatic mutation in *FLT3* (Chang *et al.*, 2013). Notably, these two last somatic mutations are in genes that are druggable targets (*SMO* and *FLT3* inhibitors). Overall, genome wide-analysis in *MLL-AF4*-positive ALL do not support a scenario of generalized genomic instability but few mutations in key player genes seem to be required for leukemogenesis.

Our group used whole-transcriptome shotgun sequencing (RNA-Seq, Illumina) approach in an attempt to investigate the complex landscape of mutations, changes in expression profiles and alternative splicing events that can occur in *BCR-ABL1*-positive ALL (Iacobucci, Ferrarini *et al.*, 2012). The incidence of the translocation t(9;22) increases with age from 2% in children to 20% in young adults (20 – 39 years) and to 40% among older adults (>40 years) (Moorman *et al.*, 2007). Historically, the presence of the t(9;22) has been associated with a dismal prognosis at all ages (Harrison, 2009). Although the advent of tyrosine kinase inhibitors (TKI) has revolutionized the treatment of all *BCR-ABL1* positive diseases, relapse is still a major obstacle to long-lasting remission. RNA-seq led to the identification of missense mutations affected genes involved in metabolic processes (*DPEP1*, *TMEM46*) and transport (*MVP*) at diagnosis and cell cycle regulation (*ABL1*) and catalytic activity (*CTSZ*) at relapse. Differences in mutational patterns of primary ALL and relapse samples suggested that the leukemia clone from which relapsed cells have been developed was not the predominant one at diagnosis or, more plausibly, that most of the relapse-specific changes are 'passenger' mutations acquired by chance during Ph+ ALL progression by the clone harboring the *BCR-ABL1* T315I mutation responsible for resistance. Point mutations in ABL kinase domain represent the Achilles' heel of therapy with TKI which warrens for sensitive screening methods able to detect small mutated clones before disease relapses. In *BCR-ABL1*-positive ALL cases with molecularly detectable disease but not yet evidence of cytogenetic or hematologic relapse, ultra-deep sequencing UDS could have identified emerging mutations 1 to 3 months before they became detectable by Sanger sequencing (Soverini *et al.*, 2013).

Next generation sequencing has been used with success in *BCR-ABL*-like ALL, an ALL subgroup lacking recurring chromosomal alterations with poor outcome and a gene expression profile significantly similar to that of *BCR-ABL1+* ALL (Den Boer *et al.*, 2009; Mulligan, Su *et al.*, 2009; Roberts *et al.*, 2014). Recently, detailed genomic analysis of 154 patients with Ph-like ALL identified kinase-activating alterations in 91% of cases (e.g. *ABL1*, *ABL2*, *CRLF2*, *CSF1R*, *EPOR*, *JAK2*, *NTRK3*, *PDGFRB*, *PTK2B*, *TSLP*, or *TYK2*). Therapeutically important, most of these alterations are amenable to inhibition with approved tyrosine kinase inhibitors (Roberts *et al.*, 2014).

The heterogeneity of ALL is confirmed by the recent studies in hypodiploid ALL showing multiple recurrent genetic alterations, distinguishing near haploid from low-hypodiploid

ALL (Holmfeldt *et al.*, 2013). Near-haploid ALL cases showed alterations targeting genes in receptor tyrosine kinase (RTK) signaling and Ras signaling (*NF1*) pathways, as well as high frequency alterations in the *IKAROS* gene family, particularly *IKZF3* which encodes for the zinc finger transcription factor AIOLOS. Low-hypodiploid cases showed genetic alterations of *TP53*, *RB1*, and *IKZF2* (Helios). In *TP53* mutated cases, non-tumor cells also harbored *TP53* mutations, suggesting an inherited basis of disease and a possible manifestation of Li-Fraumeni syndrome. Both low-hypodiploid and near-haploid ALL showed activation of RAS-signaling and PI3K signaling pathways that were sensitive to PI3K inhibitors such as rapamycin *in vitro*, suggesting that PI3K inhibitors could be explored as a therapeutic treatment option.

4   NGS and T-cell Acute Lymphoblastic Leukemia

T-cell acute lymphoblastic leukemia (T-ALL) is a less common hematologic malignancy, counting about 15% of childhood and 25% of adult ALL cases (Van Vlierberghe *et al.*, 2012). Novel intensified chemotherapeutic protocols ameliorated the outcome, with survival in children approaching 90% (Inaba *et al.*, 2013). Nevertheless, relapse is frequently observed and treatment in infants and adults needs improvement (Bassan & Hoelzer, 2011; Pui & Evans, 2006). In recent years, application of the novel whole genome scale technologies increased our knowledge about the genomic abnormalities which might sustain the onset/development of T-ALL, or which might contribute to the aggressiveness of the disease (Iacobucci, Papayannidis *et al.*, 2012). Despite that, T-ALL pathogenesis is still unclear and no effective target therapy exists. Because T-ALL is an extremely heterogeneous disease, application of NGS is further improving its characterization with novel notions translatable to clinical practice.

Through the X-chromosome DNA capture followed by NGS, Van Vlierberghe *et al.* (2010) identified a new X-linked tumor suppressor gene, *PHF6* (PHD finger protein 6 on Xq26.3) with a proposed role in controlling gene expression, and whose inactivation is already associated with Borjeson-Forssman-Lehmann syndrome (BFLS, MIM301900). In T-ALL, mutational loss of *PHF6* is a somatically acquired leukemia-associated genetic event, mainly due to widespread nonsense and frameshift mutations, and in a lower extent to missense mutations, which impair gene expression or protein function. *PHF6* mutations seem to be restricted to T-lineage ALL, are more frequent in males than females (Huh *et al.*, 2013), and prevail in adult compared to pediatric patients. Moreover, *PHF6* mutations resulted associated with the aberrant expression of *TLX1* and *TLX3* (Ferrando *et al.*, 2002), and with mutations of *NOTCH1*, *JAK1*, and *SET-NUP214* rearrangement (Wang *et al.*, 2011). Although the knowledge on PHF6 role in leukemogenesis is extremely limited and its clinical significance is still unclear (Van Vlierberghe *et al.*, 2010), this study demonstrated for the first time the power of NGS approach to further dissect T-ALL heterogeneity in order to identify novel partners that cooperate to leukemia development.

The recently identify early T-cell precursor (ETP) leukemia is a novel subtype of T-ALL which comprises up to 15% of T-ALL and confers a poor prognosis (Coustan-Smith *et al.*, 2009). ETP ALL is characterized by a peculiar immunophenotype pattern (absence of CD1a and CD8 expression, weak CD5 expression, and expression of one or more myeloid- or stem cell-associated markers such as CD13, CD33, CD34 and CD117). This pattern is similar to that of murine early T-cell precursor (Rothenberg *et al.*, 2008), the thymic progenitors that have lost B-cell potential but still retain myeloid potential (Wada *et al.*, 2008). An extensive study of pediatric ETP ALL based on WGS, RNA-seq and WES, has been conducted to define common genetic abnormalities (Zhang *et al.*, 2012). Although ETP ALL appeared as a uniform entity, no common alteration has been found. Overall, WGS analysis of 12 ETP ALL followed by a validation analysis in a recurrence cohort of 52 ETP ALL and 42 non-ETP ALL, confirmed a high degree of genetic instability (Coustan-Smith *et al.*, 2009) which induces both structural rearrangements and sequence mutations. Interestingly, among the genes involved in translocations, the authors identified *ETV6*, a transcription factor frequently altered in leukemia which is deleted or mutated in a large proportion of ETP ALL compared to non-ETP ALL (33% versus 10%) (Zhang *et al.*, 2012). In addition to genes commonly mutated in T-ALL, pediatric ETP ALL sequence mutations/indels prevalently target cytokine receptors and RAS signaling pathway (e.g. *BRAF, FLT3, IGFR1, JAK1, JAK3, KRAS, NRAS* ad *IL7R*); genes involved in hematopoietic development (e.g. *RUNX1, IKZF1, ETV6, GATA3* and *EP300*); components of the polycomb repressor complex 2 (*PRC2*) which contributes to histone modifications (e.g. *EED, EZH2* and *SUZ12*) (Zhang *et al.*, 2012). In all cases, the percentage of mutated ETP ALL were extremely higher compared to non-ETP ALL. Novel recurrent somatic mutations have been found in *DNM2, ECT2L* and *RELN*, with unknown functions in normal lymphoid or leukemic development (Zhang *et al.*, 2012). In adult ETP ALL (Neumann *et al.*, 2013), WES analysis confirmed the presence of mutations in several genes, including the novel *DNM2*, and revealed the involvement of epigenetic regulators, in particular *MLL2, DNMT3A,* and with a lower rate *PRC2*. Of note, *DNMT3A* mutations are highly recurrent in patients with de novo acute myeloid leukemia (Ley *et al.*, 2010), highlighting the premature maturational stage of ETP ALL, and encouraging the application of therapies used for AML treatment. *RUNX1* and *DNMT3A* mutations have also been identified in adult T-ALL deep sequencing studies where resulted associated with shorter overall survival (Grossmann *et al.*, 2013). The mutational spectrum of typical T-ALL has been recently analyzed with WES in a large cohort of more than 60 adult and pediatric samples (De Keersmaecker eta l., 2013). Through an accurate filtering approach, novel mutations have been detected in a set of candidate driver genes, including *CNOT3*, proposed to act as a tumor suppressor, and *RPL5* and *RPL10*, two genes encoding ribosomal proteins. Moreover, this study pointed out the clear correlation between the increase in patient age and mutation number, and the differences in mutation distribution between adult and pediatric T-ALL, with CNOT3 mutations mainly present in adults, whereas *RPL10* mutations almost exclusively found in children.

Nowadays, only one study has been conducted to compare matched diagnosis, remission and relapse samples, by means of WES (Tzoneva *et al.*, 2013): the most remarkable finding of this study was the identification of relapse-associated mutations in *NT5C2* (5'-nucleotidase, cytosolic II), involved in cellular purine metabolism. *NT5C2* mutations prevail in relapse T-ALL compared to relapsed B-ALL (19% versus 3%). These mutations affect the nucleotidase activity of *NT5C2* compared to wild-type, and confer resistance to the nucleoside analogs 6-mercaptopurine (6-MP) and 6-thioguanine (6-TG) commonly used in ALL treatment, as assessed in *in vitro* cellular models.

The sensitivity and accuracy of the high-throughput sequencing (HTS) have been translated into clinical practice through a targeted sequencing of T cell receptor (TCR) gene loci (*TCRB* and *TCRG*) by Wu *et al.*, who identified in pre-treatment samples the recombined TCR gene sequences representing the patient's clonal neoplastic T lymphoblasts, and evaluated minimal residual disease (MRD) in paired post-treatment T-ALL patients (Wu *et al.*, 2012). The importance to assess MRD in order to predict clinical outcomes of patients is broadly recognized (Flohr *et al.*, 2008). Compared to conventional multiparametric flow cytometry (mpFC) approach, there were no cases in which MRD was detected by mpFC but not by HTS. Moreover, HTS enabled detection of the clonal TCR rearrangements in post-treatment samples where mpFC failed to do it, highlighting the potential of this technology to improve clinical diagnosis, patients' stratification and subsequent MRD monitoring with lower detection thresholds.

Another analysis based on NGS technology is the targeted re-sequencing. This approach enables the investigation of a set of known cancer related genes and might provide an accurate map of genomic abnormalities useful for patient characterization, risk assessment or therapeutic approach (Kalender Atak *et al.*, 2012).

Finally, NGS has been successfully used in T-ALL murine (Bagley *et al.*, 2012) and cellular models (Zhang *et al.*, 2013). Exon capture sequencing in a murine model for heritable T-ALL, called Spontaneous dominant leukemia (Sdl), detected a spontaneously acquired dominant mutation in Mcm4 (Mcm4D573H), which encodes for a protein essential for the initiation of eukaryotic genome replication. Mcm4D573H is likely the causative tumor genetic lesion in Sdl, although the role of MCM proteins is still unclear in human cancers (Bagley *et al.*, 2012). Whole transcriptome deep sequencing of Jurkat cell line identified T-ALL-R-LncR1 as a novel long non-coding RNAs associated to T-ALL (Zhang *et al.*, 2013). LncRNAs are transcribed RNA molecules that do not encode proteins, and have an emerging role in cancer progression (Yan & Wang, 2012). T-ALL-R-LncR1 was not detected in normal tissue specimens, while its expression was confirmed in tumor tissues and T-ALL patient samples. Moreover, knockdown of T-ALL-R-LncR1 predisposed T-ALL Jurkat cells to undergo Par-4 (the proapoptotic factor prostate apoptosis response protein-4)-induced apoptosis. Although these results obtained in murine or cellular models require further investigations in human T-ALL, they provided novel findings suitable to identify innovative targeted therapies.

5   Conclusions and Future Directions

In hematopoietic malignancies, more than in any other fields, the advent of next-generation sequencing technologies coupled to functional and clinical studies has radically changed our comprehension of the genetic basis of acute lymphoblastic leukemia. This has allowed a more precise sub-classification of genetic subgroups and suggested novel targeted and more effective therapies with a profound impact on the prognosis of patients. The best example is the recent identified *EBF1-PDGFRB* fusion in BCR-ABL1-like ALL that is sensitive to TKIs in clinical settings (Weston *et al.*, 2013). Screening for the novel additional lesions targeting kinases or cytokine receptors could be important in ALL since most of these lesions have been demonstrated in *in vitro* and *ex vivo* models to be sensitive to tyrosine kinase inhibition (Roberts *et al.*, 2014). Moreover, the ability to sequence single clones and to monitor at high sensitivity minimal residual disease by NGS could guide therapeutic interventions preventing leukemia reoccurrence. Overall, the identification of novel diagnostic and prognostic biomarkers and/or genomic signatures able to recommend tailored approaches to leukemia is expected to improve both the anti-leukemia therapeutic success and the sustainability and efficiency of the healthcare system. This will result in a twofold benefit: on one hand very expensive, and in some cases useless or even harmful therapies will be removed, on the other hand new biological drugs will be specifically directed only to patients for whom they are safe and useful. A personalized medicine era is not anymore a dream but is becoming a reality.

Acknowledgement

Supported by European LeukemiaNet, AIL, AIRC, Progetto Regione-Università 2010-12 (L. Bolondi), NGS-PTL project, grant agreement number 306242, funded by the EC Seventh Framework Programme theme FP7- HEALTH-2012-INNOVATION-1.

References

A. Andersson JM, Jianmin Wang, Xiang Chen, Michael Rusch, Gang Wu, John Easton, Matthew Parker, Susana Raimondi, Linda Holmfeldt, Jared Becksfort, Pankaj Gupta, Amanda Gedman, Joy Nakitandwe, Debbie Payne-Turner, Guangchun Song, Rosemary Sutton, Nicola Venn, Albert Chetcuti, Amanda Rush, Daniel Catchpole, Jesper Heldrup, Thoas Fioretos, Charles Lu, Li Ding, Ching-Hon Pui, Sheila Shurtleff, Tanja Gruber, Charles Mullighan, Elaine Mardis, Richard Wilson, Jinghui Zhang, and James Downing. Abstract 4869: Whole genome sequence analysis of MLL rearranged infant acute lymphoblastic leukemias reveals remarkably few somatic mutations: A Report From the St Jude Children's Research Hospital - Washington University Pediatric Cancer Genome Project Cancer Research. 2012;72(8):Supplement1.

Bagley BN, Keane TM, Maklakova VI, Marshall JG, Lester RA, Cancel MM, et al. A dominantly acting murine allele of Mcm4 causes chromosomal abnormalities and promotes tumorigenesis. PLoS Genet. 2012;8(11):e1003034.

Bassan R, Hoelzer D. Modern therapy of acute lymphoblastic leukemia. J Clin Oncol. 2011 Feb 10;29(5):532-43.

Bueno C, Montes R, Catalina P, Rodriguez R, Menendez P. Insights into the cellular origin and etiology of the infant pro-B acute lymphoblastic leukemia with MLL-AF4 rearrangement. Leukemia. 2011 Mar;25(3):400-10.

Cancer Genome Atlas Research N. Genomic and epigenomic landscapes of adult de novo acute myeloid leukemia. The New England journal of medicine. 2013 May 30;368(22):2059-74.

Chang VY, Basso G, Sakamoto KM, Nelson SF. Identification of somatic and germline mutations using whole exome sequencing of congenital acute lymphoblastic leukemia. BMC Cancer. 2013;13:55.

Corces-Zimmerman MR, Hong WJ, Weissman IL, Medeiros BC, Majeti R. Preleukemic mutations in human acute myeloid leukemia affect epigenetic regulators and persist in remission. Proceedings of the National Academy of Sciences of the United States of America. 2014 Feb 18;111(7):2548-53.

Coustan-Smith E, Mullighan CG, Onciu M, Behm FG, Raimondi SC, Pei D, et al. Early T-cell precursor leukaemia: a subtype of very high-risk acute lymphoblastic leukaemia. The Lancet Oncology. 2009 Feb;10(2):147-56.

De Keersmaecker K, Atak ZK, Li N, Vicente C, Patchett S, Girardi T, et al. Exome sequencing identifies mutation in CNOT3 and ribosomal genes RPL5 and RPL10 in T-cell acute lymphoblastic leukemia. Nat Genet. 2013 Feb;45(2):186-90.

Den Boer ML, van Slegtenhorst M, De Menezes RX, Cheok MH, Buijs-Gladdines JG, Peters ST, et al. A subtype of childhood acute lymphoblastic leukaemia with poor treatment outcome: a genome-wide classification study. The Lancet Oncology. 2009 Feb;10(2):125-34.

Dobbins SE, Sherborne AL, Ma YP, Bardini M, Biondi A, Cazzaniga G, et al. The silent mutational landscape of infant MLL-AF4 pro-B acute lymphoblastic leukemia. Genes Chromosomes Cancer. 2013 Oct;52(10):954-60.

Driessen EM, van Roon EH, Spijkers-Hagelstein JA, Schneider P, de Lorenzo P, Valsecchi MG, et al. Frequencies and prognostic impact of RAS mutations in MLL-rearranged acute lymphoblastic leukemia in infants. Haematologica. 2013 Jun;98(6):937-44.

Droege M, Hill B. The Genome Sequencer FLX System--longer reads, more applications, straight forward bioinformatics and more complete data sets. Journal of biotechnology. 2008 Aug 31;136(1-2):3-10.

Fedurco M, Romieu A, Williams S, Lawrence I, Turcatti G. BTA, a novel reagent for DNA attachment on glass and efficient generation of solid-phase amplified DNA colonies. Nucleic acids research. 2006;34(3):e22.

Ferrando AA, Neuberg DS, Staunton J, Loh ML, Huard C, Raimondi SC, et al. Gene expression signatures define novel onco- genic pathways in T cell acute lymphoblastic leukemia. Cancer Cell. 2002 Feb;1(1):75-87.

Flohr T, Schrauder A, Cazzaniga G, Panzer-Grumayer R, van der Velden V, Fischer S, et al. Minimal residual disease-directed risk stratification using real-time quantitative PCR analysis of immunoglobulin and T-cell receptor gene rearrangements in the international multicenter trial AIEOP-BFM ALL 2000 for childhood acute lymphoblastic leukemia. Leukemia. 2008 Apr;22(4):771-82.

Greaves M. Pre-natal origins of childhood leukemia. Rev Clin Exp Hematol. 2003 Sep;7(3):233-45.

Grossmann V, Haferlach C, Weissmann S, Roller A, Schindela S, Poetzinger F, et al. The molecular profile of adult T-cell acute lymphoblastic leukemia: mutations in RUNX1 and DNMT3A are associated with poor prognosis in T-ALL. Genes Chro- mosomes Cancer. 2013 Apr;52(4):410-22.

Gutierrez A, Kentsis A, Sanda T, Holmfeldt L, Chen SC, Zhang J, et al. The BCL11B tumor suppressor is mutated across the major molecular subtypes of T-cell acute lymphoblastic leukemia. Blood. 2011 Oct 13;118(15):4169-73.

Harrison CJ JB. Acute Lymphoblastic Leukaemia. Cancer Cytogenetics. 2009:233–96.

Holmfeldt L, Wei L, Diaz-Flores E, Walsh M, Zhang J, Ding L, et al. The genomic landscape of hypodiploid acute lymphoblastic leukemia. Nat Genet. 2013 Mar;45(3):242-52.

Huh HJ, Lee SH, Yoo KH, Sung KW, Koo HH, Jang JH, et al. Gene mutation profiles and prognostic implications in Korean pa- tients with T-lymphoblastic leukemia. Ann Hematol. 2013 May;92(5):635-44.

Huse SM, Huber JA, Morrison HG, Sogin ML, Welch DM. Accuracy and quality of massively parallel DNA pyrosequencing. Genome biology. 2007;8(7):R143.

Iacobucci I, Ferrari A, Lonetti A, Papayannidis C, Paoloni F, Trino S, et al. CDKN2A/B alterations impair prognosis in adult BCR-ABL1-positive acute lymphoblastic leukemia patients. Clin Cancer Res. 2011 Dec 1;17(23):7413-23.

Iacobucci I, Ferrarini A, Sazzini M, Giacomelli E, Lonetti A, Xumerle L, et al. Application of the whole-transcriptome shotgun sequencing approach to the study of Philadelphia-positive acute lymphoblastic leukemia. Blood Cancer J. 2012 Mar;2(3):e61.

Iacobucci I, Iraci N, Messina M, Lonetti A, Chiaretti S, Valli E, et al. IKAROS deletions dictate a unique gene expression signa- ture in patients with adult B-cell acute lymphoblastic leukemia. PLoS One. 2012;7(7):e40934.

Iacobucci I, Lonetti A, Paoloni F, Papayannidis C, Ferrari A, Storlazzi CT, et al. The PAX5 gene is frequently rearranged in BCR-ABL1-positive acute lymphoblastic leukemia but is not associated with outcome. A report on behalf of the GIMEMA Acute Leukemia Working Party. Haematologica. 2010 Oct;95(10):1683-90.

Iacobucci I, Papayannidis C, Lonetti A, Ferrari A, Baccarani M, Martinelli G. Cytogenetic and molecular predictors of outcome in acute lymphocytic leukemia: recent developments. Curr Hematol Malig Rep. 2012 Jun;7(2):133-43.

Iacobucci I, Storlazzi CT, Cilloni D, Lonetti A, Ottaviani E, Soverini S, et al. Identification and molecular characterization of recurrent genomic deletions on 7p12 in the IKZF1 gene in a large cohort of BCR-ABL1-positive acute lymphoblastic leu- kemia patients: on behalf of Gruppo Italiano Malattie Ematologiche dell'Adulto Acute Leukemia Working Party (GIME- MA AL WP). Blood. 2009 Sep 3;114(10):2159-67.

Inaba H, Greaves M, Mulligan CG. Acute lymphoblastic leukaemia. Lancet. 2013 Jun 1;381(9881):1943-55.

Kalender Atak Z, De Keersmaecker K, Gianfelici V, Geerdens E, Vandepoel R, Pauwels D, et al. High accuracy mutation detec- tion in leukemia on a selected panel of cancer genes. PLoS One. 2012;7(6):e38463.

Kleppe M, Lahortiga I, El Chaar T, De Keersmaecker K, Mentens N, Graux C, et al. Deletion of the protein tyrosine phosphatase gene PTPN2 in T-cell acute lymphoblastic leukemia. Nat Genet. 2010 Jun;42(6):530-5.

Kraszewska MD, Dawidowska M, Szczepanski T, Witt M. T-cell acute lymphoblastic leukaemia: recent molecular biology find- ings. Br J Haematol. 2012 Feb;156(3):303-15.

Lahortiga I, De Keersmaecker K, Van Vlierberghe P, Graux C, Cauwelier B, Lambert F, et al. Duplication of the MYB oncogene in T cell acute lymphoblastic leukemia. Nat Genet. 2007 May;39(5):593-5.

Larson Gedman A, Chen Q, Kugel Desmoulin S, Ge Y, LaFiura K, Haska CL, et al. *The impact of NOTCH1, FBW7 and PTEN mutations on prognosis and downstream signaling in pediatric T-cell acute lymphoblastic leukemia: a report from the Children's Oncology Group. Leukemia. 2009 Aug;23(8):1417-25.*

Ley TJ, Ding L, Walter MJ, McLellan MD, Lamprecht T, Larson DE, et al. *DNMT3A mutations in acute myeloid leukemia. N Engl J Med. 2010 Dec 16;363(25):2424-33.*

Liang DC, Shih LY, Fu JF, Li HY, Wang HI, Hung IJ, et al. *K-Ras mutations and N-Ras mutations in childhood acute leukemias with or without mixed-lineage leukemia gene rearrangements. Cancer. 2006 Feb 15;106(4):950-6.*

Marguerat S, Wilhelm BT, Bahler J. *Next-generation sequencing: applications beyond genomes. Biochem Soc Trans. 2008 Oct;36(Pt 5):1091-6.*

Meyer C, Kowarz E, Hofmann J, Renneville A, Zuna J, Trka J, et al. *New insights to the MLL recombinome of acute leukemias. Leukemia. 2009 Aug;23(8):1490-9.*

Meyer C, Schneider B, Jakob S, Strehl S, Attarbaschi A, Schnittger S, et al. *The MLL recombinome of acute leukemias. Leukemia. 2006 May;20(5):777-84.*

Miller CA, White BS, Dees ND, Griffith M, Welch JS, Griffith OL, et al. *SciClone: inferring clonal architecture and tracking the spatial and temporal patterns of tumor evolution. PLoS computational biology. 2014 Aug;10(8):e1003665.*

Moorman AV HC, Buck GA, Richards SM, Secker-Walker LM, Martineau M, Vance GH, Cherry AM, Higgins RR, Fielding AK, Foroni L, Paietta E, Tallman MS, Litzow MR, Wiernik PH, Rowe JM, Goldstone AH, Dewald GW; . *Karyotype is an independent prognostic factor in adult acute lymphoblastic leukemia (ALL): analysis of cytogenetic data from patients treated on the Medical Research Council (MRC) UKALLXII/Eastern Cooperative Oncology Group (ECOG) 2993 trial. Blood. 2007;109(8):3189-97.*

Moorman AV. *The clinical relevance of chromosomal and genomic abnormalities in B-cell precursor acute lymphoblastic leukaemia. Blood Rev. 2012 May;26(3):123-35.*

Mullighan CG, Collins-Underwood JR, Phillips LA, Loudin MG, Liu W, Zhang J, et al. *Rearrangement of CRLF2 in B-progenitor- and Down syndrome-associated acute lymphoblastic leukemia. Nature genetics. 2009 Nov;41(11):1243-6.*

Mullighan CG, Goorha S, Radtke I, Miller CB, Coustan-Smith E, Dalton JD, et al. *Genome-wide analysis of genetic alterations in acute lymphoblastic leukaemia. Nature. 2007 Apr 12;446(7137):758-64.*

Mullighan CG, Miller CB, Radtke I, Phillips LA, Dalton J, Ma J, et al. *BCR-ABL1 lymphoblastic leukaemia is characterized by the deletion of Ikaros. Nature. 2008 May 1;453(7191):110-4.*

Mullighan CG, Su X, Zhang J, Radtke I, Phillips LA, Miller CB, et al. *Deletion of IKZF1 and prognosis in acute lymphoblastic leukemia. The New England journal of medicine. 2009 Jan 29;360(5):470-80.*

Neumann M, Heesch S, Schlee C, Schwartz S, Gokbuget N, Hoelzer D, et al. *Whole-exome sequencing in adult ETP-ALL reveals a high rate of DNMT3A mutations. Blood. 2013 Jun 6;121(23):4749-52.*

Niedringhaus TP, Milanova D, Kerby MB, Snyder MP, Barron AE. *Landscape of next-generation sequencing technologies. Anal Chem. 2011 Jun 15;83(12):4327-41.*

Palomero T, Sulis ML, Cortina M, Real PJ, Barnes K, Ciofani M, et al. *Mutational loss of PTEN induces resistance to NOTCH1 inhibition in T-cell leukemia. Nat Med. 2007 Oct;13(10):1203-10.*

Pieters R, Schrappe M, De Lorenzo P, Hann I, De Rossi G, Felice M, et al. *A treatment protocol for infants younger than 1 year with acute lymphoblastic leukaemia (Interfant-99): an observational study and a multicentre randomised trial. Lancet. 2007 Jul 21;370(9583):240-50.*

Pui CH, Campana D, Pei D, Bowman WP, Sandlund JT, Kaste SC, et al. *Treating childhood acute lymphoblastic leukemia without cranial irradiation. N Engl J Med. 2009 Jun 25;360(26):2730-41.*

Pui CH, Evans WE. *Treatment of acute lymphoblastic leukemia. N Engl J Med. 2006 Jan 12;354(2):166-78.*

Pui CH. *Recent research advances in childhood acute lymphoblastic leukemia. J Formos Med Assoc. 2010 Nov;109(11):777-87.*

Roberts KG, Li Y, Payne-Turner D, Harvey RC, Yang YL, Pei D, et al. *Targetable kinase-activating lesions in Ph-like acute lymphoblastic leukemia. The New England journal of medicine. 2014 Sep 11;371(11):1005-15.*

Roberts KG, Morin RD, Zhang J, Hirst M, Zhao Y, Su X, et al. *Genetic alterations activating kinase and cytokine receptor signaling in high-risk acute lymphoblastic leukemia. Cancer cell. 2012 Aug 14;22(2):153-66.*

Rothenberg EV, Moore JE, Yui MA. *Launching the T-cell-lineage developmental programme. Nat Rev Immunol. 2008 Jan;8(1):9-21.*

Sallan SE. *Myths and lessons from the adult/pediatric interface in acute lymphoblastic leukemia. Hematology Am Soc Hematol Educ Program. 2006:128-32.*

Shendure J, Porreca GJ, Reppas NB, Lin X, McCutcheon JP, Rosenbaum AM, et al. *Accurate multiplex polony sequencing of an evolved bacterial genome. Science. 2005 Sep 9;309(5741):1728-32.*

Silva A, Yunes JA, Cardoso BA, Martins LR, Jotta PY, Abecasis M, et al. *PTEN posttranslational inactivation and hyperactivation of the PI3K/Akt pathway sustain primary T cell leukemia viability. J Clin Invest. 2008 Nov;118(11):3762-74.*

Sive JI, Buck G, Fielding A, Lazarus HM, Litzow MR, Luger S, et al. *Outcomes in older adults with acute lymphoblastic leukaemia (ALL): results from the international MRC UKALL XII/ECOG2993 trial. Br J Haematol. 2012 May;157(4):463-71.*

Soverini S, De Benedittis C, Machova Polakova K, Brouckova A, Horner D, Iacono M, et al. *Unraveling the complexity of tyrosine kinase inhibitor-resistant populations by ultra-deep sequencing of the BCR-ABL kinase domain. Blood. 2013 Jun 21.*

Turcatti G, Romieu A, Fedurco M, Tairi AP. *A new class of cleavable fluorescent nucleotides: synthesis and optimization as reversible terminators for DNA sequencing by synthesis. Nucleic acids research. 2008 Mar;36(4):e25.*

Tzoneva G, Perez-Garcia A, Carpenter Z, Khiabanian H, Tosello V, Allegretta M, et al. *Activating mutations in the NT5C2 nucleotidase gene drive chemotherapy resistance in relapsed ALL. Nat Med. 2013 Mar;19(3):368-71.*

Van Vlierberghe P, Ferrando A. *The molecular basis of T cell acute lymphoblastic leukemia. J Clin Invest. 2012 Oct 1;122(10):3398-406.*

Van Vlierberghe P, Palomero T, Khiabanian H, Van der Meulen J, Castillo M, Van Roy N, et al. *PHF6 mutations in T-cell acute lymphoblastic leukemia. Nat Genet. 2010 Apr;42(4):338-42.*

Wada H, Masuda K, Satoh R, Kakugawa K, Ikawa T, Katsura Y, et al. *Adult T-cell progenitors retain myeloid potential. Nature. 2008 Apr 10;452(7188):768-72.*

Wang Q, Qiu H, Jiang H, Wu L, Dong S, Pan J, et al. *Mutations of PHF6 are associated with mutations of NOTCH1, JAK1 and rearrangement of SET-NUP214 in T-cell acute lymphoblastic leukemia. Haematologica. 2011 Dec;96(12):1808-14.*

Weston BW, Hayden MA, Roberts KG, Bowyer S, Hsu J, Fedoriw G, et al. *Tyrosine kinase inhibitor therapy induces remission in a patient with refractory EBF1-PDGFRB-positive acute lymphoblastic leukemia. Journal of clinical oncology: official journal of the American Society of Clinical Oncology. 2013 Sep 1;31(25):e413-6.*

Wong KM, Hudson TJ, McPherson JD. *Unraveling the genetics of cancer: genome sequencing and beyond. Annu Rev Genomics Hum Genet. 2011;12:407-30.*

Wu D, Sherwood A, Fromm JR, Winter SS, Dunsmore KP, Loh ML, et al. *High-throughput sequencing detects minimal residual disease in acute T lymphoblastic leukemia. Sci Transl Med. 2012 May 16;4(134):134ra63.*

Yan B, Wang Z. *Long noncoding RNA: its physiological and pathological roles. DNA Cell Biol. 2012 Oct;31 Suppl 1:S34-41.*

Zenatti PP, Ribeiro D, Li W, Zuurbier L, Silva MC, Paganin M, et al. *Oncogenic IL7R gain-of-function mutations in childhood T-cell acute lymphoblastic leukemia. Nature genetics. 2011 Oct;43(10):932-9.*

Zhang J, Ding L, Holmfeldt L, Wu G, Heatley SL, Payne-Turner D, et al. *The genetic basis of early T-cell precursor acute lymphoblastic leukaemia. Nature. 2012 Jan 12;481(7380):157-63.*

Zhang L, Xu HG, Lu C. *A novel long non-coding RNA T-ALL-R-LncR1 knockdown and Par-4 cooperate to induce cellular apoptosis in T-cell acute lymphoblastic leukemia cells. Leuk Lymphoma. 2013 Aug 28.*

Dynamics of VEGF-A and its Receptors in Cancer Vascularization – An Overview

Germana Domingues[*†‡], Sofia Gouveia Fernandes[*†] and Jacinta Serpa[*†]

1 Introduction

The present chapter aims to disclose the cancer vascularization processes, giving primary emphasis to the role of vascular endothelial growth factor (VEGF) and its receptors.

The formation of blood vessels can be driven by several mechanisms: 1) vasculogenesis, which defines the embryonic formation of blood vessels; 2) angiogenesis that names the *de novo* formation of blood vessels, in adults, through the proliferation of endothelial cells (ECs); 3) neovasculogenesis that defines the *de novo* formation of a primary vascular plexus from endothelial progenitor cells (EPCs), and 4) vascular mimicry, which consists of a process through which cancer cells can behave as ECs by establishing vascular structures (Figure 1).

The processes underlying blood vessels formation in cancer will be further depicted in this chapter, integrating the relevance of VEGF signaling whenever appropriated. Vasculogenesis will not be addressed, since it is a physiological mechanism occurring during the development of the embryo.

Nevertheless, it is important to refer that angiogenesis is the term often used to denote overall tumor neovascularization, though scientifically this is not fully correct. Angiogenesis and neovasculogenesis refer both to the formation of new vessels, but through different processes. However, in several circumstances, particularly when anti-vascularization therapy in cancer is addressed the designation of anti-angiogenesis therapy is often or almost exclusively used.

1.1 Angiogenesis

In healthy adults, the vasculature is mostly quiescent (Witmer *et al.*, 2003). In a few situations, however, ECs may experience some proliferation: wound healing (Paavonen *et al.*, 2000; Witmer *et al.*, 2003), skeletal growth and the female reproductive cycle (Ferrara *et al.*, 2003). Some pathophysiological processes may also encompass the *de novo* formation of new blood vessel capillaries from an existing vasculature, as result of the imbalance in the demand and supply of oxygen and nutrients (Verbridge *et al.*, 2009; Witmer *et al.*, 2003). These diseases include diabetic retinopathy (Witmer *et al.*, 2003), rheumatoid arthritis (Robinson & Stringer, 2001), pathology of the female reproductive tract and cancer (Ferrara *et al.*, 2003). The formation of new capillaries from pre-existing vessels, by their sprouting or splitting, is called angiogenesis (George *et al.*, 2011; Kovacic *et al.*, 2008; Risau, 1997).

---

[*] Faculdade de Ciências Médicas, Universidade Nova De Lisboa, Portugal

[†] Instituto Português de Oncologia de Lisboa Francisco Gentil, Portugal

[‡] Instituto de Medicina Molecular, Faculdade de Medicina, Universidade de Lisboa, Portugal

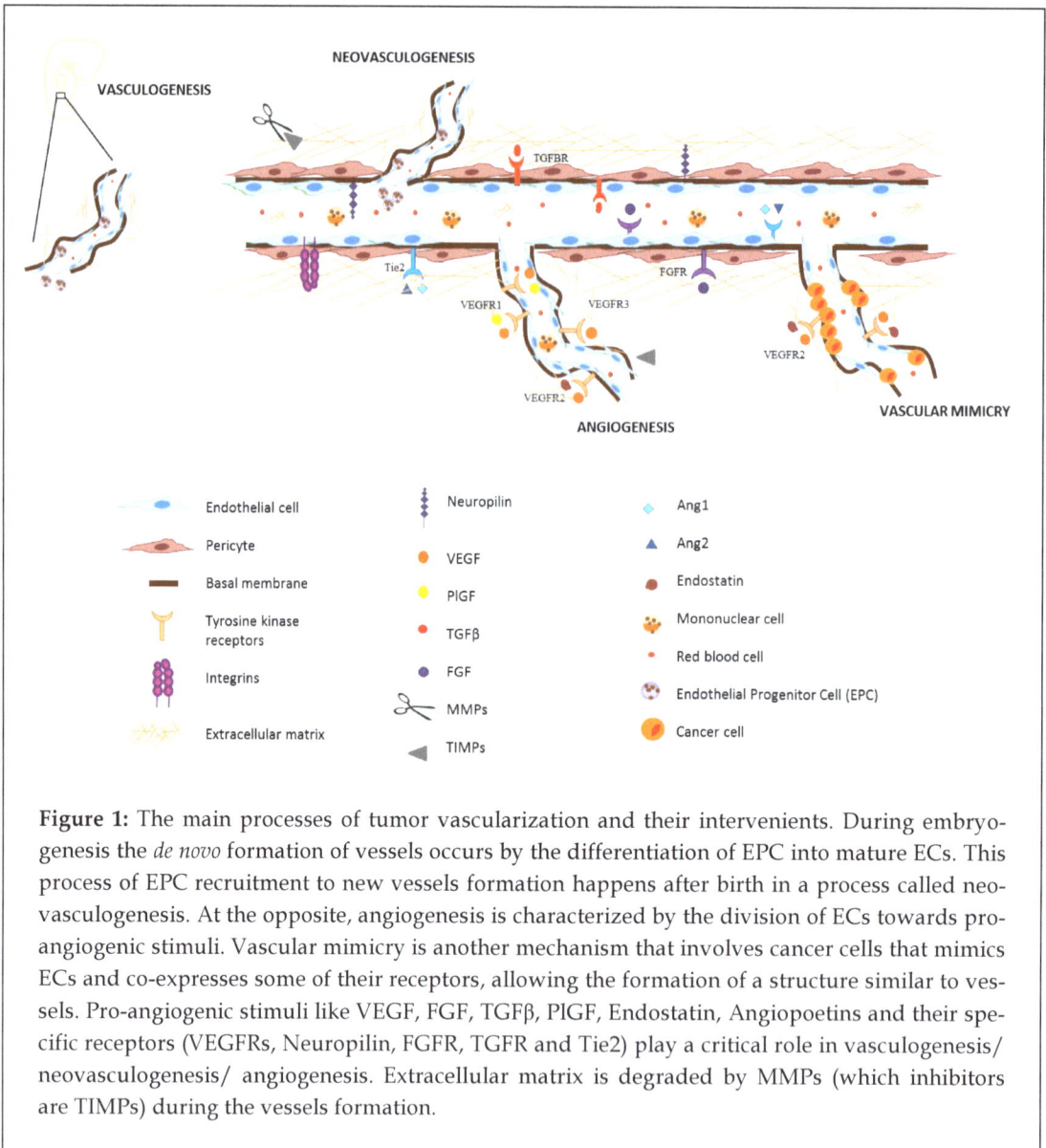

Figure 1: The main processes of tumor vascularization and their intervenients. During embryogenesis the *de novo* formation of vessels occurs by the differentiation of EPC into mature ECs. This process of EPC recruitment to new vessels formation happens after birth in a process called neovasculogenesis. At the opposite, angiogenesis is characterized by the division of ECs towards proangiogenic stimuli. Vascular mimicry is another mechanism that involves cancer cells that mimics ECs and co-expresses some of their receptors, allowing the formation of a structure similar to vessels. Pro-angiogenic stimuli like VEGF, FGF, TGFβ, PlGF, Endostatin, Angiopoetins and their specific receptors (VEGFRs, Neuropilin, FGFR, TGFR and Tie2) play a critical role in vasculogenesis/ neovasculogenesis/ angiogenesis. Extracellular matrix is degraded by MMPs (which inhibitors are TIMPs) during the vessels formation.

The switch from the normal quiescent vasculature to angiogenesis is the result of a dynamic and tightly controlled balance between angiogenic activators and inhibitors, released predominantly by surrounding pericytes and lymphocytes, and ECs themselves, which induce a number of signal transduction systems that activate ECs (Carmeliet & Jain, 2000; Folkman, 1997; Hanahan & Folkman, 1996; Robinson & Stringer, 2001). These angiogenic factors are increasingly receiving attention, especially in the field of malignant neoplastic vascularization (Nishida *et al.*, 2006).

Angiogenesis is a complex multi-step process, characterized by a cascade of events: firstly, vasodilatation of existing vessels and an increase of vascular permeability along with the localized degradation of the surrounding extracellular matrix (ECM), enabling further activation of ECs which proliferate and migrate to form tubes; subsequently, these cells undergo a maturation phase and remodel into capillary structures, and a new ECM is deposited (Hanahan & Folkman, 1996; Nishida *et al.*, 2006; Robinson & Stringer, 2001).

1.1.1 Tumor Angiogenesis

Tumor cells initially lack angiogenic ability (Folkman, 1992; Hanahan & Weinberg, 2011). In order to sustain survival and to expand in size, incipient neoplasias must develop angiogenic ability, which seems to be acquired in a discrete step during tumor development, via an "angiogenic switch" (Folkman & Hanahan, 1991; Hanahan & Folkman, 1996; Verbridge *et al.*, 2009). Tumor vessels play an essential role in supplying nutrients, oxygen and immune cells, and also in the removal of waste products, enabling tumors to grow beyond the limitations of passive diffusion. In addition, and very importantly, newly formed vessels also afford the possibility of primary tumor to invade adjacent tissues, and circulate, through bloodstream, to distant sites, where they may form secondary tumors, known as metastases (Sporn, 1996; Kawaguchi, 200; Nishida *et al.*, 2006). Angiogenesis represents, therefore, a crucial step in cancer progression.

As mentioned above, angiogenic switch is induced by several factors – Figure 1. Such angiogenic factors (positive regulators) include fibroblast growth factors (FGFs), thymidine phosphorylase (TP), transforming growth factor β (TGF-β), tumor necrosis factor α (TNF- α), platelet-derived growth factors (PDGFs), angiopoietins, interleukin-8 (IL-8) and vascular endothelial growth factors (VEGFs) (Ferrara *et al.*, 2003; Nishida *et al.*, 2006). Among these, VEGFs, particularly VEGFA (VEGF), and their receptors assume particular relevance, VEGF being the only growth factor observed almost ubiquitously at sites of angiogenesis and representing a critical rate-limiting step in physiological angiogenesis, and fundamental in pathophysiological angiogenesis as well (Robinson & Stringer, 2001; Ferrara *et al.* 2003; Gerber & Ferrara, 2003; Cebe-Suarez *et al.*, 2006). In the field of neoplastic neovascularization, VEGFs and their receptors families have received increased attention.

Angiogenesis stimulation however depends also on the downregulation of angiogenic inhibitors, besides the upregulation of angiogenic activators. Such suppressors include angiostatin, endostatin, interferon, platelet factor 4, trombospondin and tissue inhibitor of metalloproteinase-1, -2 and -3 (TIMP-1, 2 and3). Levels of expression of angiogenic factors are usually correlated to the aggressiveness of tumor cells (Nishida *et al.*, 2006)

1.2 Neovasculogenesis – Endothelial Progenitor Cells (EPCs)

Recent data have disclosed the occurrence of a new mechanism for formation of vessels in adult, different from angiogenesis, termed postnatal/adult vasculogenesis or neovasculogenesis. This mechanism differs from angiogenesis by comprising the *de novo* formation of a primary vascular plexus from EPCs (George *et al.*, 2011; Kovacic *et al.*, 2008).

The emerging evidence seems, thus, to unsettle the dogma that, for a long time, stated EPCs would contribute to vessel growth exclusively in the embryo (vasculogenesis), whereas in the adult that growth would occur only from division of differentiated ECs (angiogenesis) (Ribatti *et al.*, 2005). Both phenomena are represented in Figure 1.

EPCs are a minor population of mononuclear non-endothelial cells capable to proliferate, migrate, and differentiate into endothelial lineage cells, but have not yet acquired characteristics of mature ECs (Fadini *et al.*, 2008; Medina *et al.*, 2010; Ribatti, 2007).

Asahara *et al.* (Asahara *et al.*, 1997) was the first to isolate putative EPCs from human peripheral blood on the basis of cell surface expression of CD34 and VEGFR-2 markers, observing experimentally EPCs differentiation into ECs. Since then, increasing knowledge on EPCs has emerged. Although some questions persist regarding the precise panel of cell surface markers defining EPCs, the combinations of CD133+CD34+VEGFR-2+, CD34+VEGFR-2+, or CD114+CD34low are now widely used to define or select cells expressing properties attributed to EPCs (Peichev *et al.*, 2000; Romagnani *et al.*, 2005; Schmidt-Lucke *et al.*, 2010).

Most circulating EPCs reside in the bone marrow in close association with hematopoietic stem cells and the stroma. EPCs circulating in the peripheral blood may correspond to cells derived from the bone marrow, not yet incorporated into the vessel wall (Ribatti *et al.*, 2005).

Tumor vascularization seems also to be supported by the mobilization and functional incorporation of EPCs. A study focusing EPCs revealed the upregulation of tumor endothelial markers on EPCs, supporting the hypothesis of the involvement of EPCs in cancer (Bagley *et al.*, 2008). Moreover, increased circulating levels of EPCs have been detected in cancer patients (Ahn *et al.*, 2010; Mancuso *et al.*, 2001; Pircher *et al.*, 2008; Richter-Ehrenstein *et al.*, 2007; Sakamori *et al.*, 2012). A strong correlation has also been observed between EPCs number and tumor growth and progression in several neoplastic contexts (Gao *et al.*, 2009; Monestiroli *et al.*, 2001; Real *et al.*, 2011; Shaked *et al.*, 2005; Yu *et al.*, 2007). Tumor secretion of VEGF was also found to be correlated with EPC mobilization (Real *et al.*, 2011; Shaked *et al.*, 2005; Young *et al.*, 2002).

The recruitment of EPCs to tumors is a multistep process, involving the arrest and homing of the circulating EPCs within the vasculogenic microvasculature, transendothelial extravasation into interticial space, extravascular formation of cellular clusters, creation of vascular sprouts and cell networks and, finally, the EPCs incorporation into a functional microvasculature (Ribatti *et al.*, 2005). VEGF appears to be an inducing factor for these events (Aicher *et al.*, 2003; Ferrara *et al.*, 2003; Greenberg *et al.*, 2008; Ribatti *et al.*, 2005).

Interestingly, increasing evidence regarding neovasculogenesis and EPCs sources has now introduced the blood mononuclear cell population as a putative intervenient, both in normal and pathological conditions. Peripheral blood mononuclear cells collected from humans were shown to be enriched in EPCs after addition of VEGF, FGF-2, insulin-like growth factor (IGF) and epidermal growth factor (EGF) to the culture medium for 7-10 days. Afterwards, these cells contributed to the formation of new vessels in ischemic limbs in mice (Kalka *et al.*, 2000). Another study showed that EPCs isolated from peripheral blood mononuclear cell fraction, although unable to proliferate, contributed to vascularization by secreting angiogenic growth factors (Rehman *et al.*, 2003). Monocytes cultured under angiogenic conditions also displayed an EPC phenotype with expression of specific surface markers and even formed cord-like structures (Rohde *et al.*, 2006; Schmeisser *et al.*, 2001). The incorporation of bone marrow-derived cells displaying characteristics of macrophages has been observed in brain vascularization (Hao *et al.*, 2008). Moreover, tumor-associated macrophages, derived from circulating monocytes, have been shown to accumulate in hypoxic regions of tumors (Ribatti *et al.*, 2007; Talks *et al.*, 2000). The involvement of monocytes/macrophages in tumor blood vessels formation was observed in numerous neoplastic contexts, either directly, as EPCs, and/or indirectly by secreting angiogenic activators, such as VEGF (Barbera-Guillem *et al.*, 2002; Bingle *et al.*, 2006; Chen *et al.*, 2011; Hao *et al.*, 2008; Ribatti *et al.*, 2007; Wang *et al.*, 2013). Macrophage migration inhibitory factor (MIF), a cytokine implied, namely, in the recruitment of EPCs and macrophages activation (Asare *et al.*, 2013; Chesney *et al.*, 1999) has been presented as an important factor in tumorigenesis, its high expression being widely associated to enhanced tumor vascularization (Bacher *et al.*, 2003; Girard *et al.*, 2012; Hira *et al.*, 2005).

The rising data on EPCs seem to introduce EPCs as powerful tools for diagnostic and prognostic purposes, and, additionally, putative targets for interventive therapies.

Both angiogenesis and neovasculogenesis are known to be part of tumor vascularization. Each relative contribution might, though, vary within the various neoplastic contexts and still remains to be clarified.

1.3 Vascular Mimicry

One of the new emerging paradigms in tumor vascularization is called "vascular mimicry", which describes the *de novo* formation of perfusable, matrix-rich, vasculogenic-like networks by aggressive malignant tumors – Figure 1. This phenomenon was first characterized in human melanoma where the tumor cells were shown to co-express endothelial and tumor markers (like VEGFR-2 that has been shown to play an essential role in vascular mimicry formation) and formed channels, networks, and tubular structures rich in laminin, collagens IV and VI, and heparin sulfate proteoglycans containing plasma and red blood cells. This could be a way of tumor cells to escape from immune system, which allows a faster pathway for metastasis. The vascular mimicry is nowadays described in a variety of cancers, namely sarcomas (Ewing, mesothelial, synovial, osteosarcoma, alveolar rhabdomyosarcoma); carcinomas of the breast, ovary, lung, prostate, bladder and kidney; laryngeal squamous cell carcinoma, gliomas, glioblastoma, and astrocytoma (Kirschmann *et al.*, 2012).

Recently, epithelial-to-mesenchymal transition (EMT) has been reported to contribute to the formation of vascular mimicry and the upregulation of EMT-associated transcription factors has been demonstrated in vascular mimicry-forming tumor cells (Z. Liu *et al.*, 2012; Sun *et al.*, 2010).

Vascular mimicry has been, additionally, presented as one of the putative reasons underlying anti-angiogenic therapy resistance in cancer, once this therapy is directed to "bona-fide" epithelium (Dunleavey & Dudley, 2012) (see 3. Therapy anti-angiogenesis).

2 Vascular Endothelial Growth Factors (VEGFs)

The VEGF family includes placental growth factor (PGF), VEGF-A, VEGF-B, VEGF-C, VEGF-D and VEGF-E (viral homologue of VEGF-A). VEGF-A, also known as vascular permeability factor (VPF) or just VEGF, was the first to be discovered and has been studied most extensively (Ferrara, 1999; Ferrara *et al.*, 2003).

VEGF is produced by a broad variety of cell types, including endothelial, hematopoietic and stromal cells (Bachelder *et al.*, 2001; Bates *et al.*, 2003; Ferrara *et al.*, 2003; Mercurio *et al.*, 2005; Stuttfeld & Ballmer-Hofer, 2009). Most tumor types, solid and hematological (tumor cells and stroma), overexpress VEGF, being this expression directly correlated to regions of angiogenesis and high vascular density (Carmeliet & Jain, 2000; J. Chen *et al.*, 2014; P. Chen *et al.*, 2014; H. F. Dvorak, 2002; Ferrara, 2005; Ferrara & Davis-Smyth, 1997; Gerber & Ferrara, 2003; Obermair *et al.*, 1997; Xu *et al.*, 2013; Yuan *et al.*, 2000).

VEGF is encoded by a gene located in chromosome 6p21.3, organized in eight exons, separated by seven introns. Through alternative splicing, this gene gives rise to several distinct VEGF isoforms, which differ in their expression patterns and their biochemical and biological properties (Gerber & Ferrara, 2003; Robinson & Stringer, 2001; Vincenti *et al.*, 1996). Five human isoforms have been identified, having 121, 145, 165, 189 and 206 aminoacids, respectively VEGF$_{121}$, VEGF$_{145}$, VEGF$_{165}$, VEGF$_{189}$ and VEGF$_{206}$. Additionally, minor splice variants have been reported. The different isoforms vary in their ability to bind to heparin, which affects their diffusion rates and concentration gradients in relation to their secretor cell. VEGF$_{206}$ exhibits the strongest binding to heparin in contrast to VEGF$_{121}$, the most diffusible isoform (Ferrara *et al.*, 1992; Gerber & Ferrara, 2003; Grunstein *et al.*, 2000; Robinson & Stringer, 2001).

VEGF is a basic, heparin-binding, homodimeric glycoprotein of about 45 kDa. These properties correspond to those of VEGF$_{165}$, the most abundant isoform (Ferrara *et al.*, 1992; Gerber & Ferrara, 2003; Grunstein *et al.*, 2000).

VEGF plays several roles, important under both physiological and pathophysiological conditions. VEGF is a potent mitogen for vascular ECs and also a critical factor for their proliferation and survival (Ferrara, 2001; Leung *et al.*, 1989; Neufeld *et al.*, 1999). During embryonic development, the disruption of a single VEGF allele lead to embryonic lethality due to impaired vessel formation and function (Carmeliet *et al.*, 1996; Ferrara, 1996). *In vitro*, VEGF was shown to prevent apoptosis, by activation of phosphatidylinositol(PI)3 kinase(K)/Akt pathway (Gerber, McMurtrey, *et al.*, 1998) and induction of the expression of anti-apoptotic proteins Bcl-2 and A1 in ECs (Gerber, Dixit, *et al.*, 1998).

VEGF is also able to induce vascular permeability (hence its alternative term VPF), which appears to be mediated by the formation of vesicular-vacuolar organelles, within the ECs, that ultimately fuse with the cell membrane, creating the vascular lumen (A. M. Dvorak *et al.*, 1996; H. F. Dvorak *et al.*, 1995; George *et al.*, 2011; Risau, 1997; Witmer *et al.*, 2003).

VEGF is also implicated in the degradation of ECM, required for the proliferation and migration of ECs, and finally the establishment of new tubes. That event demands the activity of matrix degrading proteases, such as matrix metalloproteinases (MMPs) and urokinase-type plasminogen activator (uPA). VEGF acts as one of the main inducers of the expression of these proteolytic enzymes (Gerber & Ferrara, 2003; Witmer *et al.*, 2003).

The vessel formation seems to be additionally controlled by VEGF on the recruitment of bone marrow-derived cells and by increasing procoagulant activity and by recruiting pericytes (Clauss *et al.*, 1990; Ferrara *et al.*, 2003; Greenberg *et al.*, 2008). VEGF is still implicated in hematopoiesis, under both normal and neoplastic conditions (Gerber & Ferrara, 2003).

Regarding VEGF role in cancer progression, some functions may be independent of neovascularization. VEGF produced by tumor cells engages VEGF receptors on tumor cells (autocrine signaling), initiating a signaling response that promotes survival, and, thus, providing tumor cells with a degree of self-sufficiency, and, ultimately facilitating their ability to migrate and metastasize (Bachelder *et al.*, 2001; Mercurio *et al.*, 2005) (see "2.3. VEGF autocrine signaling"). Studies related this self-sufficiency to the activation of PI3-kinase (PI3K) pathway (Bachelder *et al.*, 2001; Mercurio *et al.*, 2005). This self-sufficiency seemed to rely, additionally, on the capacity of VEGF to mitigate apoptosis, that being mostly induced by the expression of the anti-apoptotic protein Bcl-2 (Mercurio *et al.*, 2005; Pidgeon *et al.*, 2001). Moreover, migration and invasion of tumor cells have also been related to VEGF signaling, likely due to regulation of the expression of C-X-C chemokine receptor type 4 (CXCR4) by VEGF (Bachelder *et al.*, 2002).

2.1   Regulation Mechanisms of VEGF Expression

The molecular mechanisms governing VEGF expression in normoxia by extracellular mediators are poorly understood. A vast body of literature has demonstrated that, in hypoxia, hypoxia-inducible factor-1 (HIF-1) is a key regulator responsible for the induction of genes that facilitate adaptation and survival of tumor cells (Semenza, 2003). As a heterodimeric complex, HIF-1 consists of a hypoxia inducible subunit HIF-1α and a constitutively expressed subunit HIF-1β. The overexpression of HIF-1α was found in various types of human and mouse cancers (Semenza, 2003). Song et al. (Song et al., 2009) showed, in ovarian cancer cells, that lysophosphatidic acid (LPA), a natural phospholipid that is a ligand for protein G coupled receptors, induces VEGF expression through c-Myc and Sp-1 transcription factors independently of HIF-1α. This mechanism can involve VEGF receptor-2 (VEGFR-2) since regulation of VEGFR-2 signal transduction also occurs through the trimeric G proteins Gaq/Ga11, which was shown to interact with VEGFR-2 in vitro (Shibuya, 2013). It was previously demonstrated, in glioblastoma, the implication of IL-6 in the regulation of VEGF expression, again through Sp1 transcription factor as a partner of signal transducer and activator of transcription 3 (STAT3) (Loeffler et al., 2005). Sp1 and STAT3, together with HIF-1α, are also involved in the expression of VEGF when the epidermal growth factor receptor (EGFR) is stimulated by the proteoglycan decorin in mouse brain ECs (Santra et al., 2008). In mouse embryonic fibroblasts NIH3T3 cell line, it was shown that PDGF (platelet-derived growth factor) pathway was important to activate VEGF expression mediated by Sp1 and Sp3 that, in these cells, are constitutively bound to VEGF promoter (Finkenzeller et al., 1997).

The expression of a constitutively active mutated form of PI3-kinase in ovarian cancer cells results in increased expression of VEGF. PKC zeta, which is the major kinase downstream of PI3-kinase, regulates VEGF expression in a phosphoinositide-dependent kinase-1 (PDK-1)-dependent manner. The inducible expression of Sp1 mutated in the two phosphorylation sites compromises VEGF expression in response to extracellular signal-regulated kinases (ERK) stimulation. This finding strongly establishes that ERK phosphorylation of Sp1 is a major determinant in VEGF expression in response to RAS activation. Sp3 is also an ubiquitous factor that is highly homologous to Sp1. Under hypoxic conditions, the expression of Sp3 decreases, whereas Sp1 is unchanged. A concomitant induction of transcription is observed in the absence of HIF-1. In this case, Sp1/Sp3 ratio represents a putative HIF-1α independent regulatory mechanism in hypoxia (Pages & Pouyssegur, 2005).

In gastric cancer, the overexpression of FoxM1b directly and significantly correlates with transactivation of VEGF expression and increased angiogenesis (Li et al., 2009).

Recent studies have indicated that cells undergoing insufficient oxygen and nutrients supply experience endoplasmic reticulum (ER) stress. ER needs energy and oxygen for the protein folding process, thus nutrient depletion and hypoxia caused by insufficient blood supply lead to inefficient protein folding and ER stress in cells, especially cells that grow and spread rapidly (Adelman et al., 2000; Drogat et al., 2007; Genbacev et al., 1997; Koumenis et al., 2007; Romero-Ramirez et al., 2004). UPR (unfolded protein response), IRE1a (Serine/threonine-protein kinase/endoribonuclease IRE1a), PERK (Proline-rich receptor-like protein kinase) and ATF6a (Activating transcription factor 6 alpha) mediate transcriptional regulation of VEGF under ER stress, during normal development of trophoblast cells in the placenta as well as in cancer cells (Ghosh et al., 2010). In ovary, carbon and energy metabolism also plays a role in the regulation of VEGF:VEGFR-2 autocrine loop. Some studies showed that glucose can increase the levels of VEGF and consequently potentiate the autocrine loop, whereas glucose depletion decreases VEGF levels and increases VEGFR-2 degradation with concomitant increase of VEGFR-2 mRNA synthesis (Adham & Coomber, 2009). This study suggests that initiation and/or progression of ovarian surface epithelial cells towards a neoplastic phenotype might be modulated by dietary conditions.

More recently, studies have been published revealing the importance of micro-RNAs (miRs) in the regulation of angiogenesis. Lei *et al.* (Lei *et al.*, 2009) and Cascio *et al.* (Cascio *et al.*, 2010) have shown a molecular mechanism of regulation of HIF-1α and VEGF, involving miR-20b through which tumor cells are able to adapt to different oxygen concentrations. This way, HIF-1α is capable of regulating VEGF expression before and after transcription, since the expression of miR-20b itself is regulated by HIF-1α. The downregulation of VEGF mRNA by miR-20b under a hypoxic environment was associated with reduced levels of nuclear HIF-1α subunit and STAT3. STAT3 is necessary for CoCl2-mediated HIF-1α nuclear accumulation and recruitment on VEGF promoter. MiR-126 is also downregulated under hypoxic conditions and may halt the hypoxia-induced neovascularization by suspending cell cycle progression and inhibiting the expression of VEGF and MMP-9 (Ye *et al.*, 2014).

It was shown that miR-126 is complementary to *VEGF* 3' UTR (untranslated region) and this interaction may inhibit the overexpression of VEGF in tumor cells both *in vitro* and *in vivo* (B. Liu *et al.*, 2009). More recently, it has been shown that this miR induces angiogenesis by activating VEGF in patients with oral cancer (Sasahira *et al.*, 2012).

In bone marrow ECs, miR-363-5p was the first miR identified. It regulates (directly and indirectly) the expression and availability of angiocrine and hematopoietic factors. Reduced miR-363-5p in ECs promotes hematopoietic precursors adhesion and expansion (Costa *et al.*, 2013)

2.2   VEGF Receptors

The biological functions of VEGF are mediated upon binding to tyrosine kinase receptors (TKRs) VEGFR-1 (FLT-1), VEGFR-2 (kinase domain region (KDR)/Flk-1) (Cebe-Suarez *et al.*, 2006; Ferrara *et al.*, 2003; Vieira *et al.*, 2010).

Similar to other TKRs, signaling by VEGFRs is initiated upon binding of a covalently linked ligand dimer to the extracelular receptor domain of the TKR. This interaction promotes receptor homo and heterodimerization followed by phosphorylation of specific tyrosine residues located in the intracellular juxtamembrane domain, the kinase insert domain, and the carboxyterminal tail of the receptor. A variety of signaling molecules is then recruited to VEGFR dimers giving rise to the assembly of large molecular complexes that activate different cellular pathways (Stuttfeld & Ballmer-Hofer, 2009). Some autophosphorylation sites have also been identified in both VEGF TKRs (Shibuya, 2006).

VEGF binding sites were initially identified on the cell surface of ECs. VEGF receptors expression is now recognized to be wider, occurring also on bone marrow-derived cells (Ferrara *et al.*, 2003), including hematopoietic stem cells (Peichev *et al.*, 2000) and circulating EPCs (Eichmann *et al.*, 1997), pericytes (Witmer *et al.*, 2002), dendritic cells (Gabrilovich *et al.*, 1996), monocytes (Barleon *et al.*, 1996; Rohde *et al.*, 2006; Sawano *et al.*, 2001; Schmeisser *et al.*, 2001), retinal progenitor cells (Suzuma *et al.*, 1998) and several types of tumor cells (Bates *et al.*, 2003; Dias *et al.*, 2001; Santos & Dias, 2004; von Marschall *et al.*, 2000).

VEGFR-1 and VEGFR-2 are 180 and 200 kDa glycoproteins, respectively (Cebe-Suarez *et al.*, 2006; Ferrara *et al.*, 2003; Vieira *et al.*, 2010). These TKRs comprise seven immunoglobulin-like domains in the extracellular domain, a single transmembrane region and a conserved intracellular tyrosine kinase sequence interrupted by a kinase-insert domain (Ferrara *et al.*, 2003; Shibuya *et al.*, 1990; Terman *et al.*, 1991).

Although both are high affinity receptors for VEGF, VEGF binds with higher affinity to VEGFR-1 than to VEGFR-2 (Cebe-Suarez *et al.*, 2006; Ferrara *et al.*, 2003; Shibuya & Claesson-Welsh, 2006; Vieira *et al.*, 2010). Another interesting feature of the two TKRs is their difference in tyrosine kinase activity in response to ligand binding: VEGFR-2 is a stronger kinase (Shibuya & Claesson-Welsh, 2006; Waltenberger *et al.*, 1994). These distinct molecular features may explain their different biological activities (Shibuya & Claesson-Welsh, 2006).

VEGFR-2 is considered to be the predominant VEGF receptor in mediating functional VEGF signaling in ECs, including mitogenesis, cytoskeleton organization and cell migration, survival, and vascular permeability (Cebe-Suarez *et al.*, 2006; Shibuya & Claesson-Welsh, 2006). VEGFR-2 is also implicated in playing a distinct role in the activation of PI3K-Akt pathway, a crucial signaling pathway in the process leading to EC survival induced by VEGF (Gerber, McMurtrey, *et al.*, 1998; Witmer *et al.*, 2003). VEGFR-2 is still involved in hematopoiesis (Gerber & Ferrara, 2003). These roles were supported by experiments in which, in VEGFR-2 knockout mice, both hematopoiesis and vasculogenesis were blocked (Shalaby *et al.*, 1995).

VEGFR-1 function in mediating effective biological responses in ECs is more elusive. In fact, in ECs, it may function as a negative regulator of VEGFR-2, at least during embryogenesis, serving a "decoy" purpose, by sequestering VEGF and thus rendering it less available to bind to VEGFR-2 (Ferrara *et al.*, 2003; Shibuya & Claesson-Welsh, 2006), as suggested by studies in which VEGFR-1 -/- mice displayed overgrowth of ECs and disorganized vascular channels (Fong *et al.*, 1995). Moreover, VEGFR-1 signaling may also be involved in hematopoiesis and EPCs recruitment (Clauss *et al.*, 1996; Hattori *et al.*, 2002).

Furthermore, synergism between the two VEGFR receptors, VEGFR-1 and VEGFR-2, enabling the modulation of a variety of VEGFR-dependent signals has been demonstrated (Carmeliet *et al.*, 2001).

VEGF-induced biological signaling is still influenced by the interaction with co-receptors, as neuropilins (NRPs, -1 and -2) and heparan sulphate proteoglycans (HSPGs), integrins and cadherins.

Neuropilins, broadly expressed transmembrane molecules, traditionally known to be involved in axonal guidance, have been identified as VEGF-binding proteins and part of the VEGF-VEGFR signaling complex (Ellis, 2006; Robinson & Stringer, 2001; Vieira *et al.*, 2010).

These receptors recognize the exon 7-encoded domain of VEGF, binding, therefore, mostly to $VEGF_{165}$ but not to $VEGF_{121}$, which misses that domain (Ellis, 2006; Soker *et al.*, 1996; Vieira *et al.*, 2010). The lack of this association has been hypothesized to be related to the lesser potency of this isoform in comparison to $VEGF_{165}$ (Ellis, 2006; Rollin *et al.*, 2004).

NRP-1 and NRP-2 are respectively 120 to 130 kDa non-tyrosine kinase receptors that share an identical structure, containing both a large N-terminal extracellular domain, a short membrane spanning domain and a small cytoplasmic domain (Ellis, 2006; Soker *et al.*, 1996; Vieira *et al.*, 2010). Their wide distribution includes, besides the developing nervous system, ECs and tumor cells (Cebe-Suarez *et al.*, 2006; Ellis, 2006; Shibuya & Claesson-Welsh, 2006).

NRP-1 and NRP-2 role in mediating VEGF signaling seems to occur mainly through association with VEGFR-2 and VEGFR-1, respectively, stimulating signaling through these TKRs (Cebe-Suarez *et al.*, 2006).

HSPGs are abundant and highly conserved components in the cell surface and ECM, playing an important function in the formation and modulation of gradients of heparin-binding growth factors, as VEGF, and they have been shown to be implicated as modulators of VEGF signaling, by interaction with VEGFR-1 and VEGFR-2 (Bernfield *et al.*, 1992; Vieira *et al.*, 2010). Besides, these molecules are still involved in the restoration of function of damaged $VEGF_{165}$, prolonging its biological activity (Gitay-Goren *et al.*, 1996; Robinson & Stringer, 2001).

Other potential co-receptors for VEGFRs include integrins, as $\alpha v\beta 3$ and $\alpha 9\beta 1$, and cell adhesion molecules, such as vascular endothelial (VE)-cadherin (Cebe-Suarez *et al.*, 2006; Shibuya, 2006; Stupack & Cheresh, 2004).

2.2.1 Regulation of VEGFR-1 Expression

VEGFR-1 mRNA and protein are specifically found in most of the vascular ECs. As an exception, VEGFR-1 mRNA is also found in human peripheral blood activated monocytes, which suggests a role in vascularization of monocyte/macrophage *in vivo* (Barleon *et al.*, 1996).

Isotope-labeled VEGF assays detect its binding sites in most of the blood vessels from embryo to adult stages. These experiments showed the higher affinity of VEGFR-1 for VEGF with more than half VEGF-binding sites being associated with VEGFR-1 (Jakeman *et al.*, 1992). However, the kinase activity of VEGFR-1 is one-tenth lower than VEGFR-2. *VEGFR-1* gene produces two proteins, a full length receptor and a soluble form (sVEGFR-1). These facts suggest that VEGFR-1 may negatively regulate angiogenesis under certain conditions (Shibuya, 2001, 2013). VEGFR-2 knockout mice exhibit a lethal phenotype due to the absence of vasculogenesis, whereas VEGFR-1 knockout mice die at the same age (E8.5-9.0) due to the overgrowth of ECs and their disorganization in blood vessels (Fong *et al.*, 1995). This indicates that during embryogenesis VEGFR-2 is a positive signal transducer and VEGFR-1 is a suppressor of VEGFR-2 signaling. There are two possible reasons: VEGFR-1 tyrosine kinase (TK) generates a negative signal against angiogenesis or the ligand-binding site of VEGFR-1 blocks VEGF activity by trapping VEGF. A VEGFR-1-TK mice was generated by Shibuya *et al.* (Shibuya, 2013) with a normal vascular growth, which demonstrates that VEGFR-1 negatively regulates vasculogenesis during early embryogenesis by trapping VEGF and decreasing provasculogenic signals from VEGFR-2.

The gene regulation of VEGFR-1 is dependent on an Ets-binding motif and on an upstream CRE/ATF-binding motif (Wakiya *et al.*, 1996). In addition, it was reported a hypoxia-response element which may be responsible for the upregulation of VEGFR-1 under hypoxic conditions (Gerber *et al.*, 1997). Zhang *et al.* (Zhang *et al.*, 2010) observed that VEGF induces potent activation of the JNK-c-Jun pathway and that JNK activity is associated with ubiquitination of VEGFR-2. At the opposite, inhibition of the ubiquitin or proteasome activity is sufficient to enhance the expression of VEGFR-1 in primary ECs. These findings suggest that ECs are continuously producing VEGFR-1 and that ubiquitin–proteosome activity is necessary to maintain its homeostatic levels. Interestingly, the regulation of VEGFR-1 protein levels is dependent on Akt and ERK1/2 phosphorylation and, since these kinases typically inhibit the degradation of proteins by the ubiquitin–proteasome system, they postulate that VEGF induces phosphorylation of Akt and ERK1/2, which in turn prevents degradation of VEGFR-1 by the ubiquitin–proteasome system. Collectively, these data suggest that VEGF orchestrates an intricate process mediated by the Akt/ERK and JNK/c-Jun that protects VEGFR-1 while VEGFR-2 is degraded, leading to rapid reversal of the protein levels of these two receptors (Zhang *et al.*, 2010).

2.2.2   Regulation of VEGFR-2 Expression

VEGFR-2 gene promoter does not have a TATA box region, but has several DNA binding sites for general and tissue-specific transcription factors. This TATA-less gene contains four upstream Sp1 sites and a single transcription start site that binds multi-functional transcription factor TFII-I for gene expression (Guo *et al.*, 2010). In large vessel ECs TFII-I is a transcription factor that regulates VEGFR-2 expression (T. A. Jackson *et al.*, 2005) and, despite TFII-I deletions being associated with cardiovascular defects (Lucena *et al.*, 2010), its function in angiogenesis remains unknown. Sp1-dependent DNA binding within −77 and −60 region of VEGFR-2 promoter seems to be essential for the regulation of both mRNA and protein in human ECs by Rac-1 (a small Rho-GTPase) (Guo *et al.*, 2010).

GATA2 is another transcription factor that regulates the activity of VEGFR-2 promoter (Minami *et al.*, 2004; Minami *et al.*, 2001) and more recently Mammoto *et al.* (Mammoto *et al.*, 2009) showed that capillary formation *in vitro* and *in vivo* is modulated by p190RhoGAP, a Rho GTPase inhibitor that controls the levels TFII-I and GATA2 antagonistic transcription factors.

Epigenetic modulation of transcription factors has been reported upon VEGF signaling; namely the binding of E2F1 to VEGFR-2, VEGFR-1 and angiopoetin-2 promoters is increased by VEGF stimulation (Pillai *et al.*, 2010) concomitantly with the acetylation of histones and E2F1. Promoter methylation is also described in VEGFR-2 promoter in cancer cell lines from stomach, colon and liver (J. Y. Kim *et al.*, 2009).

In Human Umbilical Vein ECs (HUVECs), NRP-1 si-RNA knockdown causes a marked decrease in VEGFR-2 protein levels and this change is independent of VEGFR-2 mRNA expression. Holmes *et al.* (Holmes & Zachary, 2008) concluded from these findings that NRP-1 is important for the stability of VEGFR-2 in HUVECs, the loss of NRP-1 enhances degradation of VEGFR-2 both under basal conditions and following activation of VEGFR-2 by VEGF.

Chronic hypoxia is a cause for specific downregulation of VEGFR-2 in human coronary artery endothelial (HCAE) cells due to the decrease of VEGF stimulation. The VEGF signaling seems to be affected upstream of eNOS (endothelial nitric oxide synthase) phosphorylation (Olszewska-Pazdrak *et al.*, 2009). Notch pathway is also responsible for downregulating VEGFR-2 expression in ECs mainly due to the activation of the expression of the Hesr-1 that is a negative regulator of transcription that targets VEGFR-2 (Taylor *et al.*, 2002).

Delta4-Notch signaling has been shown to significantly decrease the expression of VEGFR-2 thus inhibiting the proliferation of angiogenic cells. These two signals have opposite effects, meaning that if the concentration of one signal increases the other will decrease proportionally (Guo *et al.*, 2010).

2.2.3   Regulation of Neuropilins Expression

Neuropilins (NRPs) are mediators of neuronal guidance and angiogenesis. They are expressed is most adult tissues, including in growing blood vessels, for example on the ECs of capillaries, arteries and veins in the postnatal mouse retina and tumor cells (Soker *et al.*, 1998). The extracellular NRP-1 domain has distinct $VEGF_{165}$ and semaphoring binding domains to which these two ligands bind non-competitively. $VEGF_{165}$ is the VEGF-A isoform with the strongest affinity for NRP-1.

NRP-1 and VEGFR-2 were 50–60% colocalized even in quiescent mouse primary ECs and remained 30 min after stimulation by $VEGF-A_{165}$ (Salikhova et al., 2008). The dependence of the NRP-1-VEGFR-2 association on the binding of the PDZ (Post synaptic density protein (PSD95), Drosophila disc large tumor suppressor (Dlg1), and Zonula occludens-1 protein (Zo-1)) adaptor protein synectin suggests that the carboxy-terminus of NRP-1 is required for this association. Since VEGFR-2 is not known to bind synectin, it is not clear why synectin would be required for the association. Lanahan et al. (Lanahan et al., 2010) suggests that APPL (β amyloid protein precursor-like) binds VEGFR-2, so NRP-1 and APPL-bound synectin dimers could cross link the two receptors, thus explaining the dependence of the NRP-1-VEGFR-2 association on synectin.

Several studies suggest that NRP-1 signals are independent of VEGFRs. The contribution of NRP-1 to VEGF signaling would be mediated by the cytoplasmic domain. Since the carboxy-terminus of the same domain is used by synectin to cross-link NRP-1 to myosin VI, the molecular motor that drives NRP-1 trafficking, it is likely that NRP 1-dependent signaling is tightly coupled to NRP-1 trafficking (Horowitz & Seerapu, 2012).

In vivo studies showed that neither semaphoring-3A (SEMA3A) nor semaphorin signaling through NRP-1 and NRP-2 are essential for embryonic vasculogenesis in the mouse (Gu et al., 2003; Vieira et al., 2007). SEMA3A has been reported to also affect pathophysiological angiogenesis in mice. For example, SEMA3A prevents vascular regeneration in a mouse model of oxygen-induced retinopathy and inhibits tumor angiogenesis by eliciting EC apoptosis and normalizing the pericyte coverage of tumor vessels (Fukushima et al., 2011). SEMA3A-induced tumor vessel normalization might be indirectly caused by SEMA3A-mediated recruitment of a subset of NRP-1-expressing monocytes that secrete several factors involved in vessel maturation (Carrer et al., 2012).

2.3 VEGF Autocrine Signaling

The complex tumor microenvironment implies that cancer cells receive signals from multiple sources, which, conversely, will influence the function of other cells. This describes a paracrine signaling. However, it has become more evident the acquisition by cancer cells of a certain degree of self-sufficiency – autocrine signaling – that will favor tumor progression (Hanahan & Weinberg, 2011). In such autocrine signaling, the secreted growth factors may act on surrounding cells from same type of producing cells as well as on the secretor cells themselves. These autocrine loops may then provide a growth advantage to tumor cells, under limiting conditions (Gerber & Ferrara, 2003).

Furthermore, there is still evident that, in certain conditions, signaling pathways, such as VEGF pathway, may be transduced even without the factor secretion – internal autocrine/intracrine signaling (Gerber & Ferrara, 2003; Gerber et al., 2002).

Such profitable autocrine signaling loops have been described in both hematological and solid neoplastic contexts. Understanding the effector functions of VEGF in malignant neoplasias may be of great utility for the development of new therapeutic strategies.

In hematological malignancies, the role of VEGF/VEGFR autocrine loops is well established and coexpression of VEGF with its receptors is frequently found.

In acute myeloid primary leukemias and cell lines, previous studies have demonstrated that VEGF:VEGFR-2 autocrine loop operates both internally and externally. It was demonstrated that VEGFR-2 is constitutively phosphorylated and located in the nucleus of VEGF-producing leukemia cells. Treatment with anti-VEGF antibody blocked VEGFR-2 nuclear translocation and inhibited the NFKB pathway (Santos & Dias, 2004). *In vivo* blocking of VEGFR-2 induced long-term remission of xenotransplanted human leukaemia (Dias *et al.*, 2001). In B-cell non-Hodgkin's lymphomas the overexpression of VEGF and phosphorylated VEGFR-2 has been reported and correlates with expression of hypoxia inducible factor 1α (HIF1α) (Giatromanolaki *et al.*, 2008), the main known regulator of VEGF expression as it will be explored below. In infantile hemangioma, cell survival seems to be related to low levels of VEGFR-1 that promotes a constitutive VEGF-dependent activation of VEGFR-2 and downstream pathways (Jinnin *et al.*, 2008). In patients with multiple myeloma it was shown that bone marrow ECs (MMEC) highly expressed VEGF and VEGFR-2 at both mRNA and protein level. MMEC showed constitutive autophosphorylation in both VEGFR-2 and ERK2. Autophosphorylation, proliferation and capillarogenesis were prevented by a neutralizing antibody against VEGF and VEGFR-2. These findings suggested the existence of an autocrine loop of VEGF in MMEC (Ria *et al.*, 2004). In other study focusing hematological malignancies, VEGFR-1 expression was detected in the cytoplasm and nuclei of proliferating multiple myeloma cells. The inhibition of this receptor abrogated those cells proliferation and motility. The results suggested the contribution of an intracrine VEGF:VEGFR-1 signaling to multiple myeloma cells growth (Vincent *et al.*, 2005).

In solid tumours the role of VEGF:VEGFR autocrine loop is less clear. In breast cancer, Weigand and co-workers (Weigand *et al.*, 2005) detected VEGF levels above the range of biological activity in cell lines and primary culture media and they also verified that, in some cases, VEGFR-2 expressed on cell surface was phosphorylated, indicating its activated state. Conversely, other authors stated that in invasive breast cancer VEGFR-2 was not expressed and the VEGF receptor responsible for the autocrine loop is NRP-1 (Bachelder *et al.*, 2001; Bachelder *et al.*, 2002; Mercurio *et al.*, 2005). Intracrine signaling was also detected in human breast carcinoma cells through VEGF binding to VEGFR-1 (Lee *et al.*, 2007).

In colon cancer, a concomitant overexpression of VEGF and VEGFR-1, but not VEGFR-2, was described by Bates *et al.* (Bates *et al.*, 2003). The same authors showed, by disturbing VEGFR-1 function with VEGFR-1 blocking antibody and dominant-negative assays, that VEGFR-1 establishes an autocrine loop with VEGF in order to promote cell survival. In contrast, in another study, *in vitro* and *in vivo* colon cancer models displayed overexpression of both VEGFR-2 and VEGF in cells with an EMT phenotype and, by blocking VEGFR-2 *in vivo*, it was observed that subcutaneous xenograft colon tumors were dramatically smaller (Serpa *et al.*, 2010). Intracrine VEGF:VEGFR-2 signaling in survival and chemoresistance of human colorectal cancer cells was also observed (Samuel *et al.*, 2011). Evidence for an autocrine VEGF mitogenic loop was also pointed out in pancreatic cancer, although in some cases the VEGF receptor involved is VEGFR-2 whereas in other situations it is VEGFR-1 (von Marschall *et al.*, 2000).

In prostate cancer, Jackson *et al.* (M. W. Jackson *et al.*, 2002) published that stimulation of LNCaP cells with VEGF$_{165}$ induces DNA synthesis and recruits quiescent cells into the S-phase of the cell cycle via signaling through VEGFR-2. These findings suggest that VEGF may regulate both angiogenesis and tumor cell growth via autocrine and/or paracrine mechanisms in prostate cancer. Before that, other authors described a functional autocrine VEGF loop for cell survival but in this case signaling was performed through VEGFR-1 (Soker *et al.*, 2001). In ovarian carcinoma, an autocrine VEGF:VEGFR-2 loop was described as developing a protective role on cells from anoikis and in ascites formation (Boocock *et al.*, 1995; Sher *et al.*, 2009).

Tumor VEGF:VEGFR-2 autocrine loop signaling was shown to trigger angiogenesis in lung cancer (Chatterjee *et al.*, 2013).

3   Therapy Anti-angiogenesis

In 1971, Judah Folkman (Folkman *et al.*, 1971) was the first to postulate that the anti-angiogenic therapy against tumor growth could be clinically relevant. Since then, many studies lead to the development of highly specific therapies with anti-angiogenic factors and their tyrosine kinase receptors as targets.

Anti-angiogenic drugs can block angiogenesis, inhibit recruitment of proangiogenic bone marrow–derived cells, induce vessel regression, and promote sensitization to radio- and chemotherapy (Welti *et al.*, 2013). One of the most well established anti-angiogenic therapies is the use of VEGF inhibitors. Anti-VEGF, as the main anti-angiogenic molecule that limits tumor growth, has an essential role in pathophysiological and physiological angiogenesis (Ferrara, 2009). A lot of preclinical studies have demonstrated modest tumor-suppression effects in different types of cancers. VEGF and its receptors inhibitors-based therapies prolong progression-free survival and overall survival in a fraction of cancer patients – Table 1.

Bevacizumab is an anti-VEGF recombinant monoclonal antibody that blocks the link between all isoforms of VEGF and its receptors and it is the most used anti-angiogenic therapy. The end result is the blocking of new blood vessels formation and the subsequent nutrients supply will stop tumor growth. Nowadays, this drug is used in colorectal, kidney, non-small cell lung cancer and certain brain tumors (Ferrara, 2005; K. J. Kim *et al.*, 1993). Almost at the same time, pegaptanib which is an aptamer that blocks 165 aminoacid-VEGFA isoform, was approved for the treatment of the wet form of age-related macular degeneration, with great success (Gragoudas *et al.*, 2004). Other good examples of success using anti-VEGF therapy include the treatment of psoriatic mice, which lead to a reduction in the severity of the disease, and the treatment of hereditary hemorrhagic telangiectasia (a disease characterized by widespread hemangiomas formation) with thalidomidem, which has shown to normalize vessels and reduce episodes of epistaxis (Schonthaler *et al.*, 2009).

Multi-targeted tyrosine kinase inhibitors as imatinib, sorafenib, sunitinib or pazopanib, which block signaling pathways such as VEGF pathway, were approved for clinical use in various types of cancers including metastatic non-small cell lung cancer, metastatic breast cancer, recurrent glioblastoma, metastatic renal cell carcinoma and melanoma. A number of studies have reported their therapeutic efficacy.

Unfortunately, clinical trials of anti-VEGF monotherapy in patients with solid tumors have been disappointing. But the combination of anti-VEGF therapy with conventional chemotherapy has improved survival in cancer patients compared with chemotherapy alone. These opposite results could be explained by a normalization of tumor neovasculature by anti-VEGF therapy. Preclinical studies have shown that anti-VEGF therapy changes tumor vasculature towards a more mature/normal phenotype (Goel *et al.*, 2011). So, several questions need to be

	Mode of action	Type of cancers	PFS	Limitations	References
Bevacizumab	Monoclonal anti-VEGF antibody	Colorectal, breast, ovarian, non-small cell lung, renal, glioblastoma, pancreatic, prostate	Most of studies with improvements	No OS improvement	(Aghajanian et al., 2012; Allegra et al., 2011; Bennouna et al., 2013; Burger et al., 2011; Friedman et al., 2009; Herbst et al., 2011; Hurwitz et al., 2004; Meadows & Hurwitz, 2012; Miles et al., 2010; Miller et al., 2007; Perren et al., 2011; Rapisarda & Melillo, 2012; Reck et al., 2010; Rini et al., 2010; Saltz et al., 2012; Tol et al., 2009; von Minckwitz et al., 2012)
Aflibercept	Chimeric VEGF/PlGF neutralizing receptor	Colorectal, pancreatic, non-small cell lung, melanoma	Improvements in colorectal, non-small cell lung and melanoma	Small or no OS improvement	(Ramlau et al., 2012; Rapisarda & Melillo, 2012; Tarhini et al., 2011; Van Cutsem et al., 2012)
Sorafenib	VEGFR Tyrosine Kinase Inhibitor (TKI)	Renal, Hepatocellular, melanoma, small-cell lung	Improvements in renal and hepatocellular	No improvements in melanoma and small-cell lung	(Escudier et al., 2009; Kindler et al., 2012; Llovet et al., 2008; Ott et al., 2010; Rapisarda & Melillo, 2012)
Sunitinib	VEGFR TKI	Renal, stromal gastrointestinal, breast, hepatocellular, colorectal, pancreatic neuroendocrine, non-small cell lung, prostate, melanoma	Improvements in most studies	No OS improvements in the majority of studies	(Decoster, 2010; Goodman et al., 2007; Motzer et al., 2009; Rapisarda & Melillo, 2012; Raymond et al., 2011)
Pazopanib	VEGFR TKI	Renal, non-small cell lung, soft tissue sarcoma	Improvements	No OS improvements	(Sternberg et al., 2013; van der Graaf et al., 2012)
Vandetanib	VEGFR TKI	Non-small cell lung, medullary thyroid	Improvements in medullary thyroid cancer	No OS improvements	(Herbst et al., 2010; Rapisarda & Melillo, 2012; Wells et al., 2012)
Axitinib	VEGFR TKI	Renal, pancreatic	Improvements in renal cancer	No OS	(Motzer et al., 2013)
Ramucirumab	VEGFR TKI	Gastric, non-small cell lung, melanoma	Improvements in most studies	Little or no OS improvements	(Garon et al., 2012; Shah, 2014; Spratlin et al., 2010)

Table 1: Anti-angiogenic drugs used in therapy against cancer: mode of action, type of cancer where it is used, progression free survival (PFS) statistics and associated limitations. OS (overall survival). Table adapted from Welti, 2013 (Welti et al., 2013).

answered, namely why the preclinical models showed a good efficacy of most anti-angiogenic drugs but the clinical data has a modest response, showing an increase in the overall survival just in a few months? A possible explanation could be that several proangiogenic molecules become upregulated under selective pressure by these drug inhibitors, which can explain the poor results in overall survival.

Overall, the evidence demonstrates that antiangiogenic therapy has remarkable therapeutic effects in various types of human cancers. However, the molecular bases of cancer type-dependent resistance mechanisms against VEGF blockade, especially VEGF-independent pro-angiogenic mechanisms, need to be clarified. Targeting these mechanisms would enhance the effects and minimize the required doses of VEGF blockers. There is no doubt that further efforts in this area will yield opportunities to greatly improve anti-angiogenic treatment (Kubota, 2012). Some promising recent studies demonstrate that the combination of anti-angiogenic therapies and anti-inflammatory or immunotherapy could improve the overall response. Some of those candidates are IL-17 and a subset of T lymphocytes (cytokine-induced killer cells) that showed an improvement of efficacy in combination with anti-angiogenic drugs (Shi *et al.*, 2013; Wong, 2013).

4   Final Remarks

Overall, the present chapter was dedicated to tumor vascularization aiming to show its complexity and explaining the central role of VEGF and its receptors in this phenomenon.

The formation of blood vessels in a tumor comprises a stepwise sequence of processes accounting for the supply of signaling factors, nutrients and oxygen to sustain tumor growth. Rationally, strategies affecting tumor vessels would deadly disturb cancer cells, culminating in the regression and/or abrogation of disease. However, the therapeutic anti-angiogenesis approaches used so far did not overcome as expected, showing once again that the dynamic network involved in vessels formation into and within a malignant neoplasia is far from being completely understood.

References

Adelman, D. M., Maltepe, E., & Simon, M. C. (2000). HIF-1 is essential for multilineage hematopoiesis in the embryo. *Adv Exp Med Biol, 475,* 275-284.

Adham, S. A., & Coomber, B. L. (2009). Glucose is a key regulator of VEGFR2/KDR in human epithelial ovarian carcinoma cells. *Biochem Biophys Res Commun, 390(1),* 130-135.

Aghajanian, C., Blank, S. V., Goff, B. A., Judson, P. L., Teneriello, M. G., Husain, A., et al. (2012). OCEANS: a randomized, double-blind, placebo-controlled phase III trial of chemotherapy with or without bevacizumab in patients with platinum-sensitive recurrent epithelial ovarian, primary peritoneal, or fallopian tube cancer. *J Clin Oncol, 30(17),* 2039-2045.

Ahn, J. B., Rha, S. Y., Shin, S. J., Jeung, H. C., Kim, T. S., Zhang, X., et al. (2010). Circulating endothelial progenitor cells (EPC) for tumor vasculogenesis in gastric cancer patients. *Cancer Lett, 288(1),* 124-132.

Aicher, A., Heeschen, C., Mildner-Rihm, C., Urbich, C., Ihling, C., Technau-Ihling, K., et al. (2003). Essential role of endothelial nitric oxide synthase for mobilization of stem and progenitor cells. *Nat Med, 9(11),* 1370-1376.

Allegra, C. J., Yothers, G., O'Connell, M. J., Sharif, S., Petrelli, N. J., Colangelo, L. H., et al. (2011). Phase III trial assessing bevacizumab in stages II and III carcinoma of the colon: results of NSABP protocol C-08. *J Clin Oncol, 29(1),* 11-16.

Asahara, T., Murohara, T., Sullivan, A., Silver, M., van der Zee, R., Li, T., et al. (1997). Isolation of putative progenitor endothelial cells for angiogenesis. Science, 275(5302), 964-967.

Asare, Y., Schmitt, M., & Bernhagen, J. (2013). The vascular biology of macrophage migration inhibitory factor (MIF). Expression and effects in inflammation, atherogenesis and angiogenesis. Thromb Haemost, 109(3), 391-398.

Bachelder, R. E., Crago, A., Chung, J., Wendt, M. A., Shaw, L. M., Robinson, G., et al. (2001). Vascular endothelial growth factor is an autocrine survival factor for neuropilin-expressing breast carcinoma cells. Cancer Res, 61(15), 5736-5740.

Bachelder, R. E., Wendt, M. A., & Mercurio, A. M. (2002). Vascular endothelial growth factor promotes breast carcinoma invasion in an autocrine manner by regulating the chemokine receptor CXCR4. Cancer Res, 62(24), 7203-7206.

Bacher, M., Schrader, J., Thompson, N., Kuschela, K., Gemsa, D., Waeber, G., et al. (2003). Up-regulation of macrophage migration inhibitory factor gene and protein expression in glial tumor cells during hypoxic and hypoglycemic stress indicates a critical role for angiogenesis in glioblastoma multiforme. Am J Pathol, 162(1), 11-17.

Bagley, R. G., Rouleau, C., St Martin, T., Boutin, P., Weber, W., Ruzek, M., et al. (2008). Human endothelial precursor cells express tumor endothelial marker 1/endosialin/CD248. Mol Cancer Ther, 7(8), 2536-2546.

Barbera-Guillem, E., Nyhus, J. K., Wolford, C. C., Friece, C. R., & Sampsel, J. W. (2002). Vascular endothelial growth factor secretion by tumor-infiltrating macrophages essentially supports tumor angiogenesis, and IgG immune complexes potentiate the process. Cancer Res, 62(23), 7042-7049.

Barleon, B., Sozzani, S., Zhou, D., Weich, H. A., Mantovani, A., & Marme, D. (1996). Migration of human monocytes in response to vascular endothelial growth factor (VEGF) is mediated via the VEGF receptor flt-1. Blood, 87(8), 3336-3343.

Bates, R. C., Goldsmith, J. D., Bachelder, R. E., Brown, C., Shibuya, M., Oettgen, P., et al. (2003). Flt-1-dependent survival characterizes the epithelial-mesenchymal transition of colonic organoids. Curr Biol, 13(19), 1721-1727.

Bennouna, J., Sastre, J., Arnold, D., Osterlund, P., Greil, R., Van Cutsem, E., et al. (2013). Continuation of bevacizumab after first progression in metastatic colorectal cancer (ML18147): a randomised phase 3 trial. Lancet Oncol, 14(1), 29-37.

Bernfield, M., Kokenyesi, R., Kato, M., Hinkes, M. T., Spring, J., Gallo, R. L., et al. (1992). Biology of the syndecans: a family of transmembrane heparan sulfate proteoglycans. Annu Rev Cell Biol, 8, 365-393.

Bingle, L., Lewis, C. E., Corke, K. P., Reed, M. W., & Brown, N. J. (2006). Macrophages promote angiogenesis in human breast tumour spheroids in vivo. Br J Cancer, 94(1), 101-107.

Boocock, C. A., Charnock-Jones, D. S., Sharkey, A. M., McLaren, J., Barker, P. J., Wright, K. A., et al. (1995). Expression of vascular endothelial growth factor and its receptors flt and KDR in ovarian carcinoma. J Natl Cancer Inst, 87(7), 506-516.

Burger, R. A., Brady, M. F., Bookman, M. A., Fleming, G. F., Monk, B. J., Huang, H., et al. (2011). Incorporation of bevacizumab in the primary treatment of ovarian cancer. N Engl J Med, 365(26), 2473-2483.

Carmeliet, P., Ferreira, V., Breier, G., Pollefeyt, S., Kieckens, L., Gertsenstein, M., et al. (1996). Abnormal blood vessel development and lethality in embryos lacking a single VEGF allele. Nature, 380(6573), 435-439.

Carmeliet, P., & Jain, R. K. (2000). Angiogenesis in cancer and other diseases. Nature, 407(6801), 249-257.

Carmeliet, P., Moons, L., Luttun, A., Vincenti, V., Compernolle, V., De Mol, M., et al. (2001). Synergism between vascular endothelial growth factor and placental growth factor contributes to angiogenesis and plasma extravasation in pathological conditions. Nat Med, 7(5), 575-583.

Carrer, A., Moimas, S., Zacchigna, S., Pattarini, L., Zentilin, L., Ruozi, G., et al. (2012). Neuropilin-1 identifies a subset of bone marrow Gr1- monocytes that can induce tumor vessel normalization and inhibit tumor growth. Cancer Res, 72(24), 6371-6381.

Cascio, S., D'Andrea, A., Ferla, R., Surmacz, E., Gulotta, E., Amodeo, V., et al. (2010). miR-20b modulates VEGF expression by targeting HIF-1 alpha and STAT3 in MCF-7 breast cancer cells. J Cell Physiol, 224(1), 242-249.

Cebe-Suarez, S., Zehnder-Fjallman, A., & Ballmer-Hofer, K. (2006). The role of VEGF receptors in angiogenesis; complex partnerships. Cell Mol Life Sci, 63(5), 601-615.

Chatterjee, S., Heukamp, L. C., Siobal, M., Schottle, J., Wieczorek, C., Peifer, M., et al. (2013). Tumor VEGF:VEGFR2 autocrine feed-forward loop triggers angiogenesis in lung cancer. J Clin Invest, 123(4), 1732-1740.

Chen, J., Tang, D., Wang, S., Li, Q. G., Zhang, J. R., Li, P., et al. (2014). High expressions of galectin-1 and VEGF are associated with poor prognosis in gastric cancer patients. Tumour Biol, 35(3), 2513-2519.

Chen, P., Huang, Y., Bong, R., Ding, Y., Song, N., Wang, X., et al. (2011). Tumor-associated macrophages promote angiogenesis and melanoma growth via adrenomedullin in a paracrine and autocrine manner. Clin Cancer Res, 17(23), 7230-7239.

Chen, P., Zhu, J., Liu, D. Y., Li, H. Y., Xu, N., & Hou, M. (2014). Over-expression of survivin and VEGF in small-cell lung cancer may predict the poorer prognosis. Med Oncol, 31(1), 775.

Chesney, J., Metz, C., Bacher, M., Peng, T., Meinhardt, A., & Bucala, R. (1999). An essential role for macrophage migration inhibitory factor (MIF) in angiogenesis and the growth of a murine lymphoma. Mol Med, 5(3), 181-191.

Clauss, M., Gerlach, M., Gerlach, H., Brett, J., Wang, F., Familletti, P. C., et al. (1990). Vascular permeability factor: a tumor-derived polypeptide that induces endothelial cell and monocyte procoagulant activity, and promotes monocyte migration. J Exp Med, 172(6), 1535-1545.

Clauss, M., Weich, H., Breier, G., Knies, U., Rockl, W., Waltenberger, J., et al. (1996). The vascular endothelial growth factor receptor Flt-1 mediates biological activities. Implications for a functional role of placenta growth factor in monocyte activation and chemotaxis. J Biol Chem, 271(30), 17629-17634.

Costa, A., Afonso, J., Osorio, C., Gomes, A. L., Caiado, F., Valente, J., et al. (2013). miR-363-5p regulates endothelial cell properties and their communication with hematopoietic precursor cells. J Hematol Oncol, 6(1), 87.

Decoster, L. (2010). Activity of sunitinib in advanced maligant melanoma and its correlation with potential predictive biomarkers. Journal of Clinical Oncology, 28(Supp 15), 8518.

Dias, S., Hattori, K., Heissig, B., Zhu, Z., Wu, Y., Witte, L., et al. (2001). Inhibition of both paracrine and autocrine VEGF/VEGFR-2 signaling pathways is essential to induce long-term remission of xenotransplanted human leukemias. Proc Natl Acad Sci U S A, 98(19), 10857-10862.

Drogat, B., Auguste, P., Nguyen, D. T., Bouchecareilh, M., Pineau, R., Nalbantoglu, J., et al. (2007). IRE1 signaling is essential for ischemia-induced vascular endothelial growth factor-A expression and contributes to angiogenesis and tumor growth in vivo. Cancer Res, 67(14), 6700-6707.

Dunleavey, J. M., & Dudley, A. C. (2012). Vascular Mimicry: Concepts and Implications for Anti-Angiogenic Therapy. Curr Angiogenes, 1(2), 133-138.

Dvorak, A. M., Kohn, S., Morgan, E. S., Fox, P., Nagy, J. A., & Dvorak, H. F. (1996). The vesiculo-vacuolar organelle (VVO): a distinct endothelial cell structure that provides a transcellular pathway for macromolecular extravasation. J Leukoc Biol, 59(1), 100-115.

Dvorak, H. F. (2002). Vascular permeability factor/vascular endothelial growth factor: a critical cytokine in tumor angiogenesis and a potential target for diagnosis and therapy. J Clin Oncol, 20(21), 4368-4380.

Dvorak, H. F., Brown, L. F., Detmar, M., & Dvorak, A. M. (1995). Vascular permeability factor/vascular endothelial growth factor, microvascular hyperpermeability, and angiogenesis. Am J Pathol, 146(5), 1029-1039.

Eichmann, A., Corbel, C., Nataf, V., Vaigot, P., Breant, C., & Le Douarin, N. M. (1997). Ligand-dependent development of the endothelial and hemopoietic lineages from embryonic mesodermal cells expressing vascular endothelial growth factor receptor 2. Proc Natl Acad Sci U S A, 94(10), 5141-5146.

Ellis, L. M. (2006). The role of neuropilins in cancer. Mol Cancer Ther, 5(5), 1099-1107.

Escudier, B., Eisen, T., Stadler, W. M., Szczylik, C., Oudard, S., Staehler, M., et al. (2009). Sorafenib for treatment of renal cell carcinoma: Final efficacy and safety results of the phase III treatment approaches in renal cancer global evaluation trial. J Clin Oncol, 27(20), 3312-3318.

Fadini, G. P., Baesso, I., Albiero, M., Sartore, S., Agostini, C., & Avogaro, A. (2008). Technical notes on endothelial progenitor cells: ways to escape from the knowledge plateau. Atherosclerosis, 197(2), 496-503.

Ferrara, N. (1996). Vascular endothelial growth factor. Eur J Cancer, 32A(14), 2413-2422.

Ferrara, N. (1999). Vascular endothelial growth factor: molecular and biological aspects. Curr Top Microbiol Immunol, 237, 1-30.

Ferrara, N. (2001). Role of vascular endothelial growth factor in regulation of physiological angiogenesis. Am J Physiol Cell Physiol, 280(6), C1358-1366.

Ferrara, N. (2005). VEGF as a therapeutic target in cancer. Oncology, 69 Suppl 3, 11-16.

Ferrara, N. (2009). VEGF-A: a critical regulator of blood vessel growth. Eur Cytokine Netw, 20(4), 158-163.

Ferrara, N., & Davis-Smyth, T. (1997). The biology of vascular endothelial growth factor. Endocr Rev, 18(1), 4-25.

Ferrara, N., Gerber, H. P., & LeCouter, J. (2003). The biology of VEGF and its receptors. Nat Med, 9(6), 669-676.

Ferrara, N., Houck, K., Jakeman, L., & Leung, D. W. (1992). Molecular and biological properties of the vascular endothelial growth factor family of proteins. Endocr Rev, 13(1), 18-32.

Finkenzeller, G., Sparacio, A., Technau, A., Marme, D., & Siemeister, G. (1997). Sp1 recognition sites in the proximal promoter of the human vascular endothelial growth factor gene are essential for platelet-derived growth factor-induced gene expression. Oncogene, 15(6), 669-676.

Folkman, J. (1992). The role of angiogenesis in tumor growth. Semin Cancer Biol, 3 (2), 65-71.

Folkman, J. (1997). Angiogenesis and angiogenesis inhibition: an overview. EXS, 79, 1-8.

Folkman, J. & Hanahan, D. (1991). Switch to the angiogenic phenotyope during tumorigenesis. Princess Takamatsu Symp, 22, 339-347.

Folkman, J., Merler, E., Abernathy, C., & Williams, G. (1971). Isolation of a tumor factor responsible for angiogenesis. J Exp Med, 133(2), 275-288.

Fong, G. H., Rossant, J., Gertsenstein, M., & Breitman, M. L. (1995). Role of the Flt-1 receptor tyrosine kinase in regulating the assembly of vascular endothelium. Nature, 376(6535), 66-70.

Friedman, H. S., Prados, M. D., Wen, P. Y., Mikkelsen, T., Schiff, D., Abrey, L. E., et al. (2009). Bevacizumab alone and in combination with irinotecan in recurrent glioblastoma. J Clin Oncol, 27(28), 4733-4740.

Fukushima, Y., Okada, M., Kataoka, H., Hirashima, M., Yoshida, Y., Mann, F., et al. (2011). Sema3E-PlexinD1 signaling selectively suppresses disoriented angiogenesis in ischemic retinopathy in mice. J Clin Invest, 121(5), 1974-1985.

Gabrilovich, D. I., Chen, H. L., Girgis, K. R., Cunningham, H. T., Meny, G. M., Nadaf, S., et al. (1996). Production of vascular endothelial growth factor by human tumors inhibits the functional maturation of dendritic cells. Nat Med, 2(10), 1096-1103.

Gao, D., Nolan, D., McDonnell, K., Vahdat, L., Benezra, R., Altorki, N., et al. (2009). Bone marrow-derived endothelial progenitor cells contribute to the angiogenic switch in tumor growth and metastatic progression. Biochim Biophys Acta, 1796(1), 33-40.

Garon, E. B., Cao, D., Alexandris, E., John, W. J., Yurasov, S., & Perol, M. (2012). A randomized, double-blind, phase III study of Docetaxel and Ramucirumab versus Docetaxel and placebo in the treatment of stage IV non-small-cell lung cancer after disease progression after 1 previous platinum-based therapy (REVEL): treatment rationale and study design. Clin Lung Cancer, 13(6), 505-509.

Genbacev, O., Zhou, Y., Ludlow, J. W., & Fisher, S. J. (1997). Regulation of human placental development by oxygen tension. Science, 277(5332), 1669-1672.

George, A. L., Bangalore-Prakash, P., Rajoria, S., Suriano, R., Shanmugam, A., Mittelman, A., et al. (2011). Endothelial progenitor cell biology in disease and tissue regeneration. J Hematol Oncol, 4, 24.

Gerber, H. P., Condorelli, F., Park, J., & Ferrara, N. (1997). Differential transcriptional regulation of the two vascular endothelial growth factor receptor genes. Flt-1, but not Flk-1/KDR, is up-regulated by hypoxia. J Biol Chem, 272(38), 23659-23667.

Gerber, H. P., Dixit, V., & Ferrara, N. (1998). Vascular endothelial growth factor induces expression of the antiapoptotic proteins Bcl-2 and A1 in vascular endothelial cells. J Biol Chem, 273(21), 13313-13316.

Gerber, H. P., & Ferrara, N. (2003). The role of VEGF in normal and neoplastic hematopoiesis. J Mol Med (Berl), 81(1), 20-31.

Gerber, H. P., Malik, A. K., Solar, G. P., Sherman, D., Liang, X. H., Meng, G., et al. (2002). VEGF regulates haematopoietic stem cell survival by an internal autocrine loop mechanism. Nature, 417(6892), 954-958.

Gerber, H. P., McMurtrey, A., Kowalski, J., Yan, M., Keyt, B. A., Dixit, V., et al. (1998). Vascular endothelial growth factor regulates endothelial cell survival through the phosphatidylinositol 3'-kinase/Akt signal transduction pathway. Requirement for Flk-1/KDR activation. J Biol Chem, 273(46), 30336-30343.

Ghosh, R., Lipson, K. L., Sargent, K. E., Mercurio, A. M., Hunt, J. S., Ron, D., et al. (2010). Transcriptional regulation of VEGF-A by the unfolded protein response pathway. PLoS One, 5(3), e9575.

Giatromanolaki, A., Koukourakis, M. I., Pezzella, F., Sivridis, E., Turley, H., Harris, A. L., et al. (2008). Phosphorylated VEGFR2/KDR receptors are widely expressed in B-cell non-Hodgkin's lymphomas and correlate with hypoxia inducible factor activation. Hematol Oncol, 26(4), 219-224.

Girard, E., Strathdee, C., Trueblood, E., & Queva, C. (2012). Macrophage migration inhibitory factor produced by the tumour stroma but not by tumour cells regulates angiogenesis in the B16-F10 melanoma model. Br J Cancer, 107(9), 1498-1505.

Gitay-Goren, H., Cohen, T., Tessler, S., Soker, S., Gengrinovitch, S., Rockwell, P., et al. (1996). Selective binding of VEGF121 to one of the three vascular endothelial growth factor receptors of vascular endothelial cells. J Biol Chem, 271(10), 5519-5523.

Goel, S., Duda, D. G., Xu, L., Munn, L. L., Boucher, Y., Fukumura, D., et al. (2011). Normalization of the vasculature for treatment of cancer and other diseases. Physiol Rev, 91(3), 1071-1121.

Goodman, V. L., Rock, E. P., Dagher, R., Ramchandani, R. P., Abraham, S., Gobburu, J. V., et al. (2007). Approval summary: sunitinib for the treatment of imatinib refractory or intolerant gastrointestinal stromal tumors and advanced renal cell carcinoma. Clin Cancer Res, 13(5), 1367-1373.

Gragoudas, E. S., Adamis, A. P., Cunningham, E. T., Jr., Feinsod, M., Guyer, D. R., & Group, V. I. S. i. O. N. C. T. (2004). Pegaptanib for neovascular age-related macular degeneration. N Engl J Med, 351(27), 2805-2816.

Greenberg, J. I., Shields, D. J., Barillas, S. G., Acevedo, L. M., Murphy, E., Huang, J., et al. (2008). A role for VEGF as a negative regulator of pericyte function and vessel maturation. Nature, 456(7223), 809-813.

Grunstein, J., Masbad, J. J., Hickey, R., Giordano, F., & Johnson, R. S. (2000). Isoforms of vascular endothelial growth factor act in a coordinate fashion To recruit and expand tumor vasculature. Mol Cell Biol, 20(19), 7282-7291.

Gu, C., Rodriguez, E. R., Reimert, D. V., Shu, T., Fritzsch, B., Richards, L. J., et al. (2003). Neuropilin-1 conveys semaphorin and VEGF signaling during neural and cardiovascular development. Dev Cell, 5(1), 45-57.

Guo, S., Colbert, L. S., Fuller, M., Zhang, Y., & Gonzalez-Perez, R. R. (2010). Vascular endothelial growth factor receptor-2 in breast cancer. Biochim Biophys Acta, 1806(1), 108-121.

Hanahan, D., & Folkman, J. (1996). Patterns and emerging mechanisms of the angiogenic switch during tumorigenesis. Cell, 86(3), 353-364.

Hanahan, D., & Weinberg, R. A. (2011). Hallmarks of cancer: the next generation. Cell, 144(5), 646-674.

Hao, Q., Liu, J., Pappu, R., Su, H., Rola, R., Gabriel, R. A., et al. (2008). Contribution of bone marrow-derived cells associated with brain angiogenesis is primarily through leukocytes and macrophages. Arterioscler Thromb Vasc Biol, 28(12), 2151-2157.

Hattori, K., Heissig, B., Wu, Y., Dias, S., Tejada, R., Ferris, B., et al. (2002). Placental growth factor reconstitutes hematopoiesis by recruiting VEGFR1(+) stem cells from bone-marrow microenvironment. Nat Med, 8(8), 841-849.

Herbst, R. S., Ansari, R., Bustin, F., Flynn, P., Hart, L., Otterson, G. A., et al. (2011). Efficacy of bevacizumab plus erlotinib versus erlotinib alone in advanced non-small-cell lung cancer after failure of standard first-line chemotherapy (BeTa): a double-blind, placebo-controlled, phase 3 trial. Lancet, 377(9780), 1846-1854.

Herbst, R. S., Sun, Y., Eberhardt, W. E., Germonpre, P., Saijo, N., Zhou, C., et al. (2010). Vandetanib plus docetaxel versus docetaxel as second-line treatment for patients with advanced non-small-cell lung cancer (ZODIAC): a double-blind, randomised, phase 3 trial. Lancet Oncol, 11(7), 619-626.

Hira, E., Ono, T., Dhar, D. K., El-Assal, O. N., Hishikawa, Y., Yamanoi, A., et al. (2005). Overexpression of macrophage migration inhibitory factor induces angiogenesis and deteriorates prognosis after radical resection for hepatocellular carcinoma. Cancer, 103(3), 588-598.

Holmes, D. I., & Zachary, I. C. (2008). Vascular endothelial growth factor regulates stanniocalcin-1 expression via neuropilin-1-dependent regulation of KDR and synergism with fibroblast growth factor-2. Cell Signal, 20(3), 569-579.

Horowitz, A., & Seerapu, H. R. (2012). Regulation of VEGF signaling by membrane traffic. Cell Signal, 24(9), 1810-1820.

Hurwitz, H., Fehrenbacher, L., Novotny, W., Cartwright, T., Hainsworth, J., Heim, W., et al. (2004). Bevacizumab plus irinotecan, fluorouracil, and leucovorin for metastatic colorectal cancer. N Engl J Med, 350(23), 2335-2342.

Jackson, M. W., Roberts, J. S., Heckford, S. E., Ricciardelli, C., Stahl, J., Choong, C., et al. (2002). A potential autocrine role for vascular endothelial growth factor in prostate cancer. Cancer Res, 62(3), 854-859.

Jackson, T. A., Taylor, H. E., Sharma, D., Desiderio, S., & Danoff, S. K. (2005). Vascular endothelial growth factor receptor-2: counter-regulation by the transcription factors, TFII-I and TFII-IRD1. J Biol Chem, 280(33), 29856-29863.

Jakeman, L. B., Winer, J., Bennett, G. L., Altar, C. A., & Ferrara, N. (1992). Binding sites for vascular endothelial growth factor are localized on endothelial cells in adult rat tissues. J Clin Invest, 89(1), 244-253.

Jinnin, M., Medici, D., Park, L., Limaye, N., Liu, Y., Boscolo, E., et al. (2008). Suppressed NFAT-dependent VEGFR1 expression and constitutive VEGFR2 signaling in infantile hemangioma. Nat Med, 14(11), 1236-1246.

Kalka, C., Masuda, H., Takahashi, T., Kalka-Moll, W. M., Silver, M., Kearney, M., et al. (2000). Transplantation of ex vivo expanded endothelial progenitor cells for therapeutic neovascularization. Proc Natl Acad Sci U S A, 97(7), 3422-3427.

Kawaguchi, T. (2005). Cancer metastasis: characterization and identification of the behaviour of metastatic tumor cells and the cell adhesion molecules, including carbohydrates. Curr Drug Targets Cardiovasc Hematol Disord, 5 (1), 39-64.

Kim, J. Y., Hwang, J. H., Zhou, W., Shin, J., Noh, S. M., Song, I. S., et al. (2009). The expression of VEGF receptor genes is concurrently influenced by epigenetic gene silencing of the genes and VEGF activation. Epigenetics, 4(5), 313-321.

Kim, K. J., Li, B., Winer, J., Armanini, M., Gillett, N., Phillips, H. S., et al. (1993). Inhibition of vascular endothelial growth factor-induced angiogenesis suppresses tumour growth in vivo. Nature, 362(6423), 841-844.

Kindler, H. L., Wroblewski, K., Wallace, J. A., Hall, M. J., Locker, G., Nattam, S., et al. (2012). Gemcitabine plus sorafenib in patients with advanced pancreatic cancer: a phase II trial of the University of Chicago Phase II Consortium. Invest New Drugs, 30(1), 382-386.

Kirschmann, D. A., Seftor, E. A., Hardy, K. M., Seftor, R. E., & Hendrix, M. J. (2012). Molecular pathways: vasculogenic mimicry in tumor cells: diagnostic and therapeutic implications. Clin Cancer Res, 18(10), 2726-2732.

Koumenis, C., Bi, M., Ye, J., Feldman, D., & Koong, A. C. (2007). Hypoxia and the unfolded protein response. Methods Enzymol, 435, 275-293.

Kovacic, J. C., Moore, J., Herbert, A., Ma, D., Boehm, M., & Graham, R. M. (2008). Endothelial progenitor cells, angioblasts, and angiogenesis--old terms reconsidered from a current perspective. Trends Cardiovasc Med, 18(2), 45-51.

Kubota, Y. (2012). Tumor angiogenesis and anti-angiogenic therapy. Keio J Med, 61(2), 47-56.

Lanahan, A. A., Hermans, K., Claes, F., Kerley-Hamilton, J. S., Zhuang, Z. W., Giordano, F. J., et al. (2010). VEGF receptor 2 endocytic trafficking regulates arterial morphogenesis. Dev Cell, 18(5), 713-724.

Lee, T. H., Seng, S., Sekine, M., Hinton, C., Fu, Y., Avraham, H. K., et al. (2007). Vascular endothelial growth factor mediates intracrine survival in human breast carcinoma cells through internally expressed VEGFR1/FLT1. PLoS Med, 4(6), e186.

Lei, Z., Li, B., Yang, Z., Fang, H., Zhang, G. M., Feng, Z. H., et al. (2009). Regulation of HIF-1alpha and VEGF by miR-20b tunes tumor cells to adapt to the alteration of oxygen concentration. PLoS One, 4(10), e7629.

Leung, D. W., Cachianes, G., Kuang, W. J., Goeddel, D. V., & Ferrara, N. (1989). Vascular endothelial growth factor is a secreted angiogenic mitogen. Science, 246(4935), 1306-1309.

Li, Q., Zhang, N., Jia, Z., Le, X., Dai, B., Wei, D., et al. (2009). Critical role and regulation of transcription factor FoxM1 in human gastric cancer angiogenesis and progression. Cancer Res, 69(8), 3501-3509.

Liu, B., Peng, X. C., Zheng, X. L., Wang, J., & Qin, Y. W. (2009). MiR-126 restoration down-regulate VEGF and inhibit the growth of lung cancer cell lines in vitro and in vivo. Lung Cancer, 66(2), 169-175.

Liu, Z., Sun, B., Qi, L., Li, H., Gao, J., & Leng, X. (2012). Zinc finger E-box binding homeobox 1 promotes vasculogenic mimicry in colorectal cancer through induction of epithelial-to-mesenchymal transition. Cancer Sci, 103(4), 813-820.

Llovet, J. M., Ricci, S., Mazzaferro, V., Hilgard, P., Gane, E., Blanc, J. F., et al. (2008). Sorafenib in advanced hepatocellular carcinoma. N Engl J Med, 359(4), 378-390.

Loeffler, S., Fayard, B., Weis, J., & Weissenberger, J. (2005). Interleukin-6 induces transcriptional activation of vascular endothelial growth factor (VEGF) in astrocytes in vivo and regulates VEGF promoter activity in glioblastoma cells via direct interaction between STAT3 and Sp1. Int J Cancer, 115(2), 202-213.

Lucena, J., Pezzi, S., Aso, E., Valero, M. C., Carreiro, C., Dubus, P., et al. (2010). Essential role of the N-terminal region of TFII-I in viability and behavior. BMC Med Genet, 11, 61.

Mammoto, A., Connor, K. M., Mammoto, T., Yung, C. W., Huh, D., Aderman, C. M., et al. (2009). A mechanosensitive transcriptional mechanism that controls angiogenesis. Nature, 457(7233), 1103-1108.

Mancuso, P., Burlini, A., Pruneri, G., Goldhirsch, A., Martinelli, G., & Bertolini, F. (2001). Resting and activated endothelial cells are increased in the peripheral blood of cancer patients. Blood, 97(11), 3658-3661.

Meadows, K. L., & Hurwitz, H. I. (2012). Anti-VEGF therapies in the clinic. Cold Spring Harb Perspect Med, 2(10).

Medina, R. J., O'Neill, C. L., Sweeney, M., Guduric-Fuchs, J., Gardiner, T. A., Simpson, D. A., et al. (2010). Molecular analysis of endothelial progenitor cell (EPC) subtypes reveals two distinct cell populations with different identities. BMC Med Genomics, 3, 18.

Mercurio, A. M., Lipscomb, E. A., & Bachelder, R. E. (2005). Non-angiogenic functions of VEGF in breast cancer. J Mammary Gland Biol Neoplasia, 10(4), 283-290.

Miles, D. W., Chan, A., Dirix, L. Y., Cortes, J., Pivot, X., Tomczak, P., et al. (2010). Phase III study of bevacizumab plus docetaxel compared with placebo plus docetaxel for the first-line treatment of human epidermal growth factor receptor 2-negative metastatic breast cancer. J Clin Oncol, 28(20), 3239-3247.

Miller, K., Wang, M., Gralow, J., Dickler, M., Cobleigh, M., Perez, E. A., et al. (2007). Paclitaxel plus bevacizumab versus paclitaxel alone for metastatic breast cancer. N Engl J Med, 357(26), 2666-2676.

Minami, T., Murakami, T., Horiuchi, K., Miura, M., Noguchi, T., Miyazaki, J., et al. (2004). Interaction between hex and GATA transcription factors in vascular endothelial cells inhibits flk-1/KDR-mediated vascular endothelial growth factor signaling. J Biol Chem, 279(20), 20626-20635.

Minami, T., Rosenberg, R. D., & Aird, W. C. (2001). Transforming growth factor-beta 1-mediated inhibition of the flk-1/KDR gene is mediated by a 5'-untranslated region palindromic GATA site. J Biol Chem, 276(7), 5395-5402.

Monestiroli, S., Mancuso, P., Burlini, A., Pruneri, G., Dell'Agnola, C., Gobbi, A., et al. (2001). Kinetics and viability of circulating endothelial cells as surrogate angiogenesis marker in an animal model of human lymphoma. Cancer Res, 61(11), 4341-4344.

Motzer, R. J., Escudier, B., Tomczak, P., Hutson, T. E., Michaelson, M. D., Negrier, S., et al. (2013). Axitinib versus sorafenib as second-line treatment for advanced renal cell carcinoma: overall survival analysis and updated results from a randomised phase 3 trial. Lancet Oncol, 14(6), 552-562.

Motzer, R. J., Hutson, T. E., Tomczak, P., Michaelson, M. D., Bukowski, R. M., Oudard, S., et al. (2009). Overall survival and updated results for sunitinib compared with interferon alfa in patients with metastatic renal cell carcinoma. J Clin Oncol, 27(22), 3584-3590.

Neufeld, G., Cohen, T., Gengrinovitch, S., & Poltorak, Z. (1999). Vascular endothelial growth factor (VEGF) and its receptors. FASEB J, 13(1), 9-22.

Nishida, N., Yano, H., Nishida, T., Kamura, T., & Kojiro, M. (2006). Angiogenesis in cancer. Vasc Health Risk Manag, 2(3), 213-219.

Obermair, A., Kucera, E., Mayerhofer, K., Speiser, P., Seifert, M., Czerwenka, K., et al. (1997). Vascular endothelial growth factor (VEGF) in human breast cancer: correlation with disease-free survival. Int J Cancer, 74(4), 455-458.

Olszewska-Pazdrak, B., Hein, T. W., Olszewska, P., & Carney, D. H. (2009). Chronic hypoxia attenuates VEGF signaling and angiogenic responses by downregulation of KDR in human endothelial cells. Am J Physiol Cell Physiol, 296(5), C1162-1170.

Ott, P. A., Hamilton, A., Min, C., Safarzadeh-Amiri, S., Goldberg, L., Yoon, J., et al. (2010). A phase II trial of sorafenib in metastatic melanoma with tissue correlates. PLoS One, 5(12), e15588.

Paavonen, K., Puolakkainen, P., Jussila, L., Jahkola, T., & Alitalo, K. (2000). Vascular endothelial growth factor receptor-3 in lymphangiogenesis in wound healing. Am J Pathol, 156(5), 1499-1504.

Pages, G., & Pouyssegur, J. (2005). Transcriptional regulation of the Vascular Endothelial Growth Factor gene--a concert of activating factors. Cardiovasc Res, 65(3), 564-573.

Peichev, M., Naiyer, A. J., Pereira, D., Zhu, Z., Lane, W. J., Williams, M., et al. (2000). Expression of VEGFR-2 and AC133 by circulating human CD34(+) cells identifies a population of functional endothelial precursors. Blood, 95(3), 952-958.

Perren, T. J., Swart, A. M., Pfisterer, J., Ledermann, J. A., Pujade-Lauraine, E., Kristensen, G., et al. (2011). A phase 3 trial of bevacizumab in ovarian cancer. N Engl J Med, 365(26), 2484-2496.

Pidgeon, G. P., Barr, M. P., Harmey, J. H., Foley, D. A., & Bouchier-Hayes, D. J. (2001). Vascular endothelial growth factor (VEGF) upregulates BCL-2 and inhibits apoptosis in human and murine mammary adenocarcinoma cells. Br J Cancer, 85(2), 273-278.

Pillai, S., Kovacs, M., & Chellappan, S. (2010). Regulation of vascular endothelial growth factor receptors by Rb and E2F1: role of acetylation. Cancer Res, 70(12), 4931-4940.

Pircher, A., Kahler, C. M., Skvortsov, S., Dlaska, M., Kawaguchi, G., Schmid, T., et al. (2008). Increased numbers of endothelial progenitor cells in peripheral blood and tumor specimens in non-small cell lung cancer: a methodological challenge and an ongoing debate on the clinical relevance. Oncol Rep, 19(2), 345-352.

Ramlau, R., Gorbunova, V., Ciuleanu, T. E., Novello, S., Ozguroglu, M., Goksel, T., et al. (2012). Aflibercept and Docetaxel versus Docetaxel alone after platinum failure in patients with advanced or metastatic non-small-cell lung cancer: a randomized, controlled phase III trial. J Clin Oncol, 30(29), 3640-3647.

Rapisarda, A., & Melillo, G. (2012). Overcoming disappointing results with antiangiogenic therapy by targeting hypoxia. Nat Rev Clin Oncol, 9(7), 378-390.

Raymond, E., Dahan, L., Raoul, J. L., Bang, Y. J., Borbath, I., Lombard-Bohas, C., et al. (2011). Sunitinib malate for the treatment of pancreatic neuroendocrine tumors. N Engl J Med, 364(6), 501-513.

Real, C., Remedio, L., Caiado, F., Igreja, C., Borges, C., Trindade, A., et al. (2011). Bone marrow-derived endothelial progenitors expressing Delta-like 4 (Dll4) regulate tumor angiogenesis. PLoS One, 6(4), e18323.

Reck, M., von Pawel, J., Zatloukal, P., Ramlau, R., Gorbounova, V., Hirsh, V., et al. (2010). Overall survival with cisplatin-gemcitabine and bevacizumab or placebo as first-line therapy for nonsquamous non-small-cell lung cancer: results from a randomised phase III trial (AVAiL). Ann Oncol, 21(9), 1804-1809.

Rehman, J., Li, J., Orschell, C. M., & March, K. L. (2003). Peripheral blood "endothelial progenitor cells" are derived from monocyte/macrophages and secrete angiogenic growth factors. Circulation, 107(8), 1164-1169.

Ria, R., Vacca, A., Russo, F., Cirulli, T., Massaia, M., Tosi, P., et al. (2004). A VEGF-dependent autocrine loop mediates proliferation and capillarogenesis in bone marrow endothelial cells of patients with multiple myeloma. Thromb Haemost, 92(6), 1438-1445.

Ribatti, D. (2007). The discovery of endothelial progenitor cells. An historical review. Leuk Res, 31(4), 439-444.

Ribatti, D., Nico, B., Crivellato, E., & Vacca, A. (2005). Endothelial progenitor cells in health and disease. Histol Histopathol, 20(4), 1351-1358.

Ribatti, D., Nico, B., Crivellato, E., & Vacca, A. (2007). Macrophages and tumor angiogenesis. Leukemia, 21(10), 2085-2089.

Richter-Ehrenstein, C., Rentzsch, J., Runkel, S., Schneider, A., & Schonfelder, G. (2007). Endothelial progenitor cells in breast cancer patients. Breast Cancer Res Treat, 106(3), 343-349.

Rini, B. I., Halabi, S., Rosenberg, J. E., Stadler, W. M., Vaena, D. A., Archer, L., et al. (2010). Phase III trial of bevacizumab plus interferon alfa versus interferon alfa monotherapy in patients with metastatic renal cell carcinoma: final results of CALGB 90206. J Clin Oncol, 28(13), 2137-2143.

Risau, W. (1997). Mechanisms of angiogenesis. Nature, 386(6626), 671-674.

Robinson, C. J., & Stringer, S. E. (2001). The splice variants of vascular endothelial growth factor (VEGF) and their receptors. J Cell Sci, 114(Pt 5), 853-865.

Rohde, E., Malischnik, C., Thaler, D., Maierhofer, T., Linkesch, W., Lanzer, G., et al. (2006). Blood monocytes mimic endothelial progenitor cells. Stem Cells, 24(2), 357-367.

Rollin, S., Lemieux, C., Maliba, R., Favier, J., Villeneuve, L. R., Allen, B. G., et al. (2004). VEGF-mediated endothelial P-selectin translocation: role of VEGF receptors and endogenous PAF synthesis. Blood, 103(10), 3789-3797.

Romagnani, P., Annunziato, F., Liotta, F., Lazzeri, E., Mazzinghi, B., Frosali, F., et al. (2005). CD14+CD34low cells with stem cell phenotypic and functional features are the major source of circulating endothelial progenitors. Circ Res, 97(4), 314-322.

Romero-Ramirez, L., Cao, H., Nelson, D., Hammond, E., Lee, A. H., Yoshida, H., et al. (2004). XBP1 is essential for survival under hypoxic conditions and is required for tumor growth. Cancer Res, 64(17), 5943-5947.

Sakamori, Y., Masago, K., Ohmori, K., Togashi, Y., Nagai, H., Okuda, C., et al. (2012). Increase in circulating endothelial progenitor cells predicts response in patients with advanced non-small-cell lung cancer. Cancer Sci, 103(6), 1065-1070.

Salikhova, A., Wang, L., Lanahan, A. A., Liu, M., Simons, M., Leenders, W. P., et al. (2008). Vascular endothelial growth factor and semaphorin induce neuropilin-1 endocytosis via separate pathways. Circ Res, 103(6), e71-79.

Saltz, L., Badarinath, S., Dakhil, S., Bienvenu, B., Harker, W. G., Birchfield, G., et al. (2012). Phase III trial of cetuximab, bevacizumab, and 5-fluorouracil/leucovorin vs. FOLFOX-bevacizumab in colorectal cancer. Clin Colorectal Cancer, 11(2), 101-111.

Samuel, S., Fan, F., Dang, L. H., Xia, L., Gaur, P., & Ellis, L. M. (2011). Intracrine vascular endothelial growth factor signaling in survival and chemoresistance of human colorectal cancer cells. Oncogene, 30(10), 1205-1212.

Santos, S. C., & Dias, S. (2004). Internal and external autocrine VEGF/KDR loops regulate survival of subsets of acute leukemia through distinct signaling pathways. Blood, 103(10), 3883-3889.

Santra, M., Santra, S., Zhang, J., & Chopp, M. (2008). Ectopic decorin expression up-regulates VEGF expression in mouse cerebral endothelial cells via activation of the transcription factors Sp1, HIF1alpha, and Stat3. J Neurochem, 105(2), 324-337.

Sasahira, T., Kurihara, M., Bhawal, U. K., Ueda, N., Shimomoto, T., Yamamoto, K., et al. (2012). Downregulation of miR-126 induces angiogenesis and lymphangiogenesis by activation of VEGF-A in oral cancer. Br J Cancer, 107(4), 700-706.

Sawano, A., Iwai, S., Sakurai, Y., Ito, M., Shitara, K., Nakahata, T., et al. (2001). Flt-1, vascular endothelial growth factor receptor 1, is a novel cell surface marker for the lineage of monocyte-macrophages in humans. Blood, 97(3), 785-791.

Schmeisser, A., Garlichs, C. D., Zhang, H., Eskafi, S., Graffy, C., Ludwig, J., et al. (2001). Monocytes coexpress endothelial and macrophagocytic lineage markers and form cord-like structures in Matrigel under angiogenic conditions. Cardiovasc Res, 49(3), 671-680.

Schmidt-Lucke, C., Fichtlscherer, S., Aicher, A., Tschope, C., Schultheiss, H. P., Zeiher, A. M., et al. (2010). Quantification of circulating endothelial progenitor cells using the modified ISHAGE protocol. PLoS One, 5(11), e13790.

Schonthaler, H. B., Huggenberger, R., Wculek, S. K., Detmar, M., & Wagner, E. F. (2009). Systemic anti-VEGF treatment strongly reduces skin inflammation in a mouse model of psoriasis. Proc Natl Acad Sci U S A, 106(50), 21264-21269.

Semenza, G. L. (2003). Angiogenesis in ischemic and neoplastic disorders. Annu Rev Med, 54, 17-28.

Serpa, J., Caiado, F., Carvalho, T., Torre, C., Goncalves, L. G., Casalou, C., et al. (2010). Butyrate-rich colonic microenvironment is a relevant selection factor for metabolically adapted tumor cells. J Biol Chem, 285(50), 39211-39223.

Shah, M. A. (2014). Gastrointestinal cancer: targeted therapies in gastric cancer-the dawn of a new era. Nat Rev Clin Oncol, 11(1), 10-11.

Shaked, Y., Bertolini, F., Man, S., Rogers, M. S., Cervi, D., Foutz, T., et al. (2005). Genetic heterogeneity of the vasculogenic phenotype parallels angiogenesis; Implications for cellular surrogate marker analysis of antiangiogenesis. Cancer Cell, 7(1), 101-111.

Shalaby, F., Rossant, J., Yamaguchi, T. P., Gertsenstein, M., Wu, X. F., Breitman, M. L., et al. (1995). Failure of blood-island formation and vasculogenesis in Flk-1-deficient mice. Nature, 376(6535), 62-66.

Sher, I., Adham, S. A., Petrik, J., & Coomber, B. L. (2009). Autocrine VEGF-A/KDR loop protects epithelial ovarian carcinoma cells from anoikis. Int J Cancer, 124(3), 553-561.

Shi, S., Wang, R., Chen, Y., Song, H., Chen, L., & Huang, G. (2013). Combining antiangiogenic therapy with adoptive cell immunotherapy exerts better antitumor effects in non-small cell lung cancer models. PLoS One, 8(6), e65757.

Shibuya, M. (2001). Structure and dual function of vascular endothelial growth factor receptor-1 (Flt-1). Int J Biochem Cell Biol, 33(4), 409-420.

Shibuya, M. (2006). Differential roles of vascular endothelial growth factor receptor-1 and receptor-2 in angiogenesis. J Biochem Mol Biol, 39(5), 469-478.

Shibuya, M. (2013). Vascular endothelial growth factor and its receptor system: physiological functions in angiogenesis and pathological roles in various diseases. J Biochem, 153(1), 13-19.

Shibuya, M., & Claesson-Welsh, L. (2006). Signal transduction by VEGF receptors in regulation of angiogenesis and lymphangiogenesis. Exp Cell Res, 312(5), 549-560.

Shibuya, M., Yamaguchi, S., Yamane, A., Ikeda, T., Tojo, A., Matsushime, H., et al. (1990). Nucleotide sequence and expression of a novel human receptor-type tyrosine kinase gene (flt) closely related to the fms family. Oncogene, 5(4), 519-524.

Soker, S., Fidder, H., Neufeld, G., & Klagsbrun, M. (1996). Characterization of novel vascular endothelial growth factor (VEGF) receptors on tumor cells that bind VEGF165 via its exon 7-encoded domain. J Biol Chem, 271(10), 5761-5767.

Soker, S., Kaefer, M., Johnson, M., Klagsbrun, M., Atala, A., & Freeman, M. R. (2001). Vascular endothelial growth factor-mediated autocrine stimulation of prostate tumor cells coincides with progression to a malignant phenotype. Am J Pathol, 159(2), 651-659.

Soker, S., Takashima, S., Miao, H. Q., Neufeld, G., & Klagsbrun, M. (1998). Neuropilin-1 is expressed by endothelial and tumor cells as an isoform-specific receptor for vascular endothelial growth factor. Cell, 92(6), 735-745.

Song, Y., Wu, J., Oyesanya, R. A., Lee, Z., Mukherjee, A., & Fang, X. (2009). Sp-1 and c-Myc mediate lysophosphatidic acid-induced expression of vascular endothelial growth factor in ovarian cancer cells via a hypoxia-inducible factor-1-independent mechanism. Clin Cancer Res, 15(2), 492-501.

Sporn, M.B. (1996). The war on cancer. Lancet, 347(9012), 1377-1381.

Spratlin, J. L., Cohen, R. B., Eadens, M., Gore, L., Camidge, D. R., Diab, S., et al. (2010). Phase I pharmacologic and biologic study of ramucirumab (IMC-1121B), a fully human immunoglobulin G1 monoclonal antibody targeting the vascular endothelial growth factor receptor-2. J Clin Oncol, 28(5), 780-787.

Sternberg, C. N., Hawkins, R. E., Wagstaff, J., Salman, P., Mardiak, J., Barrios, C. H., et al. (2013). A randomised, double-blind phase III study of pazopanib in patients with advanced and/or metastatic renal cell carcinoma: final overall survival results and safety update. Eur J Cancer, 49(6), 1287-1296.

Stupack, D. G., & Cheresh, D. A. (2004). Integrins and angiogenesis. Curr Top Dev Biol, 64, 207-238.

Stuttfeld, E., & Ballmer-Hofer, K. (2009). Structure and function of VEGF receptors. IUBMB Life, 61(9), 915-922.

Sun, T., Zhao, N., Zhao, X. L., Gu, Q., Zhang, S. W., Che, N., et al. (2010). Expression and functional significance of Twist1 in hepatocellular carcinoma: its role in vasculogenic mimicry. Hepatology, 51(2), 545-556.

Suzuma, K., Takagi, H., Otani, A., Suzuma, I., & Honda, Y. (1998). Increased expression of KDR/Flk-1 (VEGF-2) in murine model of ischemia-induced retinal neovascularization. Microvasc Res, 56(3), 183-191.

Talks, K. L., Turley, H., Gatter, K. C., Maxwell, P. H., Pugh, C. W., Ratcliffe, P. J., et al. (2000). The expression and distribution of the hypoxia-inducible factors HIF-1alpha and HIF-2alpha in normal human tissues, cancers, and tumor-associated macrophages. Am J Pathol, 157(2), 411-421.

Tarhini, A. A., Frankel, P., Margolin, K. A., Christensen, S., Ruel, C., Shipe-Spotloe, J., et al. (2011). Aflibercept (VEGF Trap) in inoperable stage III or stage iv melanoma of cutaneous or uveal origin. Clin Cancer Res, 17(20), 6574-6581.

Taylor, K. L., Henderson, A. M., & Hughes, C. C. (2002). Notch activation during endothelial cell network formation in vitro targets the basic HLH transcription factor HESR-1 and downregulates VEGFR-2/KDR expression. Microvasc Res, 64(3), 372-383.

Terman, B. I., Carrion, M. E., Kovacs, E., Rasmussen, B. A., Eddy, R. L., & Shows, T. B. (1991). Identification of a new endothelial cell growth factor receptor tyrosine kinase. Oncogene, 6(9), 1677-1683.

Tol, J., Koopman, M., Cats, A., Rodenburg, C. J., Creemers, G. J., Schrama, J. G., et al. (2009). Chemotherapy, bevacizumab, and cetuximab in metastatic colorectal cancer. N Engl J Med, 360(6), 563-572.

Van Cutsem, E., Tabernero, J., Lakomy, R., Prenen, H., Prausova, J., Macarulla, T., et al. (2012). Addition of aflibercept to fluorouracil, leucovorin, and irinotecan improves survival in a phase III randomized trial in patients with metastatic colorectal cancer previously treated with an oxaliplatin-based regimen. J Clin Oncol, 30(28), 3499-3506.

van der Graaf, W. T., Blay, J. Y., Chawla, S. P., Kim, D. W., Bui-Nguyen, B., Casali, P. G., et al. (2012). Pazopanib for metastatic soft-tissue sarcoma (PALETTE): a randomised, double-blind, placebo-controlled phase 3 trial. Lancet, 379(9829), 1879-1886.

Verbridge, S. S., Choi, N. W., Zheng, Y., Brooks, D. J., Stroock, A. D., & Fischbach, C. (2009). Oxygen-controlled three-dimensional cultures to analyze tumor angiogenesis. Tissue Eng Part A, 16(7), 2133-2141.

Vieira, J. M., Ruhrberg, C., & Schwarz, Q. (2010). VEGF receptor signaling in vertebrate development. Organogenesis, 6(2), 97-106.

Vieira, J. M., Schwarz, Q., & Ruhrberg, C. (2007). Selective requirements for NRP1 ligands during neurovascular patterning. Development, 134(10), 1833-1843.

Vincent, L., Jin, D. K., Karajannis, M. A., Shido, K., Hooper, A. T., Rashbaum, W. K., et al. (2005). Fetal stromal-dependent paracrine and intracrine vascular endothelial growth factor-a/vascular endothelial growth factor receptor-1 signaling promotes proliferation and motility of human primary myeloma cells. Cancer Res, 65(8), 3185-3192.

Vincenti, V., Cassano, C., Rocchi, M., & Persico, G. (1996). Assignment of the vascular endothelial growth factor gene to human chromosome 6p21.3. Circulation, 93(8), 1493-1495.

von Marschall, Z., Cramer, T., Hocker, M., Burde, R., Plath, T., Schirner, M., et al. (2000). De novo expression of vascular endothelial growth factor in human pancreatic cancer: evidence for an autocrine mitogenic loop. Gastroenterology, 119(5), 1358-1372.

von Minckwitz, G., Eidtmann, H., Rezai, M., Fasching, P. A., Tesch, H., Eggemann, H., et al. (2012). Neoadjuvant chemotherapy and bevacizumab for HER2-negative breast cancer. N Engl J Med, 366(4), 299-309.

Wakiya, K., Begue, A., Stehelin, D., & Shibuya, M. (1996). A cAMP response element and an Ets motif are involved in the transcriptional regulation of flt-1 tyrosine kinase (vascular endothelial growth factor receptor 1) gene. J Biol Chem, 271(48), 30823-30828.

Waltenberger, J., Claesson-Welsh, L., Siegbahn, A., Shibuya, M., & Heldin, C. H. (1994). Different signal transduction properties of KDR and Flt1, two receptors for vascular endothelial growth factor. J Biol Chem, 269(43), 26988-26995.

Wang, X., Zhao, X., Wang, K., Wu, L., & Duan, T. (2013). Interaction of monocytes/macrophages with ovarian cancer cells promotes angiogenesis in vitro. Cancer Sci, 104(4), 516-523.

Weigand, M., Hantel, P., Kreienberg, R., & Waltenberger, J. (2005). Autocrine vascular endothelial growth factor signalling in breast cancer. Evidence from cell lines and primary breast cancer cultures in vitro. Angiogenesis, 8(3), 197-204.

Wells, S. A., Jr., Robinson, B. G., Gagel, R. F., Dralle, H., Fagin, J. A., Santoro, M., et al. (2012). Vandetanib in patients with locally advanced or metastatic medullary thyroid cancer: a randomized, double-blind phase III trial. J Clin Oncol, 30(2), 134-141.

Welti, J., Loges, S., Dimmeler, S., & Carmeliet, P. (2013). Recent molecular discoveries in angiogenesis and antiangiogenic therapies in cancer. J Clin Invest, 123(8), 3190-3200.

Witmer, A. N., Dai, J., Weich, H. A., Vrensen, G. F., & Schlingemann, R. O. (2002). Expression of vascular endothelial growth factor receptors 1, 2, and 3 in quiescent endothelia. J Histochem Cytochem, 50(6), 767-777.

Witmer, A. N., Vrensen, G. F., Van Noorden, C. J., & Schlingemann, R. O. (2003). Vascular endothelial growth factors and angiogenesis in eye disease. Prog Retin Eye Res, 22(1), 1-29.

Wong, W. (2013). Combining anti-inflammatory and anti-angiogenic therapy. Science Signalling, 6(294), ec224.

Xu, X. L., Ling, Z. Q., Chen, W., Xu, Y. P., & Mao, W. M. (2013). The overexpression of VEGF in esophageal cancer is associated with a more advanced TMN stage: a meta-analysis. Cancer Biomark, 13(2), 105-113.

Ye, P., Liu, J., He, F., Xu, W., & Yao, K. (2014). Hypoxia-induced deregulation of miR-126 and its regulative effect on VEGF and MMP-9 expression. Int J Med Sci, 11(1), 17-23.

Young, P. P., Hofling, A. A., & Sands, M. S. (2002). VEGF increases engraftment of bone marrow-derived endothelial progenitor cells (EPCs) into vasculature of newborn murine recipients. Proc Natl Acad Sci U S A, 99(18), 11951-11956.

Yu, D., Sun, X., Qiu, Y., Zhou, J., Wu, Y., Zhuang, L., et al. (2007). Identification and clinical significance of mobilized endothelial progenitor cells in tumor vasculogenesis of hepatocellular carcinoma. Clin Cancer Res, 13(13), 3814-3824.

Yuan, A., Yu, C. J., Chen, W. J., Lin, F. Y., Kuo, S. H., Luh, K. T., et al. (2000). Correlation of total VEGF mRNA and protein expression with histologic type, tumor angiogenesis, patient survival and timing of relapse in non-small-cell lung cancer. Int J Cancer, 89(6), 475-483.

Zhang, Z., Neiva, K. G., Lingen, M. W., Ellis, L. M., & Nor, J. E. (2010). VEGF-dependent tumor angiogenesis requires inverse and reciprocal regulation of VEGFR1 and VEGFR2. Cell Death Differ, 17(3), 499-512.

Laser Capture Microdissection in Tumor Angiogenesis Research related to Bcl-2 Expression on Endothelial Cells: A Review

Tomoatsu Kaneko[*], Yukiko Sueyama[*], Takashi Okiji[†] and Jacques E. Nör[‡]

1   Introduction

Laser capture microdissection (LCM) is a powerful methodology that allows us to retrieve specific types of normal and diseased cells from tissue sections. The dissected tissue sections can then be used for DNA, RNA or protein expression analysis. Thus, in accordance with the recent LCM technological/methodological advancement, LCM also has been applied to tumor angiogenesis research.

Angiogenesis is the growth of new blood vessels from pre-existing vasculature in response to interactions between tumor cells and endothelial cells, growth factors, and extracellular matrix components. Tumor angiogenesis is an absolute requirement for tumor growth and development. In recent years, the effect of Bcl-2 (B-cell lymphoma 2) expression on endothelial cells during tumor angiogenic events is one that is recognized. First, Bcl-2 is shown to be upregulated in endothelial cells exposed to VEGF and that upregulation of Bcl-2 in these cells is sufficient to enhance tumor angiogenesis and tumor growth. More recently, it has been demonstrated that Bcl-2 functions as a pro-angiogenic signaling molecule in endothelial cells through a pathway that involves activation of the canonical NF-kB pathways resulting in the upregulation of angiogenic chemokines CXCL1 and CXCL8. Moreover, Bcl-2 also activates the STAT3 signaling pathway in endothelial cells resulting in the upregulation of VEGF secretion and induction of Bcl-2 expression in tumor cells via VEGFR1. Thus, the effect of Bcl-2 expression on endothelial cells during tumor angiogenic events becomes more importance.

To quantify the Bcl-2 expression on tumor-associated endothelial cells, LCM is also a powerful methodology. Thus, in the present review, we focus on the presentation and discussion of existing literature in the field of Bcl2 and tumor angiogenesis, and especially provide an overview of the field of tumor angiogenesis research assisted with LCM. In addition, we present a brief protocol of cDNA synthesis following immune-LCM from paraffin-embedded tissue sections.

2   The Bcl-2 Family

[*] Division of Cariology, Operative Dentistry and Endodontics, Niigata University Graduate School of Medical and Dental Sciences, Niigata, Japan

[†] Department of Pulp Biology and Endodontics, Graduate School of Medical and Dental Sciences, Tokyo Medical and Dental University, Tokyo, Japan

[‡] Cariology, Restorative Sciences and Endodontics, University of Michigan, Ann Arbor, MI, USA

2.1 Generalities

The Bcl-2 family shows diverse family protein members that originates from their first identi-fied member, Bcl-2, in 1984. The Bcl-2 was discovered by the observation of t(14;18) chromo-somal translocation in follicular lymphoma to evaluate the pathogenesis of B-cell neoplasms carrying the translocation (Erikson *et al.*, 1984; Tsujimoto *et al.*, 1984). Bcl-2 gene has been shown to promote hematopoietic cell survival and to cooperate with c-myc to immortalize pre-B cells (Vaux *et al.* 1988). If the BCL-2 protein is overproduced, the growth of Epstein-Barr virus-immortalized B cells is enhanced (Tsujimoto Y, 1989).

Bcl-2 is localized to the inner mitochondrial membrane that blocks programmed cell death (Hockenbery *et al.*, 1990). Bcl-2 also localizes to the nuclear envelope, and endoplasmic reticulum (Krajewski *et al.*, 1993). Overexpression of Bcl-2 in lymphoid tissues of Bcl-2-immunoglobulin transgenic mice develops a polyclonal expansion of small resting B cells. Thus the transgenic mice that overexpress Bcl-2 display extended survival of resting B cells (Nuñez *et al.*, 1990). Bcl-2 also confers an antidote to apoptosis that aids malignant transfor-mation (Hockenbery *et al.* 1991). Thus, Bcl-2 functions to inhibit apoptosis in a variety of in vitro and in vivo experiments, suggesting interference with a central mechanism of apoptosis (Hockenbery D.M., 1992).

Human Bcl-2 is a 26 kDa integral membrane oncoprotein consisting of five domains. The domains consist of four Bcl-2 homology (BH) domains named BH1, BH2, BH3 and BH4, and one transmembrane domain (Brunelle and Letai, 2009).

Apoptosis is a regulated process that is designed to eliminate cells with damage, super-fluousness, and senescence (Glucksmann A., 1951, Kerr *et al.*, 1972, Wyllie *et al.*, 1980). To date, Bcl-2 family consists of 25 pro- and anti-apoptotic members, and is grouped into three classes, according to their pro- and anti-apoptotic effects and the presence of Bcl-2 homology (BH) domains. The first class of the Bcl-2 family proteins such as Bcl-2, Bcl-2 related gene long isoform (Bcl-xL), Bcl-w, myeloid cell leukemia-1 (Mcl-1), and Bcl-2 related gene A1 (A1) inhib-it apoptosis. These anti-apoptotic proteins have similar 3D structures and four BH domains. The BH domains that are possessed by the anti-apoptotic Bcl-2 family proteins (Brunelle and Letai, 2009) are crucial for the function of apoptotic control. The second class of the Bcl-2 fami-ly proteins are divided into multi-domain 'effectors' such as Bcl-2-associated-x protein (Bax), Bcl-2 homologuous agonist killer (Bak) and Bcl-2 related ovarian killer (Bok). They are pro-apoptosis proteins that contain up to 3 BH domains (Letai, 2008; Skommer *et al.*, 2007; Youle and Strasser, 2008). If these effecter proteins are once activated, Bax and Bak promote apopto-sis by enabling pore formation within the mitochondrial outer membrane (Lindsten T., 2000). The third class of the Bcl-2 family proteins are divided into the BH3-only 'facilitators' such as BH3 interacting-domain death agonist (Bid), Bcl-2-associated death promotorBad, Bcl-2 inter-acting mediator of cell death (Bim), Bcl-2-interacting killer (Bik), NOXA and p53-upregulated modulator of apoptosis (PUMA). The BH3-only group members inhibit the function of the anti-apoptotic members or promote the function of the multi-domain pro-apoptotic members (Letai, 2008; Skommer *et al.*, 2007; Youle and Strasser, 2008). BH3-only protein signaling is essential for the initiation of the mitochondrial apoptotic pathway, but MOMP requires the presence of either Bax or Bak (Weyhenmeyer *et al.*, 2012). Thus, regulation of apoptosis is rec-ognized as an important function of Bcl-2 family proteins.

2.2   Bcl-2 and Endothelial Cell Survival

In 1994, Kondo *et al.* first showed a role for Bcl-2 in endothelial cell survival. In the study, they showed that apoptosis of murine aortic endothelial (MAE) cells was induced by deprivation of basic fibroblast growth factor (bFGF) but required new RNA and protein synthesis. Furthermore, enforced expression of Bcl-2 gene in MAE cells using gene transfer techniques decreased apoptosis induced by the deprivation of bFGF. Thus, Bcl-2 proteins protect endothelial cells against death induced by the removal of growth factors such as bFGF (Kondo *et al.*, 1994).

In endothelial cells, Bcl-2 has an important correlation with vascular endothelial growth factor (VEGF). VEGF is a survival factor for endothelial cells and a key positive regulator of normal and pathological angiogenesis (Ferrara and Davis-Smyth, 1997), and Bcl-2 is one of the novel target genes of VEGF (Gerber et al, 1998). Overexpression of Bcl-2 by means of transient biolistic transfection experiments of primary human umbilical vein endothelial cells prevents from apoptotic cell death in the absence of VEGF (Gerber HP, 1998). Thus, Bcl-2 is sufficient to inhibit endothelial cell apoptosis.

On the other hand, Nör et al showed another role for Bcl-2 in endothelial cell survival. In the analysis, they demonstrated that implantation of Bcl-2-incorporated polylactic acid sponges into SCID mice exhibited an increase in the number of microvessels and a decrease in the number of apoptotic cells (Nör *et al.*, 1999). The induction of Bcl-2 expression inhibits endothelial cell apoptosis mediated by thrombospondin-1, which inhibits angiogenesis in association with increased expression of Bax (Nör *et al.*, 2000).

2.3   Bcl-2 and Angiogenesis

Angiogenesis is the growth of new blood vessels from pre-existing vasculature. It is an essential feature of pathological and physiological processes such as granulation tissue development, tissue repair and wound healing (Folkman, 1972; DeLisser *et al.*, 1997). On the other hand, the effect of Bcl-2 proteins on angiogenic events is recently becoming more recognized as another major function of this molecule. For example, in tumor angiogenesis, a constitutive upregulation of Bcl-2, the first class of the Bcl-2 family proteins, in vascular endothelial cells is sufficient to enhance angiogenesis (Nör *et al.*, 2001). The up-regulation of Bcl-2 in microvascular endothelial cells that constitute tumor microvessels accelerates tumor growth (Nör *et al.*, 2001). In tumor cell lines, Bcl-2 expression is also an important factor of angiogenic potential. For example, xenograft tumors derived from Bcl-2-overexpressing prostate carcinoma cell lines that express high levels of VEGF display an increased angiogenic potential and grow more aggressively than tumors derived from control cell lines (Fernandez *et al.*, 2001). Thus, Bcl-2 is a novel factor for tumor progression not only by the inhibition of apoptosis, but also by the induction of angiogenesis.

3   LCM-based Tumor Angiogenesis Research related to Bcl-2 Expression

LCM was first introduced as a system that is able to retrieve defined cell population from human tissue samples and developed during the mid-1990s by Dr. Emmert-Buck and colleagues at the National Institutes of Health (NIH), Bethesda, ML, USA (Emmert-Buck *et al.*, 1996). Nowadays a variety of LCM apparatus are available such as the PixCell system (Arcturus, MDS Analytical Technology, California), Zeiss's PALM system (a subsidiary of Carl Zeiss MicroImaging, Jana, Germany), Leica LMD system (Mannheim, Germany), and mmi CellCut Plus syatem (Molecular Machines & Industries (MMI), Switzerland). Their major differences relate to how they collect dissected cells.

Three types of LCM systems are currently available. The first type is the infrared (IR)-laser based LCM system such as the PixCell II and AutoPix. The IR laser-based LCM damages the tissue very little and is good for small targets, whereas it is not suitable for dissection of thicker samples, as compared with the ultraviolet (UV)-laser based LCM system mentioned below. The PixCell system was originated in a Cooperative Research and Development Agreement between NIH, the National Cancer Institute, and the National Institute for the Child and Human Development, and was manufactured/marketed by Arcturus.

The second type is the UV-laser based LCM system such as the Zeiss PALM, Leica LMD, and mmi CellCut. The UV-laser based LCM is suitable for clusters of cells and big areas of target tissues and possible to dissect thick sections such as those at 30 µm (Yamanaka *et al.*, 2012). The Zeiss PALM system (Carl Zeiss, City, Germany) uses a pulsed UV-A laser to collect samples by photonic pressure termed laser pressure catapulting. The Leica LMD system (Leica, Mannheim, Germany) uses a UV laser to cut and then dissected cells fall into a collecting tube by gravity. The mmi CellCut Plus system uses a solid-state UV laser and manufactured/marketed by MMI, which was founded in 1998 by Prof. Stefan Seeger from University of Zurich, Switzerland.

The third type is the combined IR-UV laser system such as the Arcturus Veritas, and Arcturus XT (Arcturus). These systems use IR laser capture microdissection and UV laser cutting in one single instrument. A solid-state IR laser delivers a capture technique, which preserves biomolecular integrity and is ideal for single cells or a small number of cells. The solid-state UV laser delivers unprecedented speed and precision, suited for micro dissecting dense tissue structures and for rapidly capturing large numbers of cells.

4   Immnue-LCM Analysis

To date, formaldehyde as a 10% neutral buffered formalin is most widely used as a fixative for various human tissues. The sections from formalin fixed samples normally show better preservation of tissue architecture, as compared with cryosections from frozen samples. As with DNA, formaldehyde reacts with RNA forming an N-methylol (N-CH2OH) followed by an electrophilic attack to form a methylene bridge between amino groups. Adenine is the most susceptible nucleotide to electrophilic attack and it is likely that the adenines within the mRNA sequence and the poly(A) tail of mRNA will be modified in the formaldehyde-fixated paraffin embedded sections to varying degrees. It is normally considered that RNA isolated from formaldehyde-fixated, paraffin embedded sections are less suitable for reverse transcription (cDNA synthesis), as compared to RNA isolated frozen tissue sections (Srinivasan *et al.*, 2002). Thus, cryo-tissue sections are commonly used for gene expression analysis using LCM (Curino *et al.*, 2004; Gandini *et al.*, 2012) and immune-LCM. However a recent report has suggested that it is possible to perform gene expression analysis from approximately one-year-old formaldehyde-fixated paraffin embedded tissue sections from human crista ampullaris (Pagedar *et al.*, 2006).

We have further developed a methodology of immune-LCM of formaldehyde fixed, paraffin embedded HNSCC (head and neck squarmous cell carcinoma) specimens that were immunostained for coagulation factor VIII (a marker of human endothelial cells), using the Leica AS LMD, which utilizes a pulsed 337 nm UV laser on an upright microscope (kaneko *et al.*, 2011). The laser beam can be moved with a software-controlled mirror system, which allows us to select target cells and tissues: following selection of a target area on a monitor by a freehand drawing tool, the computer-controlled mirror moves the laser beam along the preselected path and the laser beam cuts the target tissue. The dissected tissue sections fall into a cap of PCR tube by their gravity. The collection by gravity is very fast and it is easy to transfer the dissected tissue sections to reaction buffer. The thickness and width of the cutting line can be controlled for each tissue. Thus, this method allows us to collect good quality RNA of factor VIII-positive endothelial cells retrieved from the tumor mass.

4.1 Immnue-LCM Analysis for Bcl-2 Expression

By immune-LCM using formaldehyde-fixated paraffin embedded samples, we have reported that the crosstalk between dermal micro-vascular endothelial cells and tumor cells plays an important role in oral squamous cell carcinoma (OSCC) growth and angiogenesis, and that Bcl-2 is a key regulator of this crosstalk. Thus, a novel role for Bcl-2 in endothelial cells as a pro-angiogenic signaling molecule has been presented (Kaneko *et al.*, 2007). Our immune-LCM analysis has also demonstrated that oral administration of a small-molecule inhibitor of VEGF receptors (PTK/ZK) is anti-angiogenic in early stage head and neck tumors, which are accompanied by quantifiable inhibition of the VEGF-Bcl-2-CXCL8 signaling axis (Miyazawa *et al.*, 2008). In another immune-LCM analysis, we investigated signaling pathways involved in the regulation of Bcl-2 in lymphatic endothelial cells, and the impact of endothelial cell Bcl-2 expression in primary tumors on six cases of lymph node metastasis. In the analysis, we have further reported that Bcl-2 in endothelial cells contributes to lymph node metastasis in patients with OSCC (Tarquinio *et al.*, 2012). Thus, this method using formaldehyde-fixated paraffin embedded samples may be better suited for the analysis of relatively rare cell types within a tissue, and may improve our ability to perform differential diagnosis of pathologies as compared to conventional LCM (Kaneko *et al.*, 2009).

Recently, another immnue-LCM analysis of endothelial cells in angioimmunoblastic T-cell lymphoma has been reported (Ratajczak *et al.*, 2012). In the analysis, immune-LCM was performed for 7 μm-thick lymph node frozen sections following immunofluorescent staining of CD34- or CD105-expressing endothelial cells, and showed a significant relationship between Bcl-2 and VEGFA mRNA levels in CD34-expressing endothelial cells.

4.2 Immune-LCM from Formaldehyde-fixated, Paraffin-embedded Oral Cancer Tissues

This protocol is modified from our previous report (Kaneko *et al.*, 2011, 2013). Protocols of measurement of RNA concentration and real-time PCR experiments are newly added, and some reagents (cDNA reverse transcription reagents) are changed. Disposable gloves should always be worn as skin often contains bacteria and molds that can be a source of contaminating RNA and RNases, The use of sterile, disposable plastic ware and filtered pipette tips is recommended for RNA work to prevent cross-contamination with RNases from shared equipment.

4.2.1 Tissue Fixation, Paraffin Embedding

1. Fix tissues with 10% neutral buffered formaldehyde for 8 – 16 hours at 4 °C.
2. Dehydrated for 30 minutes in 70% ethanol, for 1 hour in 90% ethanol, and for 30 minutes in 95% ethanol at 4 °C.
3. Dehydrated 3 times for 1 hour in 100% ethanol at room temperature.
4. Immersed 2 times in xylene for 1 hour at room temperature.
5. Immersed 4 times in paraffin for 30 minutes at 58 °C.
6. The specimen is embedded in paraffin and blocked.

4.2.2 Paraffin block storage

1. We recommend that the paraffin blocks be stored at 4 °C, but the paraffin blocks can be stored at room temperature until processed.
2. The blocks can be kept for 12 months, but we recommend that the blocks should be sectioned as soon as possible.

4.2.3 Sectioning and mounting

1. Cut sections on a microtome with a new sterile disposable blade (8 – 10 μm thick).
2. Float paraffin ribbons on 43 °C nuclease-free water (diethylpyrocarbonate (DEPC)-treated water).
3. Mount the section on poly-L-lysine coated glass foiled polyethylene naphthalate (PEN) slides for LCM (Leica)
4. Dry slides in a 35 °C incubator for 6 hours.

4.2.4 Slide storage

1. We recommend that the slides be stored at 4 °C and LCM should be performed as soon as possible. Slides should be used within a week after preparation.

4.2.5 Staining: nuclear staining by hematoxylin

1. Deparaffinize the slides 3 times with 2 minutes xylene washes at room temperature.
2. 100% ethanol washes 3 times for 20 seconds at 4 °C.
3. 90% ethanol wash for 30 seconds at 4 °C.
4. 70% ethanol wash for 1 minute at 4 °C.
5. DEPC-treated water wash for 30 seconds at 4 °C.
6. Gill No.3' hematoxylin (Sigma-Aldrich, Deisenhofen, Germany) for 5 – 10 seconds at room temperature.

7. DEPC-treated water wash for 30 seconds at 4 °C.

8. Air dry the slide for 1 – 3 hours at 4 °C.

4.2.6 Staining: immunostainig

Avidine-biotin-peroxidase complex (ABC) method is employed. 2 ~ 4 slides per session is easy to manageable.

1. Deparaffinize the slides twice with 3 minutes xylene washes at room temperature.

2. 100% ethanol washes 3 times for 30 seconds at 4 °C.

3. 90% ethanol wash for 30 seconds at 4 °C.

4. 70% ethanol wash for 1 minute at 4 °C.

5. RNase-free phosphate buffered saline (PBS) washes 3 times for 30 seconds at 4 °C.

6. Pre-treat these sections with 0.125% trypsin for 5 ~ 30 minutes at room temperature. To avoid RNA degradation (Vrtacnik et al., 2014), pre-treatment of trypsin should be performed at room temperature.

7. RNase-free PBS washes 3 times for 30 seconds at 4 °C.

8. Endogenous peroxidase activity blockage with 0.3% hydrogen peroxide in methanol for 3 minutes at 4 °C.

9. RNase-free PBS washes 3 times for 30 seconds at 4 °C.

10. Incubation with a primary antibody for 16 h at 4 °C, or for 30 minutes at room temperature.

11. RNase-free PBS washes 3 times for 30 seconds at 4 °C.

12. Incubation with biotinylated secondary antibody (Vector laboratories, Burlingame, CA; diluted 1:500) for 1 hour at 4 °C.

13. RNase-free PBS washes 3 times for 30 seconds at 4 °C.

14. Incubation with avidine-biotine-peroxidase complex (Elite ABC kit; Vector) for 1 hour at 4 °C.

15. RNase-free PBS washes 3 times for 30 seconds at 4 °C.

16. Development in diaminobenzidine-H_2O_2 solution (DAB substrate kit; Vector) for 3 minutes at room temperature.

17. RNase-free PBS washes 3 times for 30 seconds at 4 °C.

18. Air dry the stained slides for 1 – 3 hours at 4 °C.

19. Store at –70 °C ~ 4 °C until ready to perform LCM.

4.2.7 LCM (Leica AS LMD system) and total RNA extraction by TRIZOL® Reagent (Life Technologies™ (Invitrogen™), Carlsbad, CA)

1. Dissect Factor VIII-positive endothelial cells from tumor mass (Figure 1A & B) or control normal mucosa (Figure 1C & D) by using a LCM system.

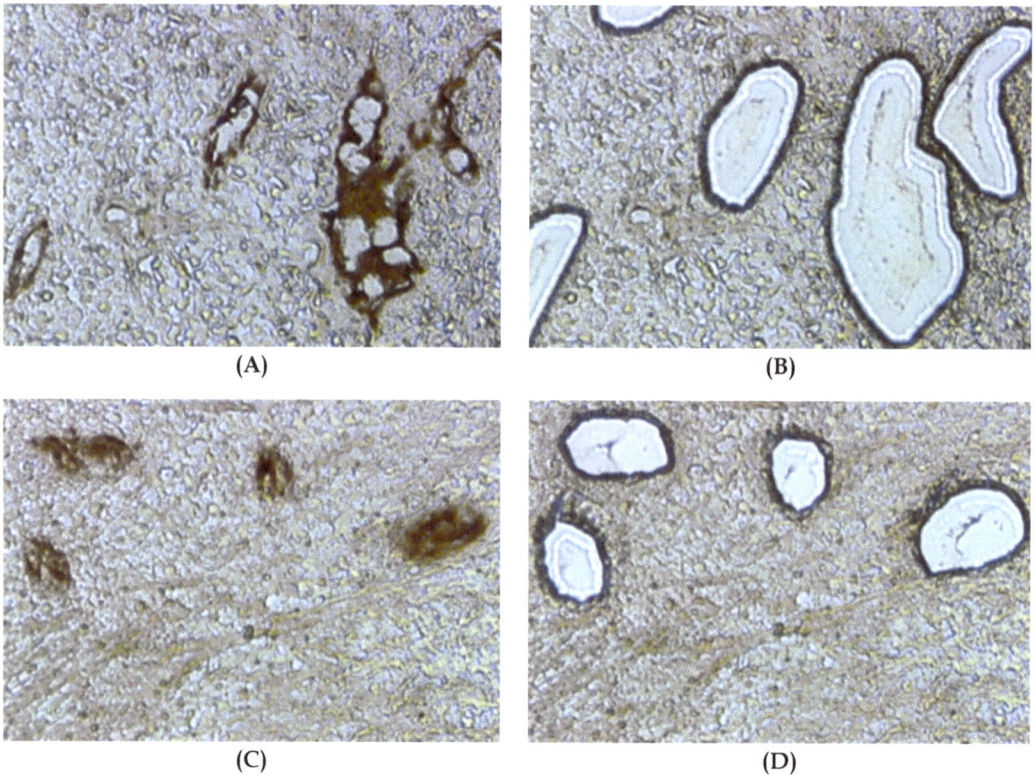

Figure 1: Retrieval of Factor VIII-positive endothelial cells by using a LCM system. **A.** Factor VIII-positive endothelial cells in a section of tumor mass. **B.** Retrieval of Factor VIII-positive endothelial cells in a section of (A). **C.** Factor VIII-positive endothelial cells in a section of control normal mucosa. **D.** Retrieval of Factor VIII-positive endothelial cells in a section of (C).

2. Collect dissected endothelial cells (approximately 400 cells) into individual tubes filled with 20 µl TRIZOL® Reagent. Tubes should be immediately placed on ice.

3. Close the tubes securely. Centrifuge the samples at 14,000 rpm for 10 seconds at 4 °C.

4. Add TRIZOL® Reagent to sufficient to 30 – 100 µl.

5. Incubate the samples for 5 minutes at room temperature.

6. Add chloroform in the same amount as TRIZOL® Reagent used.

7. Close sample tubes securely. Shake tubes briefly for 30 – 60 seconds and incubate them for 5 minutes on ice.

8. Centrifuge the samples at 14,000 rpm for 15 minutes at 4 °C.

9. Transfer the aqueous phase to a fresh tube. (Following centrifugation, the mixture separates into three layers; a lower red phenol-chloroform phase, an interphase, and a colorless upper aqueous phase. RNA is contained exclusively in the aqueous phase.)

10. Add isopropyl alcohol (RNA precipitant) to the tube in the same amount as the aqueous phase transferred. Incubate the samples at 4 °C for 10 minutes. Centrifuge at 13,000 rpm

for 15 minutes at 4 °C. RNA will be precipitate under the tube. The RNA precipitate forms a white small dotted pellet on the side and bottom of the tube. The RNA precipitate is sometimes invisible after centrifugation,

11. Discard the supernatant gently.

12. Add 70 – 75% ethanol in DEPC-treated water to the RNA pellet and mix the sample by vortex.

13. Centrifuge at 6000 – 7500 rpm for 5 minutes at 4 °C.

14. Discard the supernatant gently.

15. Add 70 – 75% ethanol in DEPC-treated water to the RNA pellet,

16. The RNA pellet can be stored at –20 °C.

4.2.8   RNA clean up by RNeasy Mini Kit (Qiagen, Frederick, ML)

All processes of RNA clean up by RNeasy Mini Kit can be performed at room temperature.

1.   Add 10 µl β-Mercaptoethanol per 1 ml Buffer RLT.

2.   Adjust the sample to a volume of 100 µl with RNase-free water. Add 350 µl Buffer RLT, and mix briefly.

3.   Add 250 µl of 100% ethanol to the diluted RNA, and mix by pipetting without centrifuge.

4.   Transfer the sample (total 700 µl) to an RNeasy Mini spin column placed in a 2 ml supplied collection tube. Centrifuge for 15 seconds at 8000 x g. Discard the flow-through.

5.   Reuse the collection tube.

6.   Add 350 µl Buffer RW1 to the RNeasy spin column. Close the lid gently, and centrifuge for 15 seconds at 10000 rpm to wash the spin column membrane and discard the flow-through.

7.   Reuse the collection tube in step 4.

8.   Add 10 µl DNase I stock solution to 70 µl Buffer RDD that is supplied with the RNase-Free DNase Set. Mix by gently inverting the tube, and centrifuge briefly to collect residual liquid from the sides of the tube.

9.   Add the DNase I incubation mix (80 µl) directly to the RNeasy spin column membrane, and place at room temperature for 15 minutes.

10. Add 350 µl Buffer RW1 to the RNeasy spin column. Close the lid gently, and centrifuge for 15 seconds at 10,000 rpm. Discard the flow-through.

11. Add 500 µl Buffer RPE to the RNeasy spin column, and centrifuge for 15 seconds at 10,000 rpm and discard the flow-through.

12. Reuse the collection tube.

13. Add 500 µl Buffer RPE to the RNeasy spin column, and centrifuge for 2 minutes at 10,000 rpm.

14. Place the RNeasy spin column in a new 2 ml collection tube, and discard the old collection tube with the flow-through, and centrifuge at 13,000 rpm for 1 minute.

15. Place the RNeasy spin column in a new 1.5 ml collection tube. Add 10 – 20 µl RNase-free water directly to the spin column membrane, and centrifuge for 1 minute at 10,000 rpm to elute the RNA.

16. Store at –70 °C until ready to perform single-stranded cDNA synthesis.

4.2.9 Measurement of RNA concentration and absorbance value by a photometer

1. Add 1 ~ 2 µl of RNA into DEPC-treated water to sufficient to 100 µl.

2. Prepare blank solution (100 µl DEPC-treated water).

3. Fill a disposable rectangular plastic cuvette (Eppendorf UVette) with blank solution.

4. Insert the filled cuvette with the blank solution into a cuvette shaft of photometer (Bio-Photometer plus, Eppendorf). Measure the blank solution.

5. Insert the filled cuvette with sample solution into a cuvette shaft of photometer. Measure the concentration result and absorbance value of the sample solution.

4.2.10 Single-stranded cDNA synthesis

1. Add 1 µg of total RNA (up to 10 µl) into 10 µl 2X master mix (High Capacity cDNA Reverse Transcription Kits, Life Technologies™ (Applied Biosystems ®)).

2. Add DEPC-treated water to sufficient to 20 µl.

3. Seal PCR tubes securely, centrifuge briefly and centrifuge the tubes to eliminate air bubbles for 10 seconds at 4 °C.

4. Place the tubes on ice until ready to load a thermal cycler (TaKaRa PCR Thermal Cycler Dice®, Takara BIO INC, Siga, Japan).

5. Program the thermal cycler (set the cycler program at the reaction volume of 20 µl).

6. cDNA synthesis and pre-denaturation: perform 1 cycle at: 25 °C for 10 minutes, 37 °C for 120 minutes 85 °C for 5 minutes.

7. Start the reverse transcription of the cycler run.

8. Add DEPC-treated water to sufficient to 100 µl.

9. Store at –70 °C until ready to perform real-time PCR (or other PCR applications).

4.2.11 Real-time PCR experiments (StepOne™, Applied Biosystems ®)

1. Add 1 µl of TaqMan Gene Expression Assay (Bcl-2, Hs00608023_m1 or 18S, Hs99999901_s1) and 1 µl of cDNA template into 10 µl 2X TaqMan Gene Expression Master Mix (Applied Biosystems ®).

2. Add 8 µl of DEPC-treated water to sufficient to 20 µl.

3. Seal a 48-well clear optical reaction plate securely, centrifuge briefly and centrifuge the tubes to eliminate air bubbles for 10 seconds at 4 °C.

4. Program the thermal cycler (set the cycler program at the reaction volume of 20 µl)

5. PCR: perform 1 cycle at: 50 °C for 2 minutes and 95 °C for 10 minutes, and perform 35 ~ 40 cycles at: 95 °C for 15 seconds and 60 °C for 1 minutes.

Figure 2 shows a graph of Statistical comparison of two experimental groups (endothelial cells retrieved from control normal mucosa vs. endothelial cells retrieved from inside the tumor mass from the same tissue arrays. Data presented from real-time PCR experiments reflect the expression level of Bcl-2 normalized by 18S.

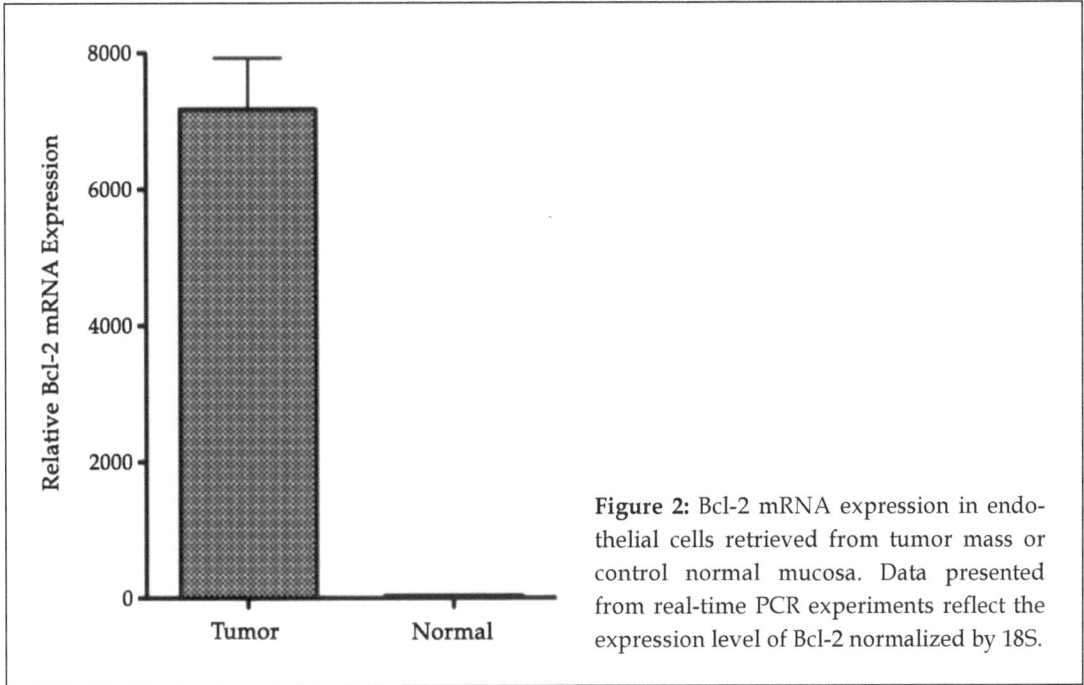

Figure 2: Bcl-2 mRNA expression in endothelial cells retrieved from tumor mass or control normal mucosa. Data presented from real-time PCR experiments reflect the expression level of Bcl-2 normalized by 18S.

5   Conclusion

Tissue based LCM is a powerful technique that combines morphology, histopathology and molecular biological analysis. The ability of LCM to retrieve specific populations of interested cells, combined with the analysis of gene sequencing and gene expression in these sub-population of cells, has made LCM a critical strategy in tumor angiogenesis research related to Bcl-2 expression.

References

Brunelle, J.K., Letai, A. (2009). Control of mitochondrial apoptosis by the Bcl-2 family. Journal of Cell Science 122,437–441.

DeLisser, H.M., Christofidou-Solomidou, M., Strieter, R.M., Burdick, M.D., Robinson, C.S., Wexler, R.S., Kerr, J.S., Garlanda, C., Merwin, J.R., Madri, J.A., Albelda, S.M. (1997). Involvement of endothelial PECAM-1/CD31 in angiogenesis. American Journal of Pathology, 151,671-677.

Emmert-Buck, M.R., Bonner, R.F., Smith, P.D., Chuaqui, R.F., Zhuang, Z., Goldstein, S.R., Weiss, R.A., Liotta, L.A. (1996). Laser capture microdissection. Science, 274, 998-1001.

Erikson, J., Finan, J., Tsujimoto, Y., Nowell, P.C., Croce, C.M. (1984). The chromosome 14 breakpoint in neoplastic B cells with the t(11;14) translocation involves the immunoglobulin heavy chain locus. Proceedings of the National Academy of Sciences of the United States of America, 81,4144–4148.

Fernandez, A., Udagawa, T., Schwesinger, C., Beecken, W., Achilles-Gerte, E., McDonnell, T., D'Amato, R. (2001). Angiogenic potential of prostate carcinoma cells overexpressing bcl-2. Journal of the National Cancer Institute, 93,208-213.

Ferrara, N., Davis-Smyth, T. (1997). The biology of vascular endothelial growth factor. Endocrine Reviews, 18,4-25.

Folkman, J. (1972). Anti-angiogenesis: new concept for therapy of solid tumors. Annals of Surgery. 175,409-416.

Gerber, H.P., Dixit, V., Ferrara, N. (1998). Vascular endothelial growth factor induces expression of the antiapoptotic proteins Bcl-2 and A1 in vascular endothelial cells. The Journal of Biological Chemistry, 273,13313-13316.

Glucksmann, A. (1951). Cell deaths in normal vertebrate ontogeny. Biological reviews of the Cambridge Philosophical Society, 26,59-86.

Hockenbery, D.M. (1992). The bcl-2 oncogene and apoptosis. Seminars in Immunology 4,413-420.

Hockenbery, D.M, Nuñez, G., Milliman, C., Schreiber, R.D., Korsmeyer, S.J. (1990). Bcl-2 is an inner mitochondrial membrane protein that blocks programmed cell death. Nature, 348,334–336.

Hockenbery, D.M., Zutter, M., Hickey, W., Nahm, M., Korsmeyer, S.J. (1991). BCL2 protein is topographically restricted in tissues characterized by apoptotic cell death. Proceedings of the National Academy of Sciences of the United States, 88,6961–6965.

Kaneko, T., Okiji, T., Kaneko, R., Suda, H., Nör, J.E. (2009). Gene expression analysis of immunostained endothelial cells isolated from formalin-fixated paraffin embedded tumors using laser capture microdissection--a technical report. Microscopy Research and Technique, 72,908-912.

Kaneko, T., Okiji, T., Kaneko, R., Suda, H., Nör, J.E. (2011). Laser-capture microdissection for Factor VIII-expressing endothelial cells in cancer tissues. Methods in Molecular Biology, 755, 395-403.

Kaneko,T., Okiji,T., Nör, J.E.(2013). Laser capture microdissection in oral cancer research: a review. The Research and Biology of Cancer II. EDt. iConcept Press, 19-32.

Kaneko, T., Zhang, Z., Mantellini, M.G., Karl, E., Zeitlin, B., Verhaegen, M., Soengas, M.S., Lingen, M., Strieter, R.M., Nunez, G., Nör, J.E. (2007). Bcl-2 orchestrates a cross-talk between endothelial and tumor cells that promotes tumor growth. Cancer Research, 67,9685-9693.

Kerr, J.F., Wyllie, A.H., Currie, A.R. (1972). Apoptosis: a basic biological phenomenon with wide-ranging implications in tissue kinetics. British Journal of Cancer, 26,239-257.

Kondo, S., Yin, D., Aoki, T., Takahashi, J.A., Morimura, T., Takeuchi, J. (1994). Bcl-2 gene prevents apoptosis of basic fibroblast growth factor-deprived murine aortic endothelial cells. Experimental Cell Research, 213,428-432.

Krajewski, S., Tanaka, S., Takayama, S., Schibler, M.J., Fenton, W., Reed, J.C. (1993). Investigation of the subcellular distribution of the bcl-2 oncoprotein: residence in the nuclear envelope, endoplasmic reticulum, and outer mitochondrial membranes. Cancer Research, 53,4701-4714.

Letai, A.G. (2008). Diagnosing and exploiting cancer's addiction to blocks in apoptosis. Nature Reviews Cancer, 8,121–132.

Lindsten, T., Ross, A.J., King, A., Zong, W.X., Rathmell, J.C., Shiels, H.A., Ulrich, E., Waymire, K.G., Mahar, P., Frauwirth, K., Chen, Y., Wei, M., Eng, V.M., Adelman, D.M., Simon, M.C., Ma, A., Golden, J.A., Evan, G., Korsmeyer, S.J., MacGregor, G.R., Thompson, C.B. (2000). The combined functions of proapoptotic Bcl-2 family members bak and bax are essential for normal development of multiple tissues.Molecular cell, 6,1389-1399.

Miyazawa, M., Dong, Z., Zhang, Z., Neiva, K.G., Cordeiro, M.M., Oliveira, D.T., Nör, J.E. (2008). Effect of PTK/ZK on the angiogenic switch in head and neck tumors. Journal of Dental Research, 87,1166-1171.

Nor, J.E., Christensen, J., Liu, J., Peters, M., Mooney, D.J., Strieter, R.M., Polverini, P.J. (2001). Up-Regulation of Bcl-2 in microvascular endothelial cells enhances intratumoral angiogenesis and accelerates tumor growth. Cancer Research. 61,2183–2188.

Nor, J.E, Christensen, J., Mooney, D.J., Polverini, P.J. (1999).Vascular endothelial growth factor (VEGF)-mediated angiogenesis is associated with enhanced endothelial cell survival and induction of Bcl-2 expression. American Journal of Pathology, 154,375–384.

Nör, J.E., Mitra, R.S., Sutorik, M.M., Mooney, D.J., Castle, V.P., Polverini, P.J. (2000). Thrombospondin-1 induces endothelial cell apoptosis and inhibits angiogenesis by activating the caspase death pathway. Journal of Vascular Research, 37,209-218.

Nuñez, G., London, L., Hockenbery, D., Alexander, M., McKearn, J.P., Korsmeyer, S.J. (1990). Deregulated Bcl-2 gene expression selectively prolongs survival of growth factor-deprived hemopoietic cell lines. The Journal of Immunology, 44,3602–3610.

Ratajczak, P., Leboeuf, C., Wang, L., Brière, J., Loisel-Ferreira, I., Thiéblemont, C., Zhao, W.L., Janin, A. (2012). BCL2 expression in CD105 positive neoangiogenic cells and tumor progression in angioimmunoblastic T-cell lymphoma. Modem Pathology, 25,805-814.

Skommer, J., Wlodkowic, D., Deptala, A. (2007). Larger than life: Mitochondria and the Bcl-2 family. Leukemia Research, 31,277–286.

Srinivasan, M., Sedmak, D., Jewell, S. (2002). Effect of fixatives and tissue processing on the content and integrity of nucleic acids. American Journal of Pathology, 161, 1961-1971.

Tarquinio, S.B., Zhang, Z., Neiva, K.G., Polverini, P.J., Nör, J.E. (2012). Endothelial cell Bcl-2 and lymph node metastasis in patients with oral squamous cell carcinoma. Journal of Oral Pathology & Medicine, 41, 124-130.

Tsujimoto, Y. (1989). Overexpression of the human BCL-2 gene product results in growth enhancement of Epstein-Barr virus-immortalized B cells. Proceedings of the National Academy of Sciences of the United States, 86,1958-1962.

Tsujimoto, Y., Yunis, J., Onorato-Showe, L., Erikson, J., Nowell, P.C., Croce, C.M. (1984). Molecular cloning of the chromosomal breakpoint of B-cell lymphomas and leukemias with the t(11;14) chromosome translocation. Science. 224,1403–1406.

Vaux, D.L., Cory, S., Adams, J.M. (1988). Bcl-2 gene promotes haemopoietic cell survival and cooperates with c-myc to immortalize pre-B cells. Nature. 335,440–442.

Vrtacnik, P., Kos, S., Bustin, S.A., Marc, J., Ostanek, B. (2014). Influence of trypsinization and alternative procedures for cell preparation before RNA extraction on RNA integrity. Anal Biochem. 15,463:38-44.

Weyhenmeyer, B., Murphy, A.C., Prehn, J.H., Murphy, B.M. (2012). Targeting the anti-apoptotic Bcl-2 family members for the treatment of cancer. Experimental oncology, 34,192-199.

Wyllie, A.H., Kerr, J.F., Currie, A.R. (1980). Cell death: the significance of apoptosis. International Review of Cytology, 68,251-306.

Yamanaka, Y., Kaneko, T., Yoshiba, K., Kaneko, R., Yoshiba, N., Shigetani, Y., Nör, J.E., Okiji, T. (2012). Expression of angiogenic factors in rat periapical lesions. Journal of Endodontics, 38, 313-317.

Youle, R.J., Strasser, A. (2008). The BCL-2 protein family: opposing activities that mediate cell death. Nature Reviews Molecular Cell Biology, 9,47–59.

Effects of Co-Transplantation of Thymus and Stem Cells on Treatment of Malignant Tumors

Ming Li[*], Kequan Guo[†], Xu Meng[†] and Susumu Ikehara[*]

1 Introduction

There has recently been a rapid increase in cancer, and inflammation has been shown to play an important role in its development (Ahmad *et al.*, 2009). Inflammatory cells produce cytokines such as TNF IL and IL which promote tumor growth, and tumor cells also produce macrophage colony-stimulating factor (M-CSF), which accelerates the immune response (Marx, 2004; Borrello *et al.*, 2008). Aging leads to a marked malfunction of multiple cellular and molecular events that ultimately get translated into various chronic ailments and diseases such as Type 2 diabetes mellitus (T2DM), Alzheimer's disease (AD), and osteoporosis, Parkinson's disease, atherosclerosis, and an increased risk of cancer (Caruso *et al.*, 2004). Aging leads to decreases in humoral and cellular immune responses, aged dendritic cells (DCs) being less able to activate T and B cells, and aged-natural killer (NK) cells being less efficient at killing tumor cells (Frasca *et al.*, 2008).

Based on histological type, cancer can be classified into five major categories: carcinoma, sarcoma, myeloma, lymphoma and mixed types. Treatment mainly includes surgery, radiotherapy, chemotherapy, immunotherapy, and stem cell transplantation. Radiotherapy and chemotherapy play a role in preventing cancer development, but cause adverse side effects. Immunotherapy is an effective method that aims to harness the body's own immune system to fight the cancer. Using this approach, T cells are more able to recognize aberrant proteins from tumor cells, and either destroy the tumor cells or inhibit their growth (Schreiber *et al.*, 2011; McNutt, 2013). The first to report a strong correlation between tumor-infiltrating T cells and patient survival in human colorectal cancer was Naito et al in 1998 (Naito *et al.*, 1998). Moreover, it has been shown that increased CD8[+] T cells infiltrate non-small-cell lung cancers, and may thus improve patient survival (Zhuang *et al.*, 2010). In terms of immunotherapy, the most successful cancer vaccine has been described by Kenter et al, who suggest that complete responses are correlated with the induction of human papillomavirus type 16-specific immunity (Kenter *et al.*, 2009). Recently, we have seen the development of new immunotherapies such as vaccination approaches and the use of monoclonal antibodies for tumors (Davies, 2014). For example, melanoma-associated antigen A3 (MAGE-A3) gene is expressed during embryogenesis and in a wide variety of tumors (Van den Eynde and van der Bruggen, 1997), and one report has shown that MAGE-A3 may facilitate antigen uptake by antigen-presenting cells, promoting T-cell responses, although it

[*] Department of Stem Cell Disorders, Kansai Medical University, Hirakata City, Osaka, Japan
[†] Department of Cardiac Surgery, Beijing Institute of Heart Lung & Blood Vessel Disease, Beijing Anzhen Hospital affiliated to Capital Medical University, Beijing, China

did not directly kill the tumor cells (Moeller *et al.*, 2012). The programmed death 1 (PD-1) receptor is a negative regulator of T-cells controlling immune responses to cancer, and anti-PD-L1 monoclonal antibodies have been shown to prevent tumor growth in patients with advanced melanoma (Hamid *et al.*, 2013). DCs are antigen presenting cells that actively promote T-cell tolerance to self-tumor antigens in tumor-bearing hosts (Chaput *et al.*, 2008). Thus, DC-based vaccines such as Sipuleucel-T have been used for patients with asymptomatic or minimally symptomatic metastatic hormone-refractory prostate cancer. Antibodies potentially exert antineoplastic effects, and have been used in cancer treatment in preclinical and clinical trials (Galluzzi *et al.*, 2012; Vacchelli *et al.*, 2013). For example, brentuximab vedotin, an anti-CD30 monomethyl auristatin E (MMAE) conjugate, has been approved to treat relapsed Hodgkin lymphoma (Younes *et al.*, 2012). Denosumab, a receptor activator of NFκB ligand (RANKL)- targeting antibody has been used to treat osteoporosis, and also to increase bone mass in patients with breast cancer (Coleman, 2012).

There have been rapid developments into research in the clinical use of stem cells. Allogeneic stem cell transplantation (ASCT) has been proven to be a useful method of treating hematological malignancies via donor-derived lymphocytes, which are used to eradicate residual tumor cells (Parmar and Ritchie, 2014). ASCT has also been shown to be an effective immunotherapy for leukemia (Oliansky *et al.*, 2007). Intra bone marrow-bone marrow transplantation has proven to be a valuable method for allogeneic BMT (ABMT), since intra bone marrow-bone marrow transplantation only requires low-dose irradiation as a preconditioning regimen and suppresses graft versus host disease (GVHD) (Kushida *et al.*, 2000; Nishida *et al.*, 2009). The thymus is a lymphoid organ in which T cells develop and then migrate to the peripheral blood. In this chapter, we focus on intra bone marrow-bone marrow transplantation + thymus transplantation (TT) to treat cancer in tumor-bearing mice.

2 Physiology of the Thymus

The thymus develops from both ectoderm and endoderm, reaches its peak weight in adolescence, and starts to atrophy with aging, starting to weigh significantly less and to produce significantly fewer thymocytes. The thymus mainly includes thymic epithelial cells (TECs), which consist of medullary TECs (mTECs) and cortical TECs (cTECs), thymocytes, and DCs. TECs shape T cell receptor (TCR) repertoire via negative and positive selection (Anderson *et al.*, 2009). Autoimmune Regulator (Aire) plays an important role in the induction of central tolerance, and Aire+mTECs are important in elucidating the stages and the checking points that regulate the formation of the thymic microenvironment. Moreover, the receptor activator of NF-kB (RANK) expression on the mTECs has been shown to be directly responsible for Aire+mTEC differentiation (Rossi *et al.*, 2007). The cytokine RANK ligand (RANKL) was produced by positively selected thymocytes and regulated the cellularity of mTECs by interacting with RANK and osteoprotegerin. Forced expression of RANKL restored thymic medulla in mice lacking positive selection, whereas RANKL perturbation impaired medulla formation, suggesting that RANKL is related to the establishment of central tolerance by promoting thymic medulla formation (Hikosaka *et al.*, 2008). One report has shown that Aire controls thymic negative selection, and mediates tolerance by direct presentation of Aire-regulated antigens to both CD4+ and CD8+ T cells. In contrast, cTECs are required for positive selection of CD4+ and CD8+ T cells (Hubert *et al.*, 2011). Thymic involution is accompanied by a drop in the number of TECs, and specifically in the number of cTECs after adolescence (Gray *et al.*, 2006), cTECs being responsible for supporting the early stage of T cell development and determining the overall lymphopoietic capacity of the thymus (Rode and Boehm, 2012). Wnt signaling controls TEC development and consequent T cell lymphopoiesis, and decreased Wnt expression leads to reduced naïve T cell output with aging (Balciunaite *et al.*, 2002; Varecza *et al.*, 2011). Mouse embryonic stem cell-derived thymic epithelial cell progenitors can enhance thymopoiesis and increase the number of peripheral T cells after BMT, and this approach could thus be used to reverse thymic involution with aging (Lai *et al.*, 2011). Human ESCs have been shown to differentiate into epithelial progenitor-like cells, and to promote T cell generation *in vivo* (Sun *et al.*, 2013).

Our previous report showed the existence of donor-type stromal cells in the thymus of mice when treated with ABMT + bone. The bone (femurs and tibias) was simultaneously engrafted subcutaneously and under the renal capsules when allogeneic BMT was carried out. These findings strongly suggest that stromal cells can migrate from the BM to the thymus, where they participate in the positive selection of thymocytes (Y. Li *et al.*, 2000). Donor- derived TECs were found in both the medullary and the cortical areas of the thymus in MRL/lpr mice treated with allogeneic intra bone marrow-bone marrow transplantation. Furthermore, bone marrow (BM) cells contain the precursors of functional TECs, and they can differentiate into TECs, which results in the correction of thymic function (Takaki *et al.*, 2008).

BM-derived common lymphoid progenitors enter the thymus and differentiate into T lymphocytes upon receiving various signals in the thymic microenvironments (Petrie and Zuniga-Pflucker, 2007). Thymus involution results in decreased migration of naïve T cells to the periphery, which is associated with lowered immune function, which in turn increases the susceptibility to infection and cancer (Lynch *et al.*, 2009). One report has shown a difference between the lymphoid progenitors in aged BM and those in young BM, and that there is a loss of T cell function in aged BM progenitors (Zediak *et al.*, 2007). Another report has indicated that thymic involution is also induced by enhancing the contribution of memory cells to the peripheral T cell pool (Hale *et al.*, 2006). Moreover, the ratio of CD4/CD8 in recent thymic emigrants (RTEs) in mice also decreased with aging, and the RTEs of old mice secrete less IL-2 than young mice (Hale *et al.*, 2006).

3 Tumors Accelerate Thymic Atrophy

Thymic atrophy can be induced by aging and tumor development, which induces impaired T cell development via the impaired maturation of thymocytes, increased apoptosis, and decreased proliferation. Vascular endothelial growth factor, hepatocyte growth factor, and IL-7 and IL-5 play important roles in thymic atrophy, and it has also been reported that increased leukemia inhibitory factor, IL-6 and stem cell factors, as well as decreased growth hormone and insulin-like growth factor induce thymic atrophy with aging (Sempowski *et al.*, 2000; Chen *et al.*, 2010). T cell maturation was blocked at the negative selection, and the percentage of CD4+ or CD8+ single positive cells within the CD3- population increased, while CD4+CD8+ double-positive cells decreased in the tumor bearing mice. Moreover, apoptosis of thymocytes was also observed to increase (Carrio and Lopez, 2009b). And, furthermore, the number of Treg increased as a result of the apoptosis of thymocytes in the thymus by inducing the production of TGFβ from TECs and macrophages (Konkel *et al.*, 2014). Thymic atrophy associated with tumor development resulted from increased CD4+ and CD8+ single-positive cells and CD4-CD8- double-negative cells in tumor-bearing mice (Y. Fu *et al.*, 1989a; Y. X. Fu *et al.*, 1989b). IFN- modulates a variety of cellular responses, including cell growth and apoptosis, and the IFN- level was increased in tumor-bearing mice, suggesting that the IFN- level is related to thymocyte apoptosis. Furthermore, it has been shown that the regulation of T cell responses by cytokines is via Jak/Stats signaling pathways. Reduced expression of Jak/Stats-related mRNA has been reported in the thymus of tumor-bearing mice, suggesting that tumor development impaired the Jak/Stat signaling pathways, and then impaired the T cell response (Carrio *et al.*, 2009a; Carrio *et al.*, 2011).

4   Intra Bone Marrow-bone Marrow Transplantation + TT Prevents Tumor Growth

Hematopoietic stem cell transplantation (HSCT) is a useful therapy for hematological malignancies, but this intervention also induces GVHD, which injures the thymus, including inducing the apoptosis of TECs and delaying T cell recovery, and thereby injuring the immune system (Toubert *et al.*, 2012). Allogeneic HSCT is a general therapy for cancer and immunodeficiency disorders that works by reconstituting the immune system. Human leukocyte antigen (HLA), which is the human version of major histocompatibility complex (MHC), helps the immune system distinguish between self-and non-self-derived proteins or cells. Specifically, T cell reconstitution is affected not only by aging but also by HLA, which is mismatched after allogeneic HSCT (Seggewiss and Einsele, 2010). Fetal thymus-derived CD4+ cells produced higher levels of IFN-γ and IL-4 than adult-derived cells, and showed different responses to antigen stimulation (Adkins, 2003). Neonatal T cells respond more rapidly to antigen stimulation than adult-derived T cells, and the activation of T cells results in cellular proliferation (Adkins *et al.*, 2003). Transplanted thymus may regulate the homeostasis of T cells, and TT is thus a simple and effective method of supplying T cells that are differentiated and regulated to treat tumors without acute rejection or infection (Ikehara, 2011). TT has also been used to treat DiGeorge syndrome and immune deficiency (Chinn and Markert, 2011). Moreover, renal allografts were accepted without immunosupressants when renal allografts and lobes of thymus were transplanted simultaneously, suggesting that TT across a fully MHC-mismatched barrier induces tolerance in a large-animal model. TT is thus a potential strategy for tolerance induction in clinical transplantation (Kamano *et al.*, 2004). Our previous studies showed that intra bone marrow-bone marrow transplantation + TT improved hyperglycemia in type 2 diabetes model mice by increasing heme oxygenase-1 expression and insulin receptor activity (M. Li *et al.*, 2010).

Intra bone marrow-bone marrow transplantation has been shown to suppress GVHD even when pretreatment consisted only of low-dose irradiation (Nakamura *et al.*, 2004). ABMT + TT can improve autoimmune diseases in chimeric-resistant MRL/lpr mice without GVHD (Hosaka *et al.*, 2007; Ryu *et al.*, 2008). Intra bone marrow-bone marrow transplantation + adult TT (ATT) prevented tumor development with mild graft-versus-host reaction (GVHR) resulting from the induction of high thymopoiesis and a strong graft-versus-tumor (GVT) effect in tumor-bearing mice. Meth A sarcoma cells were subcutaneously inoculated into mice, and intra bone marrow-bone marrow transplantation + ATT was then used to treat these mice when the tumor had grown to 5mm. The number of T cell receptor rearrangement excision circles (TRECs) was higher, and the number of CD4[+] FoxP3[+] cells was lower, in the mice treated with intra bone marrow-bone marrow transplantation + ATT than in those treated with intra bone marrow-bone marrow transplantation alone. Furthermore, the number of CD8[+] cells infiltrating the tumor and the levels of IFN-γ were higher in the mice treated with intra bone marrow-bone marrow transplantation + ATT than in those treated with intra bone marrow-bone marrow transplantation alone (Miyake *et al.*, 2009). Although Tregs have been reported to suppress the GVHR induced by CD4[+]T cells, they did not reduce the GVT induced by CD8[+] T cells (Edinger *et al.*, 2003).

Leukemias are hematologic malignancies, and include acute and chronic myeloid leukemia. Some leukemia cells express CD80, CD86, and some may express MHC class I and II, which can be recognized and eradicated by T cells (Whiteway *et al.*, 2003). ABMT is an effective immunotherapy for acute leukemia in children (Oliansky *et al.*, 2007) and, from our experience, we can maximize the graft-versus-leukemic (GVL) effect with minimal GVHD. We performed experiments to treat leukemia by ABMT using leukemia-bearing mice induced by EL-4 cells. EL-4 cells are derived from the thymoma of mice, and can induce the mimicking of leukemia in mice. We compared the effects of intra bone marrow-bone marrow transplantation +donor lymphocyte infusion (DLI) with intra bone marrow-bone marrow transplantation + ATT in leukemia-bearing mice. DLI is sometimes used to treat leukemia, but there is also a risk of GVHD in the recipients (Deol and Lum, 2010). Our results showed that intra bone marrow-bone marrow transplantation + ATT prevented the growth of leukemia by improving mitogen responses to both T and B cells, and significantly increased IL-2 production, IL-2 having been reported to protect against ABMT-induced GVHD (Zhang *et al.*, 2012; Satake *et al.*, 2014). Moreover, the number of CD62L[-]CD44[+] effector memory T cells was higher in mice treated with intra bone marrow-bone marrow transplantation + TT than in those treated with intra bone marrow-bone marrow transplantation + DLI, although there was no difference in the number of CD62L[+]CD44[+] central memory or CD62L[-] CD44[-] naïve T cells between the two groups. These results showed that intra bone marrow-bone marrow transplantation + ATT induces strong GVL effects with mild GVHD, suggested that TT is useful for treating leukemia.

Our previous report showed that newborn liver cell transplantation (NLT) with newborn TT (NTT) can ameliorate intestinal injury following irradiation in supralethally irradiated mice, by increasing the number of CD4[+] T cells and B cells when compared with NLC transplantation alone. The production of interleukin (IL)-7 and keratinocyte growth factor play an important role in protection against radiation injury in the intestine, and their levels were higher in newborn thymus than fetal or adult thymus (Ryu *et al.*, 2008). We therefore compared the results of BMT+ATT, NLT+NTT, or fetal LT (FLT) + fetal TT (FTT) on tumor suppression. Our results showed that tumors were suppressed to a greater extent as a result of the increased CD4[+] and CD8[+] T cells and decreased number of Gr-1[+]/CD11b[+] myeloid suppressor cells and Foxp3[+]/CD4[+] Tregs in Meth A sarcoma-bearing mice treated with HSCT + TT than in those treated with HSCT alone. Furthermore, the tumors were suppressed in mouse Meth A sarcoma-bearing mice treated with NLT+NTT or FLT+FTT. Moreover, the production of CD62L[-]CD44[+] effector memory T cells and IFN-γ were also higher in these two groups than in the HSCT+TT group (Zhang *et al.*, 2011). Our results showed that FTT grafts showed greater growth than NTT or ATT, and some atrophic features were observed in ATT grafts, suggesting aging-related changes in the thymus. These results suggested that FLT+FTT is an effective method of treating tumors without GVHD.

5 Conclusions and Future Directions

Our previous studies showed that HSCT+TT could be a useful intervention for treating tumors. Specifically, FLT+FTT was shown to be superior for tumor therapy (Figure 1), although it may be difficult to obtain both HSCs and fetal human thymus from the same donor.

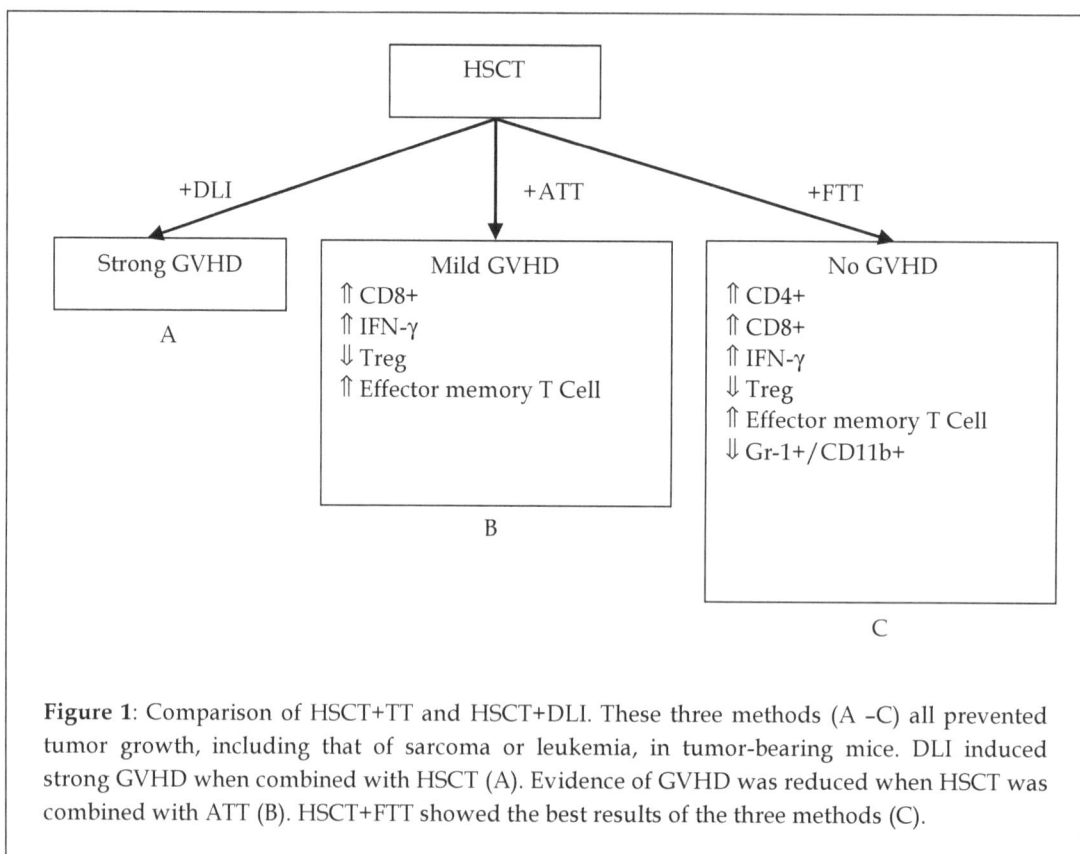

Figure 1: Comparison of HSCT+TT and HSCT+DLI. These three methods (A –C) all prevented tumor growth, including that of sarcoma or leukemia, in tumor-bearing mice. DLI induced strong GVHD when combined with HSCT (A). Evidence of GVHD was reduced when HSCT was combined with ATT (B). HSCT+FTT showed the best results of the three methods (C).

Donor thymus may be obtained from donors who donate the heart or other organs for transplantation or from aborted fetuses. Moreover, thymus can be generated from induced pluripotent stem cells (Inami *et al.*, 2011). We have, however, shown that triple chimeric mice survived for a long period with sufficient T-cell functions, and almost all the hematolymphoid cells were derived from donor bone marrow cells that showed tolerance to all three types of MHC determinants with donor-derived thymic dendritic cells, suggesting third-party fetal thymus can be used to induce tolerance in elderly recipients with low thymic function (Cui *et al.*, 2008). Future studies will further clarify the mechanism of TT in cancer therapy in tumor-bearing mice.

Tracking the fate of transplanted stem cells is important in order to analyze the molecular pathways and control the stem cell migration. Molecular imaging is a noninvasive method of tracking stem cell migration, survival, and differentiation, and for monitoring the transplanted cells in the live recipient (Gu *et al.*, 2012). Molecular imaging may allow treatments to be modified to maximize their efficacy for brain tumors. Moreover, stem cells are of great interest as they show a tropism to tumor cells and will even migrate long distances to track down single tumor cells (Aboody *et al.*, 2000). The identification of genetic and biochemical mechanisms underlying tumor growth and progression, along with the unraveling of the human genome, has provided a plethora of new targets for cancer detection, treatment and monitoring. The biological processes and target expression can be visualized by positron emission tomography or single photon emission computed tomography. Molecular imaging may help us understand the mechanisms by which stem cells migrate toward invasive tumors and to identify appropriate tissue sources when stem cells are used to treat brain tumors (Sandu *et al.*, 2012a; Sandu and Schaller, 2012b; Spiriev *et al.*, 2013). Similarly, molecular imaging will likely play an important role in tracking stem cell migration and in continuously observing the effects of stem cells when used in other cancer therapies.

Acknowledgments

We would like to thank Mr. Hilary Eastwick-Field and Ms. Keiko Ando for their help in the preparation of the manuscript.

References

Aboody, K. S., Brown, A., Rainov, N. G., Bower, K. A., Liu, S., Yang, W., Small, J. E., Herrlinger, U., Ourednik, V., Black, P. M., Breakefield, X. O., and Snyder, E. Y.(2000). Neural stem cells display extensive tropism for pathology in adult brain: evidence from intracranial gliomas. Proc Natl Acad Sci U S A 97, 12846-12851.

Adkins, B.(2003). Peripheral CD4+ lymphocytes derived from fetal versus adult thymic precursors differ phenotypically and functionally. J Immunol 171, 5157-5164.

Adkins, B., Williamson, T., Guevara, P., and Bu, Y.(2003). Murine neonatal lymphocytes show rapid early cell cycle entry and cell division. J Immunol 170, 4548-4556.

Ahmad, A., Banerjee, S., Wang, Z., Kong, D., Majumdar, A. P., and Sarkar, F. H.(2009). Aging and inflammation: etiological culprits of cancer. Curr Aging Sci 2, 174-186.

Anderson, G., Jenkinson, E. J., and Rodewald, H. R.(2009). A roadmap for thymic epithelial cell development. Eur J Immunol 39, 1694-1699.

Balciunaite, G., Keller, M. P., Balciunaite, E., Piali, L., Zuklys, S., Mathieu, Y. D., Gill, J., Boyd, R., Sussman, D. J., and Hollander, G. A.(2002). Wnt glycoproteins regulate the expression of FoxN1, the gene defective in nude mice. Nat Immunol 3, 1102-1108.

Borrello, M. G., Degl'innocenti, D., and Pierotti, M. A.(2008). Inflammation and cancer: the oncogene-driven connection. Cancer Lett 267, 262-270.

Carrio, R., Altman, N. H., and Lopez, D. M.(2009a). Downregulation of interleukin-7 and hepatocyte growth factor in the thymic microenvironment is associated with thymus involution in tumor-bearing mice. Cancer Immunol Immunother 58, 2059-2072.

Carrio, R., and Lopez, D. M.(2009b). Impaired thymopoiesis occurring during the thymic involution of tumor-bearing mice is associated with a down-regulation of the antiapoptotic proteins Bcl-XL and A1. Int J Mol Med 23, 89-98.

Carrio, R., Torroella-Kouri, M., Iragavarapu-Charyulu, V., and Lopez, D. M.(2011). Tumor-induced thymic atrophy: alteration in interferons and Jak/Stats signaling pathways. Int J Oncol 38, 547-553.

Caruso, C., Lio, D., Cavallone, L., and Franceschi, C.(2004). Aging, longevity, inflammation, and cancer. Ann N Y Acad Sci 1028, 1-13.

Chaput, N., Conforti, R., Viaud, S., Spatz, A., and Zitvogel, L.(2008). The Janus face of dendritic cells in cancer. Oncogene 27, 5920-5931.

Chen, B. J., Deoliveira, D., Spasojevic, I., Sempowski, G. D., Jiang, C., Owzar, K., Wang, X., Gesty-Palmer, D., Cline, J. M., Bourland, J. D., Dugan, G., Meadows, S. K., Daher, P., Muramoto, G., Chute, J. P., and Chao, N. J.(2010). Growth hormone mitigates against lethal irradiation and enhances hematologic and immune recovery in mice and nonhuman primates. PLoS One 5, e11056.

Chinn, I. K., and Markert, M. L.(2011). Induction of tolerance to parental parathyroid grafts using allogeneic thymus tissue in patients with DiGeorge anomaly. J Allergy Clin Immunol 127, 1351-1355.

Coleman, R. E.(2012). Bone cancer in 2011: Prevention and treatment of bone metastases. Nat Rev Clin Oncol 9, 76-78.

Cui, W., Hosaka, N., Miyake, T., Wang, X., Guo, K., Cui, Y., Li, Q., Song, C., Feng, W., Li, Q., Takaki, T., Nishida, T., Inaba, M., and Ikehara, S.(2008). Analysis of tolerance induction using triple chimeric mice: major histocompatibility complex-disparate thymus, hemopoietic cells, and microenvironment. Transplantation 85, 1151-1158.

Davies, M.(2014). New modalities of cancer treatment for NSCLC: focus on immunotherapy. Cancer Manag Res 6, 63-75.

Deol, A., and Lum, L. G.(2010). Role of donor lymphocyte infusions in relapsed hematological malignancies after stem cell transplantation revisited. Cancer Treat Rev 36, 528-538.

Edinger, M., Hoffmann, P., Ermann, J., Drago, K., Fathman, C. G., Strober, S., and Negrin, R. S.(2003). CD4+CD25+ regulatory T cells preserve graft-versus-tumor activity while inhibiting graft-versus-host disease after bone marrow transplantation. Nature medicine 9, 1144-1150.

Frasca, D., Landin, A. M., Riley, R. L., and Blomberg, B. B.(2008). Mechanisms for decreased function of B cells in aged mice and humans. J Immunol 180, 2741-2746.

Fu, Y., Paul, R. D., Wang, Y., and Lopez, D. M.(1989a). Thymic involution and thymocyte phenotypic alterations induced by murine mammary adenocarcinomas. J Immunol 143, 4300-4307.

Fu, Y. X., Altman, N., and Lopez, D. M.(1989b). Thymic atrophy induced by murine mammary adenocarcinoma in vivo. In Vivo 3, 1-5.

Galluzzi, L., Senovilla, L., Vacchelli, E., Eggermont, A., Fridman, W. H., Galon, J., Sautes-Fridman, C., Tartour, E., Zitvogel, L., and Kroemer, G.(2012). Trial watch: Dendritic cell-based interventions for cancer therapy. Oncoimmunology 1, 1111-1134.

Gray, D. H., Seach, N., Ueno, T., Milton, M. K., Liston, A., Lew, A. M., Goodnow, C. C., and Boyd, R. L.(2006). Developmental kinetics, turnover, and stimulatory capacity of thymic epithelial cells. Blood 108, 3777-3785.

Gu, E., Chen, W. Y., Gu, J., Burridge, P., and Wu, J. C.(2012). Molecular imaging of stem cells: tracking survival, biodistribution, tumorigenicity, and immunogenicity. Theranostics 2, 335-345.

Hale, J. S., Boursalian, T. E., Turk, G. L., and Fink, P. J.(2006). Thymic output in aged mice. Proc Natl Acad Sci U S A 103, 8447-8452.

Hamid, O., Robert, C., Daud, A., Hodi, F. S., Hwu, W. J., Kefford, R., Wolchok, J. D., Hersey, P., Joseph, R. W., Weber, J. S., Dronca, R., Gangadhar, T. C., Patnaik, A., Zarour, H., Joshua, A. M., Gergich, K., Elassaiss-Schaap, J., Algazi, A., Mateus, C., Boasberg, P., Tumeh, P. C., Chmielowski, B., Ebbinghaus, S. W., Li, X. N., Kang, S. P., and Ribas, A.(2013). Safety and tumor responses with lambrolizumab (anti-PD-1) in melanoma. N Engl J Med 369, 134-144.

Hikosaka, Y., Nitta, T., Ohigashi, I., Yano, K., Ishimaru, N., Hayashi, Y., Matsumoto, M., Matsuo, K., Penninger, J. M., Takayanagi, H., Yokota, Y., Yamada, H., Yoshikai, Y., Inoue, J., Akiyama, T., and Takahama, Y.(2008). The cytokine RANKL produced by positively selected thymocytes fosters medullary thymic epithelial cells that express autoimmune regulator. Immunity 29, 438-450.

Hosaka, N., Ryu, T., Miyake, T., Cui, W., Nishida, T., Takaki, T., Inaba, M., and Ikehara, S.(2007). Treatment of autoimmune diseases in MRL/lpr mice by allogenic bone marrow transplantation plus adult thymus transplantation. Clin Exp Immunol 147, 555-563.

Hubert, F. X., Kinkel, S. A., Davey, G. M., Phipson, B., Mueller, S. N., Liston, A., Proietto, A. I., Cannon, P. Z., Forehan, S., Smyth, G. K., Wu, L., Goodnow, C. C., Carbone, F. R., Scott, H. S., and Heath, W. R.(2011). Aire regulates the transfer of antigen from mTECs to dendritic cells for induction of thymic tolerance. Blood 118, 2462-2472.

Ikehara, S.(2011). Thymus transplantation for treatment of cancer: lessons from murine models. Expert Rev Clin Immunol 7, 205-211.

Inami, Y., Yoshikai, T., Ito, S., Nishio, N., Suzuki, H., Sakurai, H., and Isobe, K.(2011). Differentiation of induced pluripotent stem cells to thymic epithelial cells by phenotype. Immunology and cell biology 89, 314-321.

Kamano, C., Vagefi, P. A., Kumagai, N., Yamamoto, S., Barth, R. N., Lamattina, J. C., Moran, S. G., Sachs, D. H., and Yamada, K.(2004). Vascularized thymic lobe transplantation in miniature swine: thymopoiesis and tolerance induction across fully MHC-mismatched barriers. Proc Natl Acad Sci U S A 101, 3827-3832.

Kenter, G. G., Welters, M. J., Valentijn, A. R., Lowik, M. J., Berends-Van Der Meer, D. M., Vloon, A. P., Essahsah, F., Fathers, L. M., Offringa, R., Drijfhout, J. W., Wafelman, A. R., Oostendorp, J., Fleuren, G. J., Van Der Burg, S. H., and Melief, C. J.(2009). Vaccination against HPV-16 oncoproteins for vulvar intraepithelial neoplasia. N Engl J Med 361, 1838-1847.

Konkel, J. E., Jin, W., Abbatiello, B., Grainger, J. R., and Chen, W.(2014). Thymocyte apoptosis drives the intrathymic generation of regulatory T cells. Proc Natl Acad Sci U S A 111, E465-473.

Kushida, T., Inaba, M., Takeuchi, K., Sugiura, K., Ogawa, R., and Ikehara, S.(2000). Treatment of intractable autoimmune diseases in MRL/lpr mice using a new strategy for allogeneic bone marrow transplantation. Blood 95, 1862-1868.

Lai, L., Cui, C., Jin, J., Hao, Z., Zheng, Q., Ying, M., Boyd, R., and Zhao, Y.(2011). Mouse embryonic stem cell-derived thymic epithelial cell progenitors enhance T-cell reconstitution after allogeneic bone marrow transplantation. Blood 118, 3410-3418.

Li, M., Abraham, N. G., Vanella, L., Zhang, Y., Inaba, M., Hosaka, N., Hoshino, S., Shi, M., Ambrosini, Y. M., Gershwin, M. E., and Ikehara, S.(2010). Successful modulation of type 2 diabetes in db/db mice with intra-bone marrow--bone marrow transplantation plus concurrent thymic transplantation. J Autoimmun 35, 414-423.

Li, Y., Hisha, H., Inaba, M., Lian, Z., Yu, C., Kawamura, M., Yamamoto, Y., Nishio, N., Toki, J., Fan, H., and Ikehara, S.(2000). Evidence for migration of donor bone marrow stromal cells into recipient thymus after bone marrow transplantation plus bone grafts: A role of stromal cells in positive selection. Exp Hematol 28, 950-960.

Lynch, H. E., Goldberg, G. L., Chidgey, A., Van Den Brink, M. R., Boyd, R., and Sempowski, G. D.(2009). Thymic involution and immune reconstitution. Trends Immunol 30, 366-373.

Marx, J.(2004). Cancer research. Inflammation and cancer: the link grows stronger. Science 306, 966-968.

Mcnutt, M.(2013). Cancer immunotherapy. Science 342, 1417.

Miyake, T., Hosaka, N., Cui, W., Nishida, T., Takaki, T., Inaba, M., Kamiyama, Y., and Ikehara, S.(2009). Adult thymus transplantation with allogeneic intra-bone marrow-bone marrow transplantation from same donor induces high thymopoiesis, mild graft-versus-host reaction and strong graft-versus-tumour effects. Immunology 126, 552-564.

Moeller, I., Spagnoli, G. C., Finke, J., Veelken, H., and Houet, L.(2012). Uptake routes of tumor-antigen MAGE-A3 by dendritic cells determine priming of naive T-cell subtypes. Cancer Immunol Immunother 61, 2079-2090.

Naito, Y., Saito, K., Shiiba, K., Ohuchi, A., Saigenji, K., Nagura, H., and Ohtani, H.(1998). CD8+ T cells infiltrated within cancer cell nests as a prognostic factor in human colorectal cancer. Cancer Res 58, 3491-3494.

Nakamura, K., Inaba, M., Sugiura, K., Yoshimura, T., Kwon, A. H., Kamiyama, Y., and Ikehara, S.(2004). Enhancement of allogeneic hematopoietic stem cell engraftment and prevention of GVHD by intra-bone marrow bone marrow transplantation plus donor lymphocyte infusion. Stem Cells 22, 125-134.

Nishida, T., Hosaka, N., Takaki, T., Miyake, T., Cui, W., Inaba, M., Kinoshita, H., Matsuda, T., and Ikehara, S.(2009). Allogeneic intra-BM-BMT plus adult thymus transplantation from same donor has benefits for long-term survival even after sublethal irradiation or low-dose BM cell injection. Bone Marrow Transplant 43, 829-837.

Oliansky, D. M., Rizzo, J. D., Aplan, P. D., Arceci, R. J., Leone, L., Ravindranath, Y., Sanders, J. E., Smith, F. O., 3rd, Wilmot, F., Mccarthy, P. L., Jr., and Hahn, T.(2007). The role of cytotoxic therapy with hematopoietic stem cell transplantation in the therapy of acute myeloid leukemia in children: an evidence-based review. Biol Blood Marrow Transplant 13, 1-25.

Parmar, S., and Ritchie, D. S.(2014). Allogeneic transplantation as anticancer immunotherapy. Curr Opin Immunol 27C, 38-45.

Petrie, H. T., and Zuniga-Pflucker, J. C.(2007). Zoned out: functional mapping of stromal signaling microenvironments in the thymus. Annu Rev Immunol 25, 649-679.

Rode, I., and Boehm, T.(2012). Regenerative capacity of adult cortical thymic epithelial cells. Proc Natl Acad Sci U S A 109, 3463-3468.

Rossi, S. W., Kim, M. Y., Leibbrandt, A., Parnell, S. M., Jenkinson, W. E., Glanville, S. H., Mcconnell, F. M., Scott, H. S., Penninger, J. M., Jenkinson, E. J., Lane, P. J., and Anderson, G.(2007). RANK signals from CD4(+)3(-) inducer cells regulate development of Aire-expressing epithelial cells in the thymic medulla. J Exp Med 204, 1267-1272.

Ryu, T., Hosaka, N., Miyake, T., Cui, W., Nishida, T., Takaki, T., Li, M., Kawamoto, K., and Ikehara, S.(2008). Transplantation of newborn thymus plus hematopoietic stem cells can rescue supralethally irradiated mice. Bone Marrow Transplant 41, 659-666.

Sandu, N., Momen-Heravi, F., Sadr-Eshkevari, P., and Schaller, B.(2012a). Molecular imaging for stem cell transplantation in neuroregenerative medicine. Neurodegener Dis 9, 60-67.

Sandu, N., and Schaller, B.(2012b). Molecular imaging of stem cell therapy in brain tumors: a step towards personalized medicine. Arch Med Sci 8, 601-605.

Satake, A., Schmidt, A. M., Nomura, S., and Kambayashi, T.(2014). Inhibition of Calcineurin Abrogates While Inhibition of mTOR Promotes Regulatory T Cell Expansion and Graft-Versus-Host Disease Protection by IL-2 in Allogeneic Bone Marrow Transplantation. PLoS One 9, e92888.

Schreiber, R. D., Old, L. J., and Smyth, M. J.(2011). Cancer immunoediting: integrating immunity's roles in cancer suppression and promotion. Science 331, 1565-1570.

Seggewiss, R., and Einsele, H.(2010). Immune reconstitution after allogeneic transplantation and expanding options for immunomodulation: an update. Blood 115, 3861-3868.

Sempowski, G. D., Hale, L. P., Sundy, J. S., Massey, J. M., Koup, R. A., Douek, D. C., Patel, D. D., and Haynes, B. F.(2000). Leukemia inhibitory factor, oncostatin M, IL-6, and stem cell factor mRNA expression in human thymus increases with age and is associated with thymic atrophy. J Immunol 164, 2180-2187.

Spiriev, T., Sandu, N., and Schaller, B.(2013). Molecular imaging and tracking stem cells in neurosciences. Methods Mol Biol 1052, 195-201.

Sun, X., Xu, J., Lu, H., Liu, W., Miao, Z., Sui, X., Liu, H., Su, L., Du, W., He, Q., Chen, F., Shi, Y., and Deng, H.(2013). Directed differentiation of human embryonic stem cells into thymic epithelial progenitor-like cells reconstitutes the thymic microenvironment in vivo. Cell stem cell 13, 230-236.

Takaki, T., Hosaka, N., Miyake, T., Cui, W., Nishida, T., Inaba, M., and Ikehara, S.(2008). Presence of donor-derived thymic epithelial cells in [B6-->MRL/lpr] mice after allogeneic intra-bone marrow-bone marrow transplantation (IBM-BMT). J Autoimmun 31, 408-415.

Toubert, A., Glauzy, S., Douay, C., and Clave, E.(2012). Thymus and immune reconstitution after allogeneic hematopoietic stem cell transplantation in humans: never say never again. Tissue Antigens 79, 83-89.

Vacchelli, E., Eggermont, A., Galon, J., Sautes-Fridman, C., Zitvogel, L., Kroemer, G., and Galluzzi, L.(2013). Trial watch: Monoclonal antibodies in cancer therapy. Oncoimmunology 2, e22789.

Van Den Eynde, B. J., and Van Der Bruggen, P.(1997). T cell defined tumor antigens. Curr Opin Immunol 9, 684-693.

Varecza, Z., Kvell, K., Talaber, G., Miskei, G., Csongei, V., Bartis, D., Anderson, G., Jenkinson, E. J., and Pongracz, J. E.(2011). Multiple suppression pathways of canonical Wnt signalling control thymic epithelial senescence. Mech Ageing Dev 132, 249-256.

Whiteway, A., Corbett, T., Anderson, R., Macdonald, I., and Prentice, H. G.(2003). Expression of co-stimulatory molecules on acute myeloid leukaemia blasts may effect duration of first remission. Br J Haematol 120, 442-451.

Younes, A., Yasothan, U., and Kirkpatrick, P.(2012). Brentuximab vedotin. Nat Rev Drug Discov 11, 19-20.

Zediak, V. P., Maillard, I., and Bhandoola, A.(2007). Multiple prethymic defects underlie age-related loss of T progenitor competence. Blood 110, 1161-1167.

Zhang, Y., Hosaka, N., Cui, Y., Shi, M., and Ikehara, S.(2011). Effects of allogeneic hematopoietic stem cell transplantation plus thymus transplantation on malignant tumors: comparison between fetal, newborn, and adult mice. Stem Cells Dev 20, 599-607.

Zhang, Y., Hosaka, N., Cui, Y., Shi, M., Li, M., Li, Q., and Ikehara, S.(2012). *Effects of intrabone marrow-bone marrow transplantation plus adult thymus transplantation on survival of mice bearing leukemia*. Stem Cells Dev 21, 1441-1448.

Zhuang, X., Xia, X., Wang, C., Gao, F., Shan, N., and Zhang, L.(2010). *A high number of CD8+ T cells infiltrated in NSCLC tissues is associated with a favorable prognosis*. Appl Immunohistochem Mol Morphol 18, 24-28.

The Preventive and Therapeutic Effect of Coptidis Rhizoma and Berberine in Cancer

Li Lei*, Wang Ning* and Feng Yibin*

1 Introduction

Coptidis Rhizoma (Huanglian in Chinese) has been widely prescribed by Chinese Medicine physician for treating damp-heat syndromes for more than two thousand years (J. Tang *et al.*, 2009). Berberine (Figure 1) is an isoquinoline alkaloid in *Coptidis Rhizoma*, which is also a major active compound in *Coptidis Rhizoma* (Enk *et al.*, 2007). Many studies have confirmed that *Coptidis Rhizoma* is a good producer of berberine. High yield of berberine can also be isolated and purified from various medical plants like Berberidaceae Ranunculaceae and Papaveraceae (Galle, Blodt, & Wagner, 1994; Grycová, Dostál, & Marek, 2007) via genetic engineering (Sato *et al.*, 2001) and now can be totally synthesized. It is found that in dried herb of *Coptidis Rhizoma*, the most abundant alkaloid is berberine (5.20 – 7.69%, w/w) (Iizuka *et al.*, 2003).

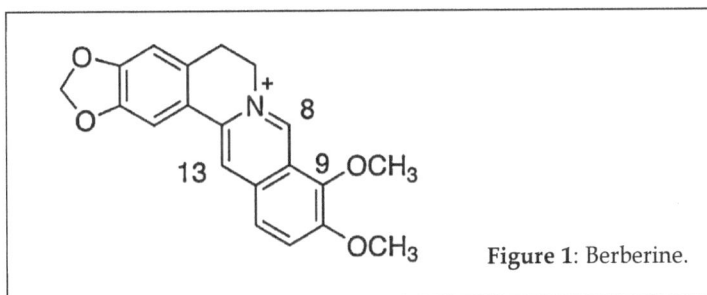

Figure 1: Berberine.

In clinic, *Coptidis Rhizoma* and berberine are commonly used for the treatment of gastrointestinal infection including acute gastroenteritis, cholera and bacillary dysentery. Since last century, *Coptidis Rhizoma* and berberine have been widely investigated for their pharmacological and biological activities. The major pharmacological properties of berberine and *Coptidis Rhizoma* include anti-microbial, anti-inflammatory, anti-oxidative and anti-tumor effect (Dharmananda, 2005; Hayashi, Minoda, Nagaoka, Hayashi, & Uesato, 2007). The purification of berberine from *Coptidis Rhizoma* has greatly facilitated investigation studies into the therapeutic effects of *Coptidis Rhizoma*.

The anti-cancer effect of berberine was first highlighted in 1959 (Hano, 1959). In1990s, Studies focusing on the anti-cancer effects of *Coptidis Rhizoma* and berberine and its underlying mechanisms of anti-cancer activity in various cancer cell types have dramatically increased. Until now, the anti-cancer effects of berberine are still hitting the eyes of many re-

* School of Chinese Medicine, Li Ka Shing Faculty of Medicine, The University of Hong Kong, Hong Kong, China

searchers. Moreover, some studies have obtained promising and interesting results. In this review, the anti-cancer effect and cancer preventative effect of *Coptidis Rhizoma* and berberine (especially berberine) in recent publications will be discussed in detail.

2   Anti-cancer Effect of Coptidis Rhizoma and Berberine

2.1   Prevent Carcinogenesis

In view of cancer etiology, pathogenic microorganism has a close relationship with carcinogenesis and it's one of the major factors that causes certain types of cancer. For example, long-term *Helicobacter pylori* infection is strongly associated with chronic gastritis and peptic ulcer disease, which might gradually develop into gastric cancer (Takahashi, 2002; Uemura *et al.*, 2001). Also, two hepatitis viruses, HBV and HCV, are confirmed to be the major factor that causes HCC (Lavanchy, 2004). Thus, the antimicrobial activity of berberine might contribute to its anticancer effect.

The antimicrobial activity of berberine was first reported in 1960s (Amin, Subbaiah, & Abbasi, 1969). Many studies showed that berberine exhibited a broad spectrum of anti-microorganism effect. Berberine could inhibit the growth of various kinds of bacterial and fungi *in vitro* including *Staphylococci* (Kowalewski, Kedzia, & Mirska, 1972), *Klebsiellapneumoniae, Proteusvulgaris, Mycobacterium smegmatis, Candida albicans*(Franzblau & Cross, 1986), *Heliobacter pylori* (L. Zhang, Yang, & Zheng, 1997), *Mycobacterium tuberculosis*(Gentry *et al.*, 1998), *Candida rugosa* (Grippa *et al.*, 1999), and *tetrahymenathermophila (T. thermophila) BF(5)* (Kong, Li, Xiao, & Zhao, 2010). At a minimum inhibitory concentration of 12.5 mg/ml, berberine could inhibited the growth of *Helicobacter pylori in vitro* (Mahady, Pendland, Stoia, & Chadwick, 2003). Berberine could reduce viral production as well as inducing toxicity in hepatitis B virus permanently transfected HepG2 2.2.15 cells (H. L. Li *et al.*, 2008). Mechanisms in the antimicrobial effect of berberine included suppressing the biofilm formation in *Staphylococcus epidermidis* (X. Q. Wang *et al.*, 2009), inhibiting the cell division protein FtsZ (Boberek, Stach, & Good, 2010) and blocking microbial adhesion to the epithelial host cells (D. Sun, Courtney, & Beachey, 1988).

The synergistic activities of berberine with other natural or synthetic anti-microbial agents were conducted in many studies. One study revealed that berberine may be the substrate of MDR enzymes due to multidrug resistance inhibitor (MDR inhibitor) sensitizing the human pathogen *Staphylococcus aureus* to berberine treatment (Stermitz, Lorenz, Tawara, Zenewicz, & Lewis, 2000). In another study, berberine could sensitize Methicillin-resistant *Staphylococcus aureus* (MRSA) bacteria to ampicillin and oxacillin treatment (H. H. Yu *et al.*, 2005). Furthermore, synergistic activity with anti-fungi agent fluconazole, strobilurin orfludi-oxonil was found in berberine (J. H. Kim *et al.*, 2007; Quan *et al.*, 2006). The underling mechanism of berberine's synergistic activity may be induction of inducing reactive oxygen species (ROS) production (Xu *et al.*, 2009).

2.2   Suppress Cancer Cell Proliferation

Berberine exhibited cytotocicity effect on different cancer cell lines in a dose- and time-dependent manner and the studied cell lines included HeLa (cervical carcinoma) (Kettmann,

Kostalova, Jantova, Cernakova, & Drimal, 2004), HepG2 (hepatocellular carcinoma) (Hwang, Kuo, Tseng, Liu, & Chu, 2006), HONE 1 (nasopharyngeal carcinoma) and HK1 (nasopharyngeal carcinoma) (Tsang *et al.*, 2009a). At a relatively low IC50, berberine could inhibit the growth of a wide range of cancer cell types including both hematological and non-hematological cancers arising from leucocytes, liver, lung, stomach, colon, skin, oral, esophagus, brain, bone, breast and sexual organs (either hormone-dependent or independent) (Y. Y. Sun, Xun, Wang, & Chen, 2009). In some cases, the IC50 of berberine was lower than 4 µg/mL, which is below the safety limit established by National Cancer Institute (NCI), suggesting the antineoplastic potential of berberine on some human cancers such as cervical cancer, leukemia and colon cancer (Letasiova, Jantova, Cipak, & Muckova, 2006). The effect of berberine on cell cycle redistribution in numerous cancer cells has been reported in many studies and contributes the broad spectrum of antineoplastic activity. In human epidermoid carcinoma cell lines, berberine inhibited cyclin-dependent kinase CDK1 and CDK2, induced G2/M cell cycle arrest, and up-regulated CDK inhibitor of p27 (Roublevskaia, Polevoda, Ludlow, & Haake, 2000). Berberine showed a similar effect on cell cycle of esophageal cancer(Iizuka *et al.*, 2000), glioblastoma (Gagliano *et al.*, 2007), hepatocellular carcinoma (X. N. Wang *et al.*, 2008), neuroblastoma (Choi *et al.*, 2008), osteosarcoma cells (Liu *et al.*, 2009), breast cancer (J. B. Kim *et al.*, 2010), cervical cancer (Lu *et al.*, 2010), pancreatic cancer (Pinto-Garcia *et al.*, 2010), colon cancer (Hu *et al.*, 2011), bladder cancer (Yan *et al.*, 2011), human cholangio carcinoma (W. He *et al.*, 2012), ovarian carcinoma (Park *et al.*, 2012b), thyroid cancer (Park *et al.*, 2012a) and colon cancer (L. Wang *et al.*, 2013). Berberine could induce apoptosis via G2 arrest on human nasopharyngeal carcinoma cells (HONE1 cells) by increasing levels of cleaved-PARP, cleaved caspase 3 and cleaved caspase 9 (Tsang *et al.*, 2009a). The induction of cell-cycle arrest was determined by the presence of p53 in some cases, for example, G1 arrest was induced in p53 functional HCO and U2OS cells while G2/M arrest in p53-deficient Saos-2 cells (Z. J. Liu *et al.*, 2009). In p53 expressing SK–N–SH cells, cell-cycle arrest in G0/G1 phase was much higher than those in p53-deficientSK–N–MC cells (Choi *et al.*, 2008). It was the same case when comparing p53 positive LNCaP prostate cells with p53 negative PC-3 cells (Choi *et al.*, 2009). Targeting multiple aspects of cellular metabolism, such as both aerobic glycolysis and mitochondrial oxidative phosphorylation (OXPHOS), has the potential to improve cancer therapeutics. A recent study showed that berberine combined with 2-deoxy-d-glucose synergistically enhanced cancer cell proliferation inhibition via energy depletion and unfolded protein response disruption (Fan *et al.*, 2013). In human multiple myeloma U266 cells, berberine suppressed cell proliferation in dose- and time-dependent manners by suppressing NF-kappa B nuclear translocation via Set9-mediated lysine methylation and reducing miR21 and Bcl-2 level, which induced ROS generation and apoptosis (Hu *et al.*, 2013). Berberine inhibited the proliferation of colon cancer cells by inactivating Wnt/beta-catenin signaling, which indicated the potential of berberine as chemoprevention and chemotherapy agent human colon cancer in human (K. Wu *et al.*, 2012).

2.3   Induce Cancer Cell Apoptosis

The ability of berberine to induce apoptotic cell death has been widely reported in various kinds of human cancer cell lines including leukemia (Jantova, Cipak, Cernakova, & Kost'alova, 2003),melanoma (Burgeiro *et al.*, 2011; Letasiova *et al.*, 2006), Ehrlich ascites carcinoma (Letasiova *et al.*, 2006), prostate carcinoma (Mantena, Sharma, & Katiyar, 2006b), epidermoid carcinoma (Mantena, Sharma, & Katiyar, 2006a), glioblastoma (Gagliano *et al.*, 2007), breast cancer (J. B. Kim *et al.*, 2010; Pazhang, Ahmadian, Javadifar, & Shafiezadeh, 2012), hepatocellular carcinoma (X. N. Wang *et al.*, 2008), neuroblastoma (Choi *et al.*, 2008), osteosarcoma cells (Z. J. Liu *et al.*, 2009), cervical cancer (Lu *et al.*, 2010; Mahata *et al.*, 2011), colon cancer (W. C. Hu, L. L. Yu, & M. H. Wang, 2011; L. Wang *et al.*, 2012), pancreatic cancer (Pinto-Garcia *et al.*, 2010), bladder cancer (K. Q. Yan *et al.*, 2011), human erythro-myeloblastoid leukemia (Pazhang, Ahmadian, Mahmoudian, & Shafiezadeh, 2011a), and myeloma (Hu *et al.*, 2013).

The underline mechanisms of berberine inducing cell apoptosis were also extensively studied in numerous cancer cell lines. In human gastric cancer cells, berberine could release cytochrome C into nuclear by up-regulating Bax expression and down-regulating Bcl-2, which would activate the cleavage of caspase-9/3 and finally induce apoptosis (J. P. Lin, Yang, Lee, Hsieh, & Chung, 2006). In human leukemia cells, berberine reduced mitochondrial membrane potential by inducing production of ROS and calcium influx and then activated the intrinsic apoptotic pathway (C. C. Lin, Kao, Chen, Ho, & Chung, 2006). Study further revealed that berberine could induce the oxidative stress and stimulates the mitochondrial permeability transition by slowing down the mitochondrial respiration (Pereira *et al.*, 2007). Another study showed that mitochondria and caspase activation were involved in the mechanism of berberine inducing apoptosis in melanoma cells, but ROS generation was not essential. The results indicated that inhibition of B-RAF/ERK survival signaling facilitated the cell death response triggered by berberine (Burgeiro *et al.*, 2011). Study demonstrated that berberine could increase the expression of FasL and phosphor-c-Jun, and the down-regulation of anti-apoptotic factors c-IAP-1, Bcl-xL, Bid and activation of JNK and p38 MAPK to initiate extrinsic apoptotic pathway (Hsu *et al.*, 2007). In human hepatocellular carcinoma, berberine induced apoptosis and activated the caspase-8/9/3 by increasing the expression of p53 and Fas (G. Y. Wang, Lv, Dong, Xu, & Dong, 2009). In another liver cancer cell line Huh7, berberine induced the apoptosis of Huh7 cells via the mitochondrial pathway (Yip & Ho, 2013). Moreover, berberine selectively inhibited the growth of human hepatocellular cancer cells by inducing AMPK mediated caspase dependent mitochondrial pathway cell apoptosis, and rarely caused cytotoxicity in normal cells (Yang & Huang, 2013). In human oral cancer cells, berberine showed its apoptotic property by down-regulating the expression ofCOX-2 to suppress the expression of Mcl-1 and activation of Akt signaling (Kuo, Chi, & Liu, 2005b). In breast cancer cell line 4T1, berberine enhanced tumor necrosis factor-related apoptosis-inducing ligand-mediated apoptosis (Refaat *et al.*, 2013). Further study showed that inhuman colorectal cancer cells, p53-inducibleATF-3 and NAG-1 were two key factors involved in berberine-driven apoptosis (Piyanuch, Sukhthankar, Wandee, & Baek, 2007). The vital role of p53 in berberine-induced apoptosis was further explained by a study demonstrating that p53-proficient cancer cells were more sensitive to berberine treatment than p53-deficient cells (Katiyar, Meeran, Katiyar, & Akhtar, 2009b). The regulating effect of berberine on p53 was further studied and the result showed that expression of MDM2 (endogenous inhibitor of p53) could be decreased by berberine treatment. The underlying mechanism may be berberine promoting MDM2 binding to death domain-associated protein (DAXX) and subsequent degradation (Li *et al.*, 2013; X. L. Zhang *et al.*, 2010). ROS-induced endoplasmic reticulum stress may contribute to berberine's pro-apoptotic action by initiating the expression of GADD153 and catalase (J. P. Lin *et al.*, 2007). Further study showed that intracellular ROS and nitric oxide (NO) were up-regulated by berberine treatment, while its anti-cancer effect were diminished by co-treatment of anti-oxidant. This study further demonstrated the role of oxidative stress in berberine-induced apoptosis (Hur, Hyun, Lim, Lee, & Kim, 2009). However, controversial result appeared in another study showing that iNOS production did not contribute to the pro-apoptotic effect of berberine, but berberine-induced survivin suppression played a more vital role (Pazhang *et al.*, 2011b). Similar result appeared in an experiment using human ductal breast epithelial tumor cell line, which indicated that the apoptotic effect of berberine may be mediated by reduction of COX-2 and survivin in T47D cell line, while the iNOS was not involved in the mechanism of apoptosis induced by berberine (Pazhang *et al.*, 2012).

2.4   Anti-angiogenesis effect

The anti-angiogenesis effect of berberine in human tumor has been reported in previous studies (Wartenberg *et al.*, 2003). In the process of tumor angiogenesis, vascular endothelial growth factor (VEGF) and hypoxia-inducible factor (HIF-1) are two key factors. In hypoxic condition, berberine could promote the binding of HIF-1α to E3 ligases and subsequent degradation instead of directly suppressing the transcription activation of HIF-1in human gastric cancer cells SC-M1. Thus, HIF-1α suppression would inhibit the transcription activation and secretion of VEGF, which is vital in tumor blood vessel formation (S. K. Lin *et al.*, 2004). Berberine could directly suppress the proliferation of VEGF-induced human umbilical vein endothelial cell (HUVEC) and berberine inhibiting VEGF-trigger Erk1/2 activation may be involved in the underline mechanism (Gao, Shi, Lee, Zhang, & Wang, 2009). In human HCC cells, berberine acted as the role of mediation between HCC cells and vascular endothelial cells by inhibiting secretion of VEGF from HCC and down-regulating VEGF mRNA expression (Jie *et al.*, 2011). In human breast cancer cells, a study suggested that berberine may suppress both TPA-induced VEGF fibronectin and VEGF-induced fibronectin through the inhibition of the PI-3K/AKT pathway, which indicated that berberine may be a potential anti-angiogeneisis candidate in human breast cancer (S. Kim *et al.*, 2013). The result of *in vivo* study suggested that the serum VEGF level in mice was significantly suppressed by berberine and the pro-angiogenic factor iNOS and COX-2 decreased when treated with berberine (Hamsa & Kuttan, 2012a).

2.5   Inhibit Cancer cell migration and invasion

Matrix metalloproteinase (MMP) is the major factors in regulating cancer cell migration and invasion. The effect of berberine in suppressing MMPs activation was demonstrated in various cancer cell models. In highlymetastatic A549 lung cancer cell line, berberine could inhibit its motility and invasion ability under noncytotoxic concentrations by suppressing uPA andMMP-2 activity and expression (Peng, Hsieh, Wang, Hsu, & Chou, 2006). In human breast cancer cells, berberine could inhibit TNF-αinduced MMP-9 expression and cell invasion by blocking the DNA-binding activity of AP-1(S. Kim, Choi, *et al.*, 2008). In human tongue cancer cells, berberine down-regulated uPA, MMP-2 and MMP-9 expression via p-JNK, p-ERK, p-p38, IkK, and NF-kB signaling pathways and thus suppress cancer cell migration (Ho, Yang, Li, *et al.*, 2009). Berberine showed metastasis inhibitory effect on mouse melanoma cells by suppressing ERK1/2, NF-αB, ATF-2 and CREB-driven MMPs expression (Hamsa & Kuttan, 2012b). Many studies also showed that berberine significantly inhibited various MMPs protein expression including MMP-1,MMP-2, MMP-9 in DU-145 prostate cancer cells (Wartenberg *et al.*, 2003), human SNU-5 gastric cancer cells (J. P. Lin *et al.*, 2008), HL-60 (S. Kim, Kim, Kim, Cho, & Chung, 2008), WEHI-3 cells(S. M. Kim & Chung, 2008), rat C6 glioma cells and U-87 human malignant glioma cells (T. H. Lin, Kuo, Chou, & Lu, 2008).

Berberine also exerted inhibitory effect on factors associated with cancer cell migration other than MMPs. Studies showed that berberine may directly suppress human HONE1cell migration by inhibiting RhoGTPase, RhoA, Rac1 andCdc42 activities (Tsang *et al.*, 2009b). Extended study found that berberine inhibited Rho-driven Ezrin phosphorylation at threonine 567 in human nasopharyngeal carcinoma (NPC) cells, and the mutation at threonine 567 of Ezrin further suppressed the anti-invasive effect (F. Q. Tang *et al.*, 2009). Epithelial to mesenchymal transition (EMT) may also be involved in the underlying mechanism of berberine's anti-invasion effect. In mouse melanoma cells, berberine could activate AMPK to inhibit the metastasis potential of cancer cells by down-regulating the Erk1/2 signaling and COX-2 expression, which may be involved in the EMT transition and tumor cell migration (H. S. Kim *et al.*, 2012). A recent study showed that berberine is an effective inhibitor of the metastatic potential of lung cancer A549 cells through suppression of TGF-beta1-induced epithelial-to-mesenchymal (Qi, Xin, Xu, Ji, & Fan, 2014). Berberine could inhibit cancer invasion by regulating expression of cell migration related genes. Studies showed that berberine could significantly increase cell migration related genes NM23-H1 and reduce SDF-1 protein level in NPC cells and leukemic cells respectively, which suppressed cancer cell motility and migration (H. Y. Li *et al.*, 2008; S. J. Liu *et al.*, 2008). Furthermore, pro-inflammatory factors play a key role in cancer cell metastasis and berberine exerted inhibitory effect on these factors in many studies. Berberine inhibited melanoma cell migration and invasion by inhibiting pro-inflammatory factors including COX-2, prostaglandin E_2 and prostaglandin E_2 (PGE) receptors, which may be related to NF-αB alteration in cancer cells with treatment of berberine (Singh, Vaid, Katiyar, Sharma, & Katiyar, 2011). Studies also showed that berberine suppressed colon cancer cells migration by reducing COX-2 expression (Fukuda *et al.*, 1999a). By suppressing AP-1 (a complex of c-fos and c-jun) activation, bebrerine could inhibit invasion of human hepatoma cells (Fukuda *et al.*, 1999b), oral cancer cells (Kuo, Chi, & Liu, 2005a) and breast cancer cells (S. Kim, Choi, *et al.*, 2008). More new mechanisms have been discovered in recent studies. Berberine inhibited the migration and invasion of T24 bladder cancer cells via reducing the expression of heparanase (L. Yan *et al.*, 2013). Berberine-induced AMPK activation inhibited the metastatic potential of colon cancer cells by decreasing integrin beta1 protein levels and downstream signaling (J. J. Park *et al.*, 2012). At noncytotoxic concentrations, berberine reduced the migration and invasion of chondrosarcoma cancer cells by modulating the alpha v beta 3 Integrin and the PKC delta , c-Src, and AP-1 Signaling Pathways (C. M. Wu, Li, Tan, Fong, & Tang, 2013). The Possible mechanism of coptis and berberine reducing COX2 expression can be referred to Figure 2.

2.6   *In-vivo* Study

The *in vivo* study of anti-cancer effect of berberine began in 1970s. Animal experiments showed that berberine has the protection effect against carcinogenesis. In mice initiated with 7,12-dimethylbenz[a]anthracene, berberine sulfate could suppress the effects of the tumor promoter 12-O-tetradecanoylphorbol-13-acetate and significantly inhibit the promoting effect of teleocidin on skin tumor formation (Nishino, Kitagawa, Fujiki, & Iwashima, 1986). The re

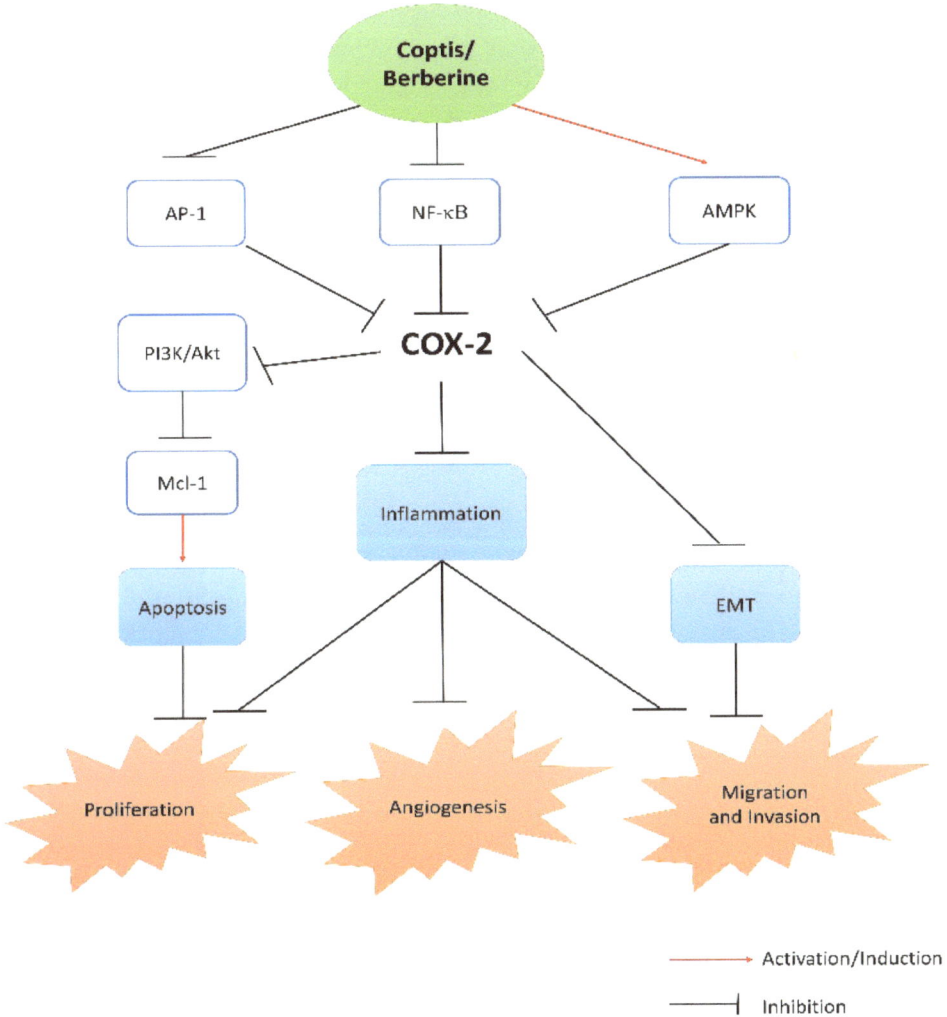

Figure 2: Possible mechanism of coptis and berberine reducing COX2 expression (Berberine inhibited migration and invasion by inhibiting pro-inflammatory factors COX-2, which may be related to NF-αB alteration. Coptis and berberine reduced the binding of AP-1 and resulted in decreased COX-2 expression. Berberine showed its apoptotic property by down-regulating the expression of COX-2 to suppress the expression of Mcl-1 and activation of PI3K/Akt signaling. Berberine could activate AMPK to inhibit the metastasis potential of cancer cells by COX-2 expression, which may be involved in the EMT transition and tumor cell migration. Berberine could also reduce pro-angiogenetic factor COX-2 expression, which may be involved in tumor angiogensis.)

sult of *Anis et al.* study suggested that carcinogenesis induced by 20-methylcholanthreneor N-nitrosodiethylamine was significantly suppressed after treated with berberine in a dose-dependent manner in both mice and rats. The incidence of tumor in animals after 20-methylcholanthrene injection significantly decreased after berberine administration. It was also observed that animals in berberine treatment group had a longer life span than those in control group. When treated with a combination of berberine and NDEA, the markers of liver injury (liver weight, aspartame aminotransferase (AST) and alanine transaminas (ALT) level), serum levels of lipid peroxide, bilirubin and glutamate pyruvate transaminase decreased compared with control group. This study revealed the potential chemical carcinogenesis protection effect of berberine (Anis, Rajeshkumar, & Kuttan, 2001).

The effect of berberine on WEHI-3 leukemia cells *in vivo* was examined in order to understand the berberine action against leukemia. The results showed that Mac-3 and CD11b markers were reduced, which suggested that differentiation inhibition of the macrophages and granulocytes precursors. There was no effect on the CD14 marker but the CD19 marker, which suggested that the promotion of the differentiation of the B-cells precursors. The weights and sizes of spleen from mice treated with berberine were found to be lower when compared to these from untreated animals (F. S. Yu *et al.*, 2007). The treatment with berberine was found to suppress the progression of leukemia induced by FMuLv, which included the effects of elevating the life span of leukemia harboring animals by more than 60 days, decreasing the anemic condition, inhibiting the massive leukemic cell infiltrations to sinusoidal spaces in spleen, decreasing the expression of Bcl-2, Raf-1, Erk-1 IFN-α receptor and erythropoietin and inducing the expression of p53 (Harikumar, Kuttan, & Kuttan, 2008).

Murine xenograft animal models are often used to study the effect of berberine on solid tumor *in vivo*. The anticancer effect of berberine *in vivo* was studied by using the transplanted B16 cancer cell line in a dose range from 1 mg/kg to 10 mg/kg. The significant reduction of tumor volume was observed on day 16 at doses of 5 and 10 mg/kg. The dose of 1 mg/kg stimulated the tumor mass, but other tested concentration, 5 and 10 mg/kg, reduced the tumor weight (Letasiova, Jantova, Muckova, & Theiszova, 2005). In SCC-4 tongue cancer bearing xenograft mice model, treatment with 10mg/kg of berberine resulted in a reduction in tumor incidence. Tumor size in xenograft mice treated with 10mg/kg berberine was significantly smaller than that in the control group. The result of the study showed that berberine may be a potential preventive drug for tongue cancer (Ho, Yang, Lu, *et al.*, 2009). The oral administration of berberine inhibited the growth of A549 (p53+/+) and H1299 (p53 -/-) lung tumors inoculated subcutaneously in athymic nude mice, especially more effective in A549 tumor xenograft mice (58% tumor volume reduction vs. 35% in H1299 at a dose of 100 mg/kg) (Katiyar, Meeran, Katiyar, & Akhtar, 2009a). Berberine also strongly suppressed the growth of human prostate cancer xenograft in mice, in which LNCaP xenografts with p53 expression were more easily affected by apoptotic cell death than those inoculated with p53-deficient PC-3 cells (Choi *et al.*, 2009). A recent study investigated the chemopreventive effects of berberine on intestinal tumor development in Apcmin/+ mice. The result showed that berberine inhibits intestinal tumor development, which is correlated with its activity to suppress tumor cell proliferation and increase apoptosis in Apcmin/+ mice. Down-regulation of Wnt and EGFR signaling pathways and COX-2 expression by berberine may be involved in its anti-tumorigenic effects (Cao *et al.*, 2013).

The anti-cancer effect of combination use of berberine and other anti-cancer drugs on tumor-bearing animal models were investigated in many studies. The chemomodulatory activity of Alstoniascholaris extract (ASE) was studied in combination with berberine hydrochloride (BCL) in Ehrlich ascites carcinoma-bearing mice. The combination of 180 mg/kg of ASE with 8 mg/kg of BCL showed the greatest antitumor effect. More tumor-free survivors and longer median survival time as well as average survival time were observed in combined treatment group (Jagetia & Baliga, 2004). It is a clinical challenge to maintain radio-sensitizing effects in lung cancer treatment. A study showed that the growth of implanted Lewis lung carcinoma inC57BL/6 mice reduced when berberine was given intraperitoneally at 2.0 mg/kg twice weekly combining with irradiation. The underlying mechanism was in consistent with the autophagy-mediated tumor diminishment. The results verified the synergistic cytotoxic effect of berberine and irradiation (Peng, Kuo, Tseng, & Chou, 2008).A study on murine melanoma B16F10 xenograft suggested that combination of berberine and doxorubicin significantly reduced tumor size and tumor weight when compare to control. This drug combination inhibited proliferation and increased apoptosis of cancer cells by reducing PCNA-positive cells and increasing cleaved caspase-3 positive cells (Mittal, Tabasum, & Singh, 2014).

3 Preventive and Curative Effects of Coptidis Rhizoma and Berberine in Hepatocellular Carcinoma: View from Our Studies

Hepatocellular carcinoma (HCC) accounts for most liver cancer. The most common risk factors for HCC include chronic hepatitis B viral (HBV) infection and chronic hepatitis C virus (HCV) infection (Rahbari *et al.*, 2011). Moreover, studies showed that chronic liver injury and live fibrosis are also involved in the progression development of HCC (Baffy, Brunt, & Caldwell, 2012; D. Y. Zhang & Friedman, 2012). However, the prognosis of HCC remains poor since the prevention and treatment for HCC are far more from effective. Our group has conducted several studies to investigate the hepatoprotective effect of *Coptidis Rhizoma* and its major active component, berberine. The anti-cancer effect of berberine was further extensively studied. From our studies, we conclude that *Coptidis Rhizoma* and berberine exhibit potential preventive and curative effects on HCC. *Coptidis Rhizoma* and berberine may prevent HCC by chronic liver injury and liver fibrosis protection, while tumor growth inhibition, anti-angiogenesis, and cancer metastasis suppression may account for their anti-cancer effect.

3.1 Effects of Coptidis Rhizoma and Berberine on Experimental Chronic Liver Injury and Liver Fibrosis

Chronic liver injury may gradually develop into HCC and may be one of the risk factors of HCC. Chronic liver injury leads to insufficiency of liver blood circulation, which is caused by gradually damage of liver blood system, and further induces hypoxia of normal hepatocytes, and then develops into genomic instability (X. Z. Wu, Xie, & Chen, 2007) and consequently leads to tumor genesis. Thus the treatment of liver injury may be an effective way to prevent HCC (Yibin Feng *et al.*, 2009). Many studies have showed that Chinese medicine has a great potential of hepatoprotective effect (Batey, Salmond, & Bensoussan, 2005; Schuppan, Jia, Brinkhaus, & Hahn, 1999) and *Coptidis Rhizoma* is one of them according to our clinical observation and lab study (YB Feng, Luo, & Zhu, 2008).

Here shows one of our experiment studies reporting on the effect and mechanism of berberine and *Coptidis Rhizoma* on chronic liver injury. In order to study the effect of *Coptidis Rhizoma* extract and berberine in diminishing hepatic damage, carbon tetrachloride (CCl4)-induced sustained chronic liver injury rats were used as *in vivo* animal model in our research. Our results indicated that Copitis and berberine acted as potential alternative therapeutic agents for chronic hepatic damage. Significant decrease of serum AST and ALT level combined with increased SOD activities were observed in *Coptidis Rhizoma* extract and berberine treatment group, which indicated that anti-oxidative action may be the underlying mechanism of *Coptidis Rhizoma* and berberine during their hepatoprotective action. Moreover, *Coptidis Rhizoma* extract and berberine significantly reduced apoptosis of hepatocyte through Erk1/2signaling inhibition. The result of our study shed light on the utilization of *Coptidis Rhizoma* and berberine for chronic liver diseases as potential complementary medication to protect hepatocyte form damage (Y. Feng *et al.*, 2010; Ye *et al.*, 2009).

Chronic liver injury, alcohol-induced liver damage, HBV infection and HCV infection are the major causes of liver fibrosis. Eliminating primary disease, modulating immune system, suppressing inflammation, inhibiting ECM protein accumulation and reducing complications are the basic principles in the treatment of liver fibrosis (Friedman, 2007). In the view of Chinese Medicine, blood and toxin stagnation and qi deficiency are the major pathological factors inducing liver fibrosis (Yibin Feng *et al.*, 2009). Chinese Medicines widely used in many Asian countries as one of the complementary and alternative treatment for liver fibrosis in clinical practice.

Our previous studies indicated that aqueous extract of *Coptidis Rhizoma* and its major active compound berberine exhibited potential therapeutic effect on CCl4-induced animal liver injury model (Y. Feng *et al.*, 2010; Ye *et al.*, 2009). The promising result provoked us to investigate the possible therapeutic effect of *Coptidis Rhizoma* extract and berberine on liver fibrosis.

In our study, two different animal models were used to imitate the process of liver fibrosis. In bile duct-ligation (BDL)-induced liver fibrosis model, extra hepatic damage was a vital factor inducing liver fibrosis. In the other alcohol-fed-induced liver fibrosis model, intrahepatic damage mainly led to liver fibrosis. The anti-fibrotic effect of *Coptidis Rhizoma* extract and its major compound berberine were determined by serum AST, ALT and total bilirubin (TBil) level. And the underlying mechanism was elaborated by serum superoxide dismutase (SOD) level. 600 mg/kg *Coptidis Rhizoma* extract and 120 mg/kg berberine were used in our study based on our preliminary observation. Animal behavior after *Coptidis Rhizoma* extract and berberine treatment was observed in the study. The results showed that both *Coptidis Rhizoma* extract and berberine diminished liver fibrosis in experimental hepatic fibrogenic model induced by either bile ductligation or alcohol. Both *Coptidis Rhizoma* extract and berberine could recover SOD activity to avoid the per-oxidation damage, protect normal liver cells from cholestatic damage and assist harmful bilious product excreting from liver. Our study suggested that *Coptidis Rhizoma* and berberine were potential complementary and alternative treatment for liver fibrosis. Results from other study also suggested that berberine exerted hepatoprotective effect. The possible mechanism may be activation of AMPK, blocking Nox4 and Akt expression (Li *et al.*, 2014). Another study showed that berberine could be effective in protecting the liver from acute CCl4-induced injury by inhibiting TNF-α, COX-2, and iNOS expression (Domitrovic, Jakovac, & Blagojevic, 2011). More detail mechanism of berberine's hepatoprotective effect can be referred to Figure 3.

3.2   Effects of Coptidis Rhizoma and Berberine on Proliferation, Angiogenesis and Metastasis in HCC

We've conducted comprehensive study to reveal the cancer cell death types induced by berberine and its underlying mechanisms in HCC. Different cell death types were examined in

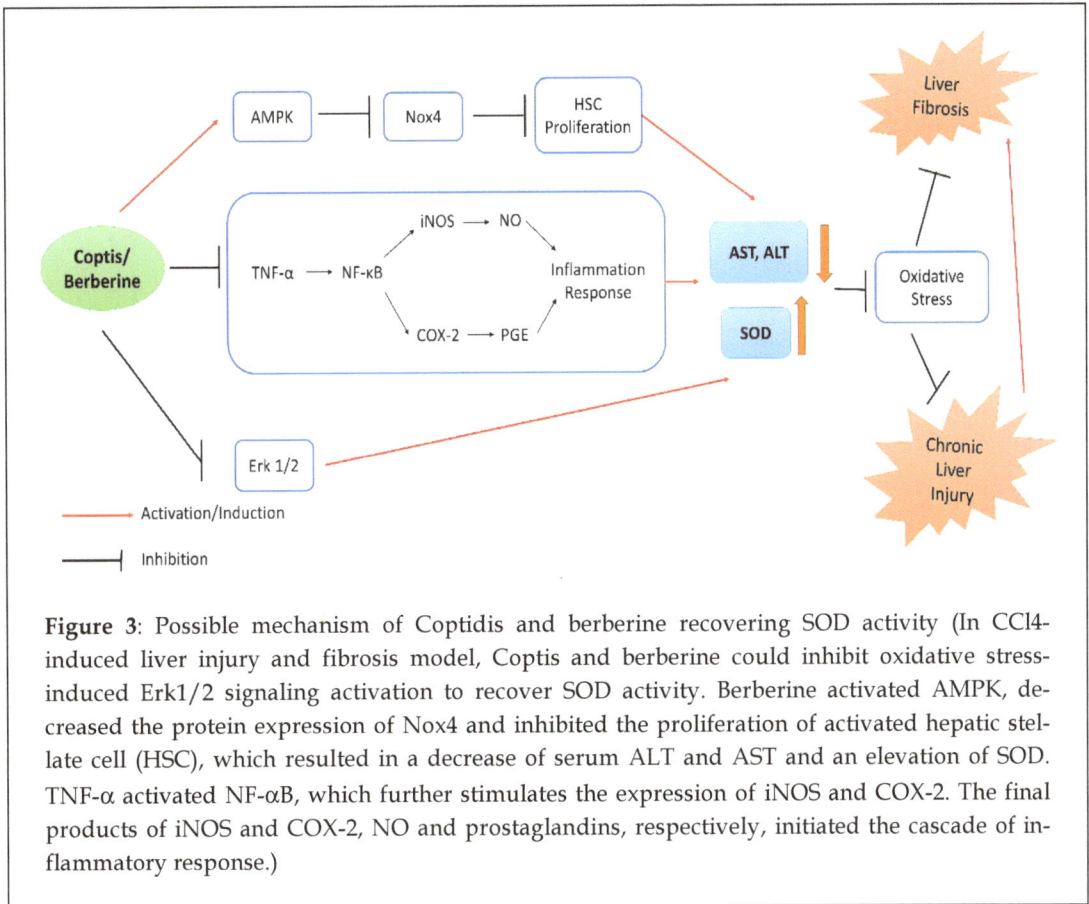

Figure 3: Possible mechanism of Coptidis and berberine recovering SOD activity (In CCl4-induced liver injury and fibrosis model, Coptis and berberine could inhibit oxidative stress-induced Erk1/2 signaling activation to recover SOD activity. Berberine activated AMPK, decreased the protein expression of Nox4 and inhibited the proliferation of activated hepatic stellate cell (HSC), which resulted in a decrease of serum ALT and AST and an elevation of SOD. TNF-α activated NF-αB, which further stimulates the expression of iNOS and COX-2. The final products of iNOS and COX-2, NO and prostaglandins, respectively, initiated the cascade of inflammatory response.)

human hepatic carcinoma cell lines HepG2 and MHCC97-L. The results of our study showed that berberine can induce both apoptosis and autophagic cell death in human hepatocellular carcinoma cells. Interference with cell death inhibitor 3-methyladenine or essential autophagy gene Atg5 diminished berberine-induced cell death in human hepatic carcinoma cells. Mechanism study showed that berberine may activate mitochondrial apoptosis in HepG2 and MHCC97-L cells by increasing Bax expression the formation of permeable transition pores, cytochrome C release to cytosol, and subsequent activation of the caspases-3 and -9 execution pathways. Berberine may also induce autophagic cell death in HepG2 and MHCC97-L cells through activation of Beclin-1 and inhibition of mTOR-signaling pathway by suppressing the activity of Akt and up-regulating P38 MAPK signaling (N. Wang, Feng, Zhu, et al., 2010; N. Wang et al., 2011). Possible mechanism of berberine-induced autophagy in cancer cells was shown in Figure 4.

Studies has showed that angiogenesis is a key factor in the progressive development from chronic liver diseases to HCC (Coulon et al., 2011). In HCC angiogenesis, HIF-1α/VEGF becomes the most common target. To verified anti-cancer effect of berberine or *Coptidis Rhizoma* on HCC, we have conducted studies to exam the action of berberine in HCC angiogenesis.

In our experiment, *Coptidis Rhizoma* aqueous extract (CRAE) was used. To further examine the effect of CRAE on tumor angiogenesis of HCC, we conducted another in-vivo ex

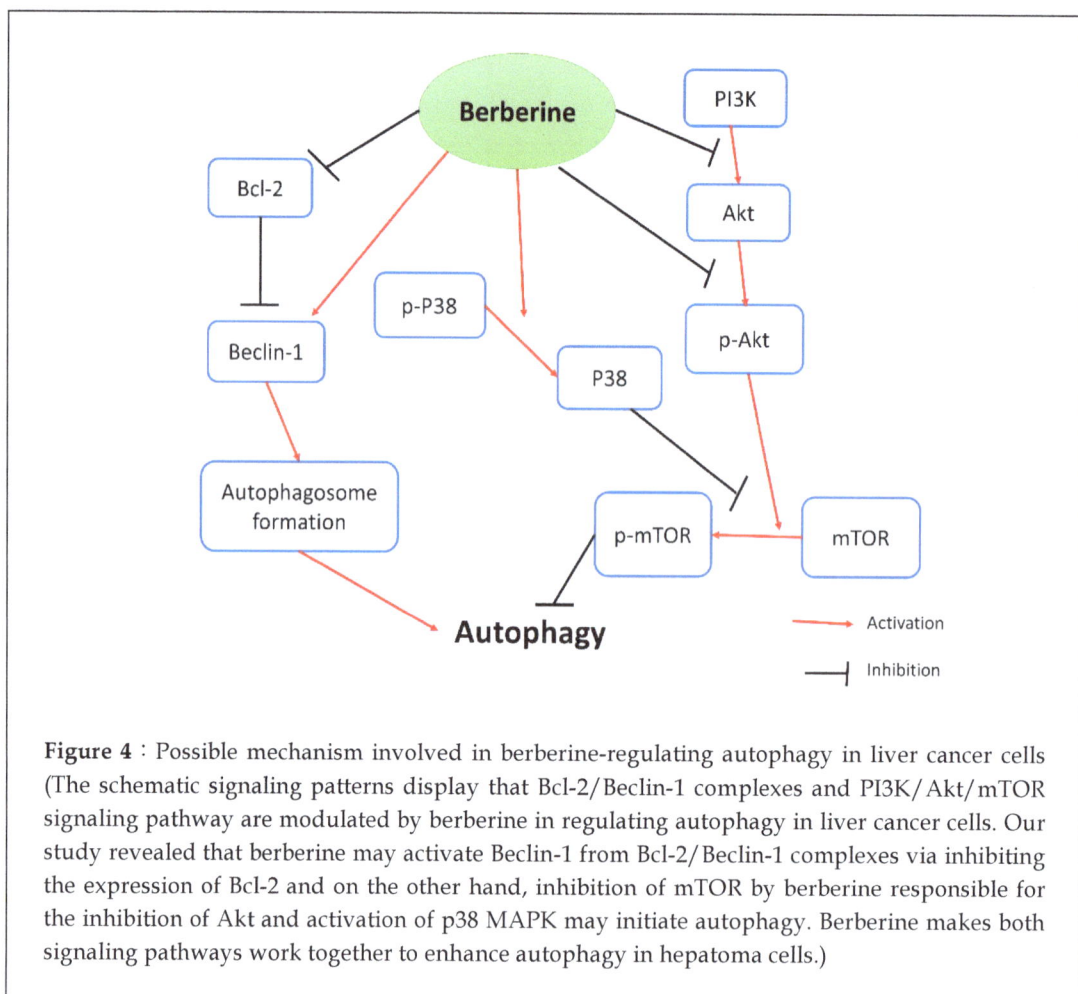

Figure 4 : Possible mechanism involved in berberine-regulating autophagy in liver cancer cells (The schematic signaling patterns display that Bcl-2/Beclin-1 complexes and PI3K/Akt/mTOR signaling pathway are modulated by berberine in regulating autophagy in liver cancer cells. Our study revealed that berberine may activate Beclin-1 from Bcl-2/Beclin-1 complexes via inhibiting the expression of Bcl-2 and on the other hand, inhibition of mTOR by berberine responsible for the inhibition of Akt and activation of p38 MAPK may initiate autophagy. Berberine makes both signaling pathways work together to enhance autophagy in hepatoma cells.)

periment focusing on VEGF. The result of our study showed that CRAE reduced subcutaneous tumor size and neovascularization in MHCC97L hepatocellular carcinoma in xenograft model. VEGF expression was blocked by CRAE at nontoxic dosage. Mechanism study showed that in HCC cells, CRAE suppressed VEGF expression by inhibiting eukaryotic elongation factor 2 (eEF2) and blocking nascent protein synthesis. Moreover, we found that CRAE exerted more inhibitory effect on eEF2 activity than berberine alone; indicating that other compounds in Coptidis Rhizoma may contribute to the inhibitory effect on eEF2.

This study revealed the new molecular mechanism of CRAE regulating VEGF expression at the posttranscriptional level by *Coptidis Rhizoma* and berberine on HCC. The study also suggested *Coptidis Rhizoma* may acts as a potential antiangiogenic agent for HCC (Tan, Wang, Tsao, Zhang, & Feng, 2013). Moreover, our preliminary study showed that Id-1 protein in HCC cells was inhibited by berberine. As previous report, Id-1 induces VEGF by enhancing the stability and activity of HIF-1alpha in human breast cancer cells (H. J. Kim *et al.*, 2007). Previous study also found that Id-1 could stabilize the HIF-1α and increase the VEGF expression in hepatocellular carcinoma cells (T. K. W. Lee *et al.*, 2003). The possible regulatory network of berberine on HCC angiogenesis is shown in Figure 5.

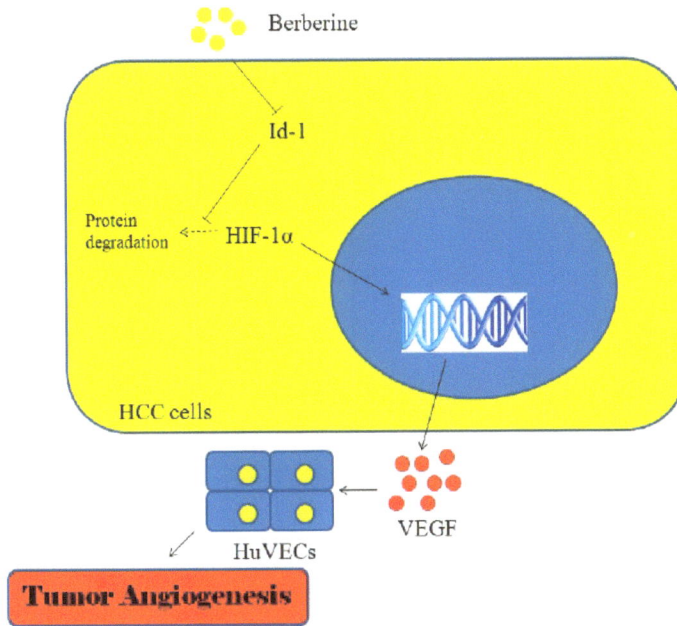

Figure 5 : The regulatory network of berberine on the tumor angiogenesis in HCC.

We also conducted study to investigate the anti-migration and anti-invasion effect of *Coptidis Rhizoma* in human HCC cell. HCC cell line with highly metastatic property, MHCC97-L cells were used in the study. 7 components were identified as berberine-like alkaloids in CRAE by high-performance liquid chromatography combined with mass spectrometry (HPLC/MS). CRAE was found to significantly inhibit cell migration and cell invasion through extracellular matrix. Mechanism study suggested that CRAE did not affect cell adhesion and attachment factors including E-cadherin/N-cadherin ratio, integrin β4 and had no effect on the expression of migration and invasion related molecules like uPA and MMPs. Interestingly, we discovered that CRAE suppressed MHCC97-L cell motility by acting on F-actin to induce filament reorganization, which may be induced by berberine's inhibitory action on RhoA/ROCK1 signaling. The inactivation of the Rho/ROCK signaling pathway involved in CRAE's inhibitory action onMHCC97-L migration indicated CRAE's role as a Rho-small GTPase inhibitor. This study sheds light on CRAE as an alternative therapy for the treatment of metastatic hepatic carcinoma (N. Wang, Feng, Lau, *et al.*, 2010).

3.3   Effect of Coptidis Rhizoma and Berberine on Epigenetics of Liver Cancer Cells

Micro RNAs (miRNAs), which was first reported in 1993 (R. C. Lee, Feinbaum, & Ambros, 1993), are single-stranded RNA molecules regulating gene expression at either the transcriptional or post-transcriptional level (Ruvkun, 2001). Studies showed that the expression patterns of microRNAs in liver tissue differ between men and women with hepatocellular carcinoma. Patients whose tumors had low miR-26 expression had shorter overall survival but a better response to interferon therapy than did patients whose tumors had high expression of the microRNA (Ji *et al.*, 2009). These finding indicates that miRNAs may play a vital role in carcinogenesis as a novel class of oncogenes or tumor-suppressor genes (L. He *et al.*, 2005). Thus, miRNAs have been considered as novel targets for cancer therapy. We have conducted a study to examine the effect of *Coptidis Rhizoma* on miRNA.

In our study, HCC MHHCC-97L cells were treated with CRAE. After treatment, a sensitive miRNA on-chip array was used to examine the variation in the miRNA expression profile. After 48h exposure to 175 µg/mlof CRAE, overexpression of miR-21 and miR-23a in MHCC-97L cells was detected. The modified expression of miRNAs affected several tumor-suppressor genes. The analysis of PicTar and TargetScan databases suggested that CRAE modified several signal transduction pathways by miRNA expression. We concluded from this study that CRAE may be a potential therapeutic agent targeting miRNAs in HCC cells (Zhu *et al.*, 2011).

4   Summary

Both *In vitro* and *in vivo* studies proved the anti-cancer properties of *Coptidis Rhizoma* and berberine in preventing carcinogenesis, inhibiting proliferation, inducing apoptosis, suppressing cancer angiogenesis and inhibiting metastasis and invasion. However, all the evidence comes from bench experiments, clinical potential of *Coptidis Rhizoma* and berberine still remains unknown. Therefore, further researches are still warranted and more advanced approaches are in need to transfer the anti-cancer properties of *Coptidis Rhizoma* and berberine from bench side to clinical practice.

Reference

Amin, A. H., Subbaiah, T. V., & Abbasi, K. M. (1969). Berberine sulfate: antimicrobial activity, bioassay, and mode of action. Can J Microbiol, 15(9), 1067-1076.

Anis, K. V., Rajeshkumar, N. V., & Kuttan, R. (2001). Inhibition of chemical carcinogenesis by berberine in rats and mice. Journal of Pharmacy and Pharmacology, 53(5), 763-768. doi: Doi 10.1211/0022357011775901

Baffy, G., Brunt, E. M., & Caldwell, S. H. (2012). Hepatocellular carcinoma in non-alcoholic fatty liver disease: an emerging menace. J Hepatol, 56(6), 1384-1391. doi: 10.1016/j.jhep.2011.10.027

Batey, R. G., Salmond, S. J., & Bensoussan, A. (2005). Complementary and alternative medicine in the treatment of chronic liver disease. Curr Gastroenterol Rep, 7(1), 63-70.

Boberek, J. M., Stach, J., & Good, L. (2010). Genetic Evidence for Inhibition of Bacterial Division Protein FtsZ by Berberine. Plos One, 5(10). doi: ARTN e13745

DOI 10.1371/journal.pone.0013745

Burgeiro, A., Gajate, C., Dakir el, H., Villa-Pulgarin, J. A., Oliveira, P. J., & Mollinedo, F. (2011). Involvement of mitochondrial and B-RAF/ERK signaling pathways in berberine-induced apoptosis in human melanoma cells. Anticancer Drugs, 22(6), 507-518. doi: 10.1097/CAD.0b013e32834438f6

Cao, H., Song, S., Zhang, H., Zhang, Y., Qu, R., Yang, B., . . . Wang, B. (2013). Chemopreventive effects of berberine on intestinal tumor development in Apcmin/+ mice. BMC Gastroenterol, 13, 163. doi: 10.1186/1471-230x-13-163

Choi, M. S., Oh, J. H., Kim, S. M., Jung, H. Y., Yoo, H. S., Lee, Y. M., . . . Hong, J. T. (2009). Berberine inhibits p53-dependent cell growth through induction of apoptosis of prostate cancer cells. International Journal of Oncology, 34(5), 1221-1230. doi: Doi 10.3892/ljo_00000250

Choi, M. S., Yuk, D. Y., Oh, J. H., Jung, H. Y., Han, S. B., Moon, D. C., & Hong, J. T. (2008). Berberine Inhibits Human

Neuroblastoma Cell Growth through Induction of p53-dependent Apoptosis. Anticancer Res, 28(6A), 3777-3784.

Coulon, S., Heindryckx, F., Geerts, A., Van Steenkiste, C., Colle, I., & Van Vlierberghe, H. (2011). *Angiogenesis in chronic liver disease and its complications. Liver International, 31(2), 146-162. doi: DOI 10.1111/j.1478-3231.2010.02369.x*

Dharmananda, S. (2005). *New Uses of Berberine: a Valuable Alkaloid from Herbs for" damp-heat" Syndromes: ITM.*

Domitrovic, R., Jakovac, H., & Blagojevic, G. (2011). *Hepatoprotective activity of berberine is mediated by inhibition of TNF-alpha, COX-2, and iNOS expression in CCl4-intoxicated mice. Toxicology, 280(1-2), 33-43. doi: DOI 10.1016/j.tox.2010.11.005*

Enk, R., Ehehalt, R., Graham, J. E., Bierhaus, A., Remppis, A., & Greten, H. J. (2007). *Differential effect of Rhizoma coptidis and its main alkaloid compound berberine on TNF-alpha induced NF kappa B translocation in human keratinocytes. J Ethnopharmacol, 109(1), 170-175. doi: DOI 10.1016/j.jep.2006.07.013*

Fan, L. X., Liu, C. M., Gao, A. H., Zhou, Y. B., & Li, J. (2013). *Berberine combined with 2-deoxy-d-glucose synergistically enhances cancer cell proliferation inhibition via energy depletion and unfolded protein response disruption. Biochim Biophys Acta, 1830(11), 5175-5183. doi: 10.1016/j.bbagen.2013.07.010*

Feng, Y., Cheung, K.-F., Wang, N., Liu, P., Nagamatsu, T., & Tong, Y. (2009). *Chinese medicines as a resource for liver fibrosis treatment.(Review)(Report). Chinese Medicine, 4, 16.*

Feng, Y., Luo, W., & Zhu, S. (2008). *[Explore new clinical application of Huanglian and corresponding compound prescriptions from their traditional use]. Zhongguo Zhong yao za zhi= Zhongguo zhongyao zazhi= China journal of Chinese materia medica, 33(10), 1221-1225.*

Feng, Y., Siu, K. Y., Ye, X., Wang, N., Yuen, M. F., Leung, C. H., . . . Kobayashi, S. (2010). *Hepatoprotective effects of berberine on carbon tetrachloride-induced acute hepatotoxicity in rats. Chin Med, 5, 33. doi: 10.1186/1749-8546-5-33*

Franzblau, S. G., & Cross, C. (1986). *Comparative in vitro antimicrobial activity of Chinese medicinal herbs. J Ethnopharmacol, 15(3), 279-288.*

Friedman, S. L. (2007). *Liver fibrosis: from mechanisms to treatment. Gastroenterol Clin Biol, 31(10), 812-814.*

Fukuda, K., Hibiya, Y., Mutoh, M., Koshiji, M., Akao, S., & Fujiwara, H. (1999a). *Inhibition by berberine of cyclooxygenase-2 transcriptional activity in human colon cancer cells. J Ethnopharmacol, 66(2), 227-233.*

Fukuda, K., Hibiya, Y., Mutoh, M., Koshiji, M., Akao, S., & Fujiwara, H. (1999b). *Inhibition of activator protein 1 activity by berberine in human hepatoma cells. Planta Medica, 65(4), 381-383. doi: 10.1055/s-2006-960795*

Gagliano, N., Moscheni, C., Torri, C., Donetti, E., Magnani, I., Costa, F., . . . Gioia, M. (2007). *Ukrain modulates glial fibrillary acidic protein, but not connexin 43 expression, and induces apoptosis in human cultured glioblastoma cells. Anticancer Drugs, 18(6), 669-676. doi: 10.1097/CAD.0b013e32808bf9ec*

Galle, K., Blodt, S., & Wagner, H. (1994). *TLC and HPLC detection of alkaloids in Mahonia aquifolium and related plants. Deutsche Apotheker Zeitung, 134, 35.*

Gao, J. L., Shi, J. M., Lee, S. M. Y., Zhang, Q. W., & Wang, Y. T. (2009). *Angiogenic Pathway Inhibition of Corydalis yanhusuo and Berberine in Human Umbilical Vein Endothelial Cells. Oncology Research, 17(11-12), 519-526.*

Gentry, E. J., Jampani, H. B., Keshavarz-Shokri, A., Morton, M. D., Velde, D. V., Telikepalli, H., . . . Baker, W. (1998). *Antitubercular natural products: berberine from the roots of commercial Hydrastis canadensis powder. Isolation of inactive 8-oxotetrahydrothalifendine, canadine, beta-hydrastine, and two new quinic acid esters, hycandinic acid esters-1 and -2. J Nat Prod, 61(10), 1187-1193. doi: 10.1021/np9701889*

Grippa, E., Valla, R., Battinelli, L., Mazzanti, G., Saso, L., & Silvestrini, B. (1999). *Inhibition of Candida rugosa lipase by berberine and structurally related alkaloids, evaluated by high-performance liquid chromatography. Biosci Biotechnol Biochem, 63(9), 1557-1562.*

Grycová, L., Dostál, J., & Marek, R. (2007). *Quaternary protoberberine alkaloids. Phytochemistry, 68(2), 150-175.*

Hamsa, T. P., & Kuttan, G. (2012a). *Antiangiogenic activity of berberine is mediated through the downregulation of hypoxia-inducible factor-1, VEGF, and proinflammatory mediators. Drug and Chemical Toxicology, 35(1), 57-70. doi: Doi 10.3109/01480545.2011.589437*

Hamsa, T. P., & Kuttan, G. (2012b). *Berberine inhibits pulmonary metastasis through down-regulation of MMP in metastatic B16F-10 melanoma cells. Phytother Res, 26(4), 568-578. doi: 10.1002/ptr.3586*

Hano, K. (1959). *The carcinostatic effects of some plant components and their related compounds. Acta-Unio Internationalis*

Contra Cancrum, 15, 122.

Harikumar, K. B., Kuttan, G., & Kuttan, R. (2008). *Inhibition of progression of erythroleukemia induced by Friend virus in BALB/c mice by natural products--berberine, curcumin and picroliv. J Exp Ther Oncol, 7(4), 275-284.*

Hayashi, K., Minoda, K., Nagaoka, Y., Hayashi, T., & Uesato, S. (2007). *Antiviral activity of berberine and related compounds against human cytomegalovirus. Bioorganic & medicinal chemistry letters, 17(6), 1562-1564.*

He, L., Thomson, J. M., Hemann, M. T., Hernando-Monge, E., Mu, D., Goodson, S., . . . Hammond, S. M. (2005). *A microRNA polycistron as a potential human oncogene. Nature, 435(7043), 828-833. doi: Doi 10.1038/Nature03552*

He, W., Wang, B., Zhuang, Y., Shao, D., Sun, K., & Chen, J. (2012). *Berberine inhibits growth and induces G1 arrest and apoptosis in human cholangiocarcinoma QBC939 cells. J Pharmacol Sci, 119(4), 341-348.*

Ho, Y. T., Yang, J. S., Li, T. C., Lin, J. J., Lin, J. G., Lai, K. C., . . . Chung, J. G. (2009). *Berberine suppresses in vitro migration and invasion of human SCC-4 tongue squamous cancer cells through the inhibitions of FAK, IKK, NF-kappa B, u-PA and MMP-2 and-9. Cancer Letters, 279(2), 155-162. doi: DOI 10.1016/j.canlet.2009.01.033*

Ho, Y. T., Yang, J. S., Lu, C. C., Chiang, J. H., Li, T. C., Lin, J. J., . . . Chung, J. G. (2009). *Berberine inhibits human tongue squamous carcinoma cancer tumor growth in a murine xenograft model. Phytomedicine, 16(9), 887-890. doi: 10.1016/j.phymed.2009.02.015*

Hsu, W. H., Hsieh, Y. S., Kuo, H. C., Teng, C. Y., Huang, H. I., Wang, C. J., . . . Kuo, W. H. (2007). *Berberine induces apoptosis in SW620 human colonic carcinoma cells through generation of reactive oxygen species and activation of JNK/p38 MAPK and FasL. Archives of Toxicology, 81(10), 719-728. doi: DOI 10.1007/s00204-006-0169-y*

Hu, H. Y., Li, K. P., Wang, X. J., Liu, Y., Lu, Z. G., Dong, R. H., . . . Zhang, M. X. (2013). *Set9, NF-kappaB, and microRNA-21 mediate berberine-induced apoptosis of human multiple myeloma cells. Acta Pharmacol Sin, 34(1), 157-166. doi: 10.1038/aps.2012.161*

Hu, W., Yu, L., & Wang, M. H. (2011). *Antioxidant and antiproliferative properties of water extract from Mahonia bealei (Fort.) Carr. leaves. Food Chem Toxicol, 49(4), 799-806. doi: 10.1016/j.fct.2010.12.001*

Hu, W. C., Yu, L. L., & Wang, M. H. (2011). *Antioxidant and antiproliferative properties of water extract from Mahonia bealei (Fort.) Carr. leaves. Food and Chemical Toxicology, 49(4), 799-806. doi: DOI 10.1016/j.fct.2010.12.001*

Hur, J. M., Hyun, M. S., Lim, S. Y., Lee, W. Y., & Kim, D. (2009). *The Combination of Berberine and Irradiation Enhances Anti-Cancer Effects Via Activation of p38 MAPK Pathway and ROS Generation in Human Hepatoma Cells. Journal of Cellular Biochemistry, 107(5), 955-964. doi: Doi 10.1002/Jcb.22198*

Hwang, J. M., Kuo, H. C., Tseng, T. H., Liu, J. Y., & Chu, C. Y. (2006). *Berberine induces apoptosis through a mitochondria/caspases pathway in human hepatoma cells. Archives of Toxicology, 80(2), 62-73. doi: DOI 10.1007/s00204-005-0014-8*

Iizuka, N., Miyamoto, K., Okita, K., Tangoku, A., Hayashi, H., Yosino, S., . . . Oka, M. (2000). *Inhibitory effect of Coptidis Rhizoma and berberine on the proliferation of human esophageal cancer cell lines. Cancer Letters, 148(1), 19-25. doi: Doi 10.1016/S0304-3835(99)00264-5*

Iizuka, N., Oka, M., Yamamoto, K., Taruoku, A., Miyamoto, K., Miyamoto, T., . . . Okita, K. (2003). *Identification of common or distinct genes related to antitumor activities of a medicinal herb and its major component by oligonucleotide microarray. International Journal of Cancer, 107(4), 666-672. doi: Doi 10.1002/Ijc.11452*

Jagetia, G. C., & Baliga, M. S. (2004). *Effect of Alstonia scholaris in enhancing the anticancer activity of berberine in the Ehrlich ascites carcinoma-bearing mice. J Med Food, 7(2), 235-244. doi: 10.1089/1096620041224094*

Jantova, S., Cipak, L., Cernakova, M., & Kost'alova, D. (2003). *Effect of berberine on proliferation, cell cycle and apoptosis in HeLa and L1210 cells. Journal of Pharmacy and Pharmacology, 55(8), 1143-1149. doi: Doi 10.1211/0022357021422*

Ji, J. F., Shi, J., Budhu, A., Yu, Z. P., Forgues, M., Roessler, S., . . . Wang, X. W. (2009). *MicroRNA Expression, Survival, and Response to Interferon in Liver Cancer. New England Journal of Medicine, 361(15), 1437-1447. doi: Doi 10.1056/Nejmoa0901282*

Jie, S. H., Li, H. Y., Tian, Y. A., Guo, D. M., Zhu, J. A., Gao, S. Y., & Jiang, L. (2011). *Berberine inhibits angiogenic potential of Hep G2 cell line through VEGF down-regulation in vitro. J Gastroenterol Hepatol, 26(1), 179-185. doi: DOI 10.1111/j.1440-1746.2010.06389.x*

Katiyar, S. K., Meeran, S. M., Katiyar, N., & Akhtar, S. (2009a). *p53 Cooperates berberine-induced growth inhibition and apoptosis of non-small cell human lung cancer cells in vitro and tumor xenograft growth in vivo. Mol Carcinog, 48(1), 24-*

37. doi: 10.1002/mc.20453

Katiyar, S. K., Meeran, S. M., Katiyar, N., & Akhtar, S. (2009b). p53 Cooperates Berberine-Induced Growth Inhibition and Apoptosis of Non-Small Cell Human Lung Cancer Cells In Vitro and Tumor Xenograft Growth In Vivo. Mol Carcinog, 48(1), 24-37. doi: Doi 10.1002/Mc.20453

Kettmann, V., Kostalova, D., Jantova, S., Cernakova, M., & Drimal, J. (2004). In vitro cytotoxicity of berberine against HeLa and L1210 cancer cell lines. Pharmazie, 59(7), 548-551.

Kim, H. J., Chung, H., Yoo, Y. G., Kim, H., Lee, J. Y., Lee, M. O., & Kong, G. (2007). Inhibitor of DNA binding 1 activates vascular endothelial growth factor through enhancing the stability and activity of hypoxia-inducible factor-1 alpha. Molecular Cancer Research, 5(4), 321-329. doi: Doi 10.1158/1541-7786.Mcr-06-0218

Kim, H. S., Kim, M. J., Kim, E. J., Yang, Y., Lee, M. S., & Lim, J. S. (2012). Berberine-induced AMPK activation inhibits the metastatic potential of melanoma cells via reduction of ERK activity and COX-2 protein expression. Biochem Pharmacol, 83(3), 385-394. doi: 10.1016/j.bcp.2011.11.008

Kim, J. B., Yu, J. H., Ko, E., Lee, K. W., Song, A. K., Park, S. Y., . . . Noh, D. Y. (2010). The alkaloid Berberine inhibits the growth of Anoikis-resistant MCF-7 and MDA-MB-231 breast cancer cell lines by inducing cell cycle arrest. Phytomedicine, 17(6), 436-440. doi: 10.1016/j.phymed.2009.08.012

Kim, J. H., Campbell, B. C., Mahoney, N., Chan, K. L., Molyneux, R. J., & May, G. S. (2007). Enhanced activity of strobilurin and fludioxonil by using berberine and phenolic compounds to target fungal antioxidative stress response. Letters in Applied Microbiology, 45(2), 134-141. doi: DOI 10.1111/j.1472-765X.2007.02159.x

Kim, S., Choi, J. H., Bin Kim, J., Nam, S. J., Yang, J. H., Kim, J. H., & Lee, J. E. (2008). Berberine Suppresses TNF-alpha-induced MMP-9 and Cell Invasion through Inhibition of AP-1 Activity in MDA-MB-231 Human Breast Cancer Cells. Molecules, 13(12), 2975-2985. doi: DOI 10.3390/molecules13122975

Kim, S., Kim, Y., Kim, J. E., Cho, K. H., & Chung, J. H. (2008). Berberine inhibits TPA-induced MMP-9 and IL-6 expression in normal human keratinocytes. Phytomedicine, 15(5), 340-347. doi: DOI 10.1016/j.phymed.2007.09.011

Kim, S., Oh, S. J., Lee, J., Han, J., Jeon, M., Jung, T., . . . Nam, S. J. (2013). Berberine Suppresses TPA-Induced Fibronectin Expression through the Inhibition of VEGF Secretion in Breast Cancer Cells. Cellular Physiology and Biochemistry, 32(5), 1541-1550. doi: Doi 10.1159/000356591

Kim, S. M., & Chung, J. H. (2008). Berberine prevents UV-induced MMP-1 and reduction of type I procollagen expression in human dermal fibroblasts. Phytomedicine, 15(9), 749-753. doi: DOI 10.1016/j.phymed.2007.11.004

Kong, W., Li, Z., Xiao, X., & Zhao, Y. (2010). Microcalorimetric investigation of the toxic action of berberine on Tetrahymena thermophila BF(5). J Basic Microbiol, 50(5), 436-441. doi: 10.1002/jobm.201000017

Kowalewski, Z., Kedzia, W., & Mirska, I. (1972). The effect of berberine sulfate on staphylococci. Arch Immunol Ther Exp (Warsz), 20(3), 353-360.

Kuo, C. L., Chi, C. W., & Liu, T. Y. (2005a). Modulation of apoptosis by berberine through inhibition of cyclooxygenase-2 and Mcl-1 expression in oral cancer cells. In Vivo, 19(1), 247-252.

Kuo, C. L., Chi, C. W., & Liu, T. Y. (2005b). Modulation of apoptosis by berberine through inhibition of cyclooxygenase-2 and Mcl-1 expression in oral cancer cells. In Vivo, 19(1), 247-252.

Lavanchy, D. (2004). Hepatitis B virus epidemiology, disease burden, treatment, and current and emerging prevention and control measures. J Viral Hepat, 11(2), 97-107.

Lee, R. C., Feinbaum, R. L., & Ambros, V. (1993). The C-Elegans Heterochronic Gene Lin-4 Encodes Small Rnas with Antisense Complementarity to Lin-14. Cell, 75(5), 843-854. doi: Doi 10.1016/0092-8674(93)90529-Y

Lee, T. K. W., Man, K., Ling, M. T., Wang, X. H., Wong, Y. C., Lo, C. M., . . . Fan, S. T. (2003). Over-expression of Id-1 induces cell proliferation in hepatocellular carcinoma through inactivation of p16(INK4a)/RB pathway. Carcinogenesis, 24(11), 1729-1736. doi: DOI 10.1093/carcin/bgg145

Letasiova, S., Jantova, S., Cipak, L., & Muckova, M. (2006). Berberine - antiproliferative activity in vitro and induction of apoptosis/necrosis of the U937 and B16 cells. Cancer Letters, 239(2), 254-262. doi: DOI 10.1016/j.canlet.2005.08.024

Letasiova, S., Jantova, S., Muckova, M., & Theiszova, M. (2005). Antiproliferative activity of berberine in vitro and in vivo. Biomed Pap Med Fac Univ Palacky Olomouc Czech Repub, 149(2), 461-463.

Li, H. L., Han, T., Liu, R. H., Zhang, C., Chen, H. S., & Zhang, W. D. (2008). Alkaloids from Corydalis saxicola and their anti-

hepatitis B virus activity. Chemistry & Biodiversity, 5(5), 777-783. doi: DOI 10.1002/cbdv.200890074

Li, H. Y., Guo, L. L., Jie, S. H., Liu, W., Zhu, J., Du, W., . . . Huang, S. (2008). *Berberine inhibits SDF-1-induced AML cells and leukemic stem cells migration via regulation of SDF-1 level in bone marrow stromal cells. Biomedicine & Pharmacotherapy, 62(9), 573-578. doi: DOI 10.1016/j.biopha.2008.08.003*

Li, J., Gu, L., Zhang, H., Liu, T., Tian, D., Zhou, M., & Zhou, S. (2013). *Berberine represses DAXX gene transcription and induces cancer cell apoptosis. Lab Invest, 93(3), 354-364. doi: 10.1038/labinvest.2012.172*

Li, J., Pan, Y., Kan, M. J., Xiao, X. N., Wang, Y. J., Guan, F. Y., . . . Chen, L. (2014). *Hepatoprotective effects of berberine on liver fibrosis via activation of AMP-activated protein kinase. Life Sci, 98(1), 24-30. doi: DOI 10.1016/j.lfs.2013.12.211*

Lin, C. C., Kao, S. T., Chen, G. W., Ho, H. C., & Chung, J. G. (2006). *Apoptosis of human leukemia HL-60 cells and murine leukemia WEHI-3 cells induced by berberine through the activation of caspase-3. Anticancer Res, 26(1A), 227-242.*

Lin, J. P., Yang, J. S., Chang, N. W., Chiu, T. H., Su, C. C., Lu, K. W., . . . Chung, J. G. (2007). *GADD153 mediates berberine-induced apoptosis in human cervical cancer Ca Ski cells. Anticancer Res, 27(5A), 3379-3386.*

Lin, J. P., Yang, J. S., Lee, J. H., Hsieh, W. T., & Chung, J. G. (2006). *Berberine induces cell cycle arrest and apoptosis in human gastric carcinoma SNU-5 cell line. World Journal of Gastroenterology, 12(1), 21-28.*

Lin, J. P., Yang, J. S., Wu, C. C., Lin, S. S., Hsieh, W. T., Lin, M. L., . . . Chung, J. G. (2008). *Berberine induced down-regulation of matrix metalloproteinase-1, -2 and -9 in human gastric cancer cells (SNU-5) in vitro. In Vivo, 22(2), 223-230.*

Lin, S. K., Tsai, S. C., Lee, C. C., Wang, B. W., Liou, J. Y., & Shyu, K. G. (2004). *Berberine inhibits HIF-1 alpha expression via enhanced proteolysis. Molecular Pharmacology, 66(3), 612-619.*

Lin, T. H., Kuo, H. C., Chou, F. P., & Lu, F. J. (2008). *Berberine enhances inhibition of glioma tumor cell migration and invasiveness mediated by arsenic trioxide. Bmc Cancer, 8. doi: Artn 58*

Doi 10.1186/1471-2407-8-58

Liu, S. J., Sun, Y. M., Tian, D. F., He, Y. C., Zeng, L., He, Y., . . . Sun, S. H. (2008). *Downregulated NM23-H1 expression is associated with intracranial invasion of nasopharyngeal carcinoma. British Journal of Cancer, 98(2), 363-369. doi: DOI 10.1038/sj.bjc.6604167*

Liu, Z. J., Liu, Q., Xu, B., Wu, J. J., Guo, C., Zhub, F. L., . . . Shao, C. S. (2009). *Berberine induces p53-dependent cell cycle arrest and apoptosis of human osteosarcoma cells by inflicting DNA damage. Mutation Research-Fundamental and Molecular Mechanisms of Mutagenesis, 662(1-2), 75-83. doi: DOI 10.1016/j.mrfmmm.2008.12.009*

Lu, B. A., Hu, M. M., Liu, K. X., & Peng, J. Y. (2010). *Cytotoxicity of berberine on human cervical carcinoma HeLa cells through mitochondria, death receptor and MAPK pathways, and in-silico drug-target prediction. Toxicology in Vitro, 24(6), 1482-1490. doi: DOI 10.1016/j.tiv.2010.07.017*

Mahady, G. B., Pendland, S. L., Stoia, A., & Chadwick, L. R. (2003). *In vitro susceptibility of Helicobacter pylori to isoquinoline alkaloids from Sanguinaria canadensis and Hydrastis canadensis. Phytother Res, 17(3), 217-221. doi: 10.1002/ptr.1108*

Mahata, S., Bharti, A. C., Shukla, S., Tyagi, A., Husain, S. A., & Das, B. C. (2011). *Berberine modulates AP-1 activity to suppress HPV transcription and downstream signaling to induce growth arrest and apoptosis in cervical cancer cells. Molecular Cancer, 10, 39. doi: 10.1186/1476-4598-10-39*

Mantena, S. K., Sharma, S. D., & Katiyar, S. K. (2006a). *Berberine inhibits growth, induces G1 arrest and apoptosis in human epidermoid carcinoma A431 cells by regulating Cdki-Cdk-cyclin cascade, disruption of mitochondrial membrane potential and cleavage of caspase 3 and PARP. Carcinogenesis, 27(10), 2018-2027. doi: 10.1093/carcin/bgl043*

Mantena, S. K., Sharma, S. D., & Katiyar, S. K. (2006b). *Berberine, a natural product, induces G1-phase cell cycle arrest and caspase-3-dependent apoptosis in human prostate carcinoma cells. Mol Cancer Ther, 5(2), 296-308. doi: 10.1158/1535-7163.MCT-05-0448*

Mittal, A., Tabasum, S., & Singh, R. P. (2014). *Berberine in combination with doxorubicin suppresses growth of murine melanoma B16F10 cells in culture and xenograft. Phytomedicine, 21(3), 340-347. doi: 10.1016/j.phymed.2013.09.002*

Nishino, H., Kitagawa, K., Fujiki, H., & Iwashima, A. (1986). *Berberine sulfate inhibits tumor-promoting activity of teleocidin in two-stage carcinogenesis on mouse skin. Oncology, 43(2), 131-134.*

Park, J. J., Seo, S. M., Kim, E. J., Lee, Y. J., Ko, Y. G., Ha, J., & Lee, M. (2012). *Berberine inhibits human colon cancer cell migration via AMP-activated protein kinase-mediated downregulation of integrin beta1 signaling. Biochem Biophys Res*

Commun, 426(4), 461-467. doi: 10.1016/j.bbrc.2012.08.091

Park, K. S., Kim, J. B., Bae, J., Park, S. Y., Jee, H. G., Lee, K. E., & Youn, Y. K. (2012a). *Berberine inhibited the growth of thyroid cancer cell lines 8505C and TPC1. Yonsei Med J, 53(2), 346-351. doi: 10.3349/ymj.2012.53.2.346*

Park, K. S., Kim, J. B., Lee, S. J., & Bae, J. (2012b). *Berberine-induced growth inhibition of epithelial ovarian carcinoma cell lines. J Obstet Gynaecol Res, 38(3), 535-540. doi: 10.1111/j.1447-0756.2011.01743.x*

Pazhang, Y., Ahmadian, S., Javadifar, N., & Shafiezadeh, M. (2012). *COX-2 and survivin reduction may play a role in berberine-induced apoptosis in human ductal breast epithelial tumor cell line. Tumour Biol, 33(1), 207-214. doi: 10.1007/s13277-011-0263-5*

Pazhang, Y., Ahmadian, S., Mahmoudian, M., & Shafiezadeh, M. (2011a). *Berberine-induced apoptosis via decreasing the survivin protein in K562 cell line. Med Oncol, 28(4), 1577-1583. doi: 10.1007/s12032-010-9586-0*

Pazhang, Y., Ahmadian, S., Mahmoudian, M., & Shafiezadeh, M. (2011b). *Berberine-induced apoptosis via decreasing the survivin protein in K562 cell line. Med Oncol, 28(4), 1577-1583. doi: DOI 10.1007/s12032-010-9586-0*

Peng, P. L., Hsieh, Y. S., Wang, C. J., Hsu, J. L., & Chou, F. P. (2006). *Inhibitory effect of berberine on the invasion of human lung cancer cells via decreased productions of urokinase-plasminogen activator and matrix metalloproteinase-2. Toxicology and Applied Pharmacology, 214(1), 8-15. doi: DOI 10.1016/j.taap.2005.11.010*

Peng, P. L., Kuo, W. H., Tseng, H. C., & Chou, F. P. (2008). *Synergistic tumor-killing effect of radiation and berberine combined treatment in lung cancer: the contribution of autophagic cell death. Int J Radiat Oncol Biol Phys, 70(2), 529-542. doi: 10.1016/j.ijrobp.2007.08.034*

Pereira, G. C., Branco, A. F., Matos, J. A. C., Pereira, S. L., Parke, D., Perkins, E. L., . . . Oliveira, P. J. (2007). *Mitochondrially targeted effects of berberine [natural yellow 18, 5,6-dihydro-9,10-dimethoxybenzo(g)-1,3-benzodioxolo(5,6-a) quinolizinium] on K1735-M2 mouse melanoma cells: Comparison with direct effects on isolated mitochondrial fractions. Journal of Pharmacology and Experimental Therapeutics, 323(2), 636-649. doi: DOI 10.1124/jpet.107.128017*

Pinto-Garcia, L., Efferth, T., Torres, A., Hoheisel, J. D., & Youns, M. (2010). *Berberine Inhibits Cell Growth and Mediates Caspase-Independent Cell Death in Human Pancreatic Cancer Cells. Planta Medica, 76(11), 1155-1161. doi: DOI 10.1055/s-0030-1249931*

Piyanuch, R., Sukhthankar, M., Wandee, G., & Baek, S. J. (2007). *Berberine, a natural isoquinoline alkaloid, induces NAG-1 and ATF3 expression in human colorectal cancer cells. Cancer Letters, 258(2), 230-240. doi: DOI 10.1016/j.canlet.2007.09.007*

Qi, H. W., Xin, L. Y., Xu, X., Ji, X. X., & Fan, L. H. (2014). *Epithelial-to-mesenchymal transition markers to predict response of Berberine in suppressing lung cancer invasion and metastasis. J Transl Med, 12, 22. doi: 10.1186/1479-5876-12-22*

Quan, H., Cao, Y. Y., Xu, Z., Zhao, J. X., Gao, P. H., Qin, X. F., & Jiang, Y. Y. (2006). *Potent in vitro synergism of fluconazole and berberine chloride against clinical isolates of Candida albicans resistant to fluconazole. Antimicrob Agents Chemother, 50(3), 1096-1099. doi: 10.1128/AAC.50.3.1096-1099.2006*

Rahbari, N. N., Mehrabi, A., Mollberg, N. M., Muller, S. A., Koch, M., Buchler, M. W., & Weitz, J. (2011). *Hepatocellular Carcinoma Current Management and Perspectives for the Future. Annals of Surgery, 253(3), 453-469. doi: Doi 10.1097/Sla.0b013e31820d944f*

Refaat, A., Abdelhamed, S., Yagita, H., Inoue, H., Yokoyama, S., Hayakawa, Y., & Saiki, I. (2013). *Berberine enhances tumor necrosis factor-related apoptosis-inducing ligand-mediated apoptosis in breast cancer. Oncol Lett, 6(3), 840-844. doi: 10.3892/ol.2013.1434*

Roublevskaia, I. N., Polevoda, B. V., Ludlow, J. W., & Haake, A. R. (2000). *Induced G2/M arrest and apoptosis in human epidermoid carcinoma cell lines by semisynthetic drug Ukrain. Anticancer Res, 20(5A), 3163-3167.*

Ruvkun, G. (2001). *Molecular biology - Glimpses of a tiny RNA world. Science, 294(5543), 797-799. doi: DOI 10.1126/science.1066315*

Sato, F., Hashimoto, T., Hachiya, A., Tamura, K.-i., Choi, K.-B., Morishige, T., . . . Yamada, Y. (2001). *Metabolic engineering of plant alkaloid biosynthesis. Proceedings of the National Academy of Sciences, 98(1), 367-372.*

Schuppan, D., Jia, J. D., Brinkhaus, B., & Hahn, E. G. (1999). *Herbal products for liver diseases: A therapeutic challenge for the new millennium. Hepatology, 30(4), 1099-1104. doi: DOI 10.1002/hep.510300437*

Singh, T., Vaid, M., Katiyar, N., Sharma, S., & Katiyar, S. K. (2011). *Berberine, an isoquinoline alkaloid, inhibits melanoma cancer cell migration by reducing the expressions of cyclooxygenase-2, prostaglandin E(2) and prostaglandin E(2) receptors. Carcinogenesis, 32(1), 86-92. doi: 10.1093/carcin/bgq215*

Stermitz, F. R., Lorenz, P., Tawara, J. N., Zenewicz, L. A., & Lewis, K. (2000). Synergy in a medicinal plant: antimicrobial action of berberine potentiated by 5'-methoxyhydnocarpin, a multidrug pump inhibitor. Proc Natl Acad Sci U S A, 97(4), 1433-1437. doi: 10.1073/pnas.030540597

Sun, D., Courtney, H. S., & Beachey, E. H. (1988). Berberine Sulfate Blocks Adherence of Streptococcus-Pyogenes to Epithelial-Cells, Fibronectin, and Hexadecane. Antimicrobial Agents and Chemotherapy, 32(9), 1370-1374.

Sun, Y. Y., Xun, K. L., Wang, Y. T., & Chen, X. P. (2009). A systematic review of the anticancer properties of berberine, a natural product from Chinese herbs. Anti-Cancer Drugs, 20(9), 757-769. doi: Doi 10.1097/Cad.0b013e328330d95b

Takahashi, S. (2002). Long-term Helicobacter pylori infection and the development of atrophic gastritis and gastric cancer in Japan. J Gastroenterol, 37 Suppl 13, 24-27.

Tan, H. Y., Wang, N., Tsao, S. w., Zhang, Z., & Feng, Y. (2013). Suppression of Vascular Endothelial Growth Factor via Inactivation of Eukaryotic Elongation Factor 2 by Alkaloids in Coptidis rhizoma in Hepatocellular Carcinoma. INTEGRATIVE CANCER THERAPIES, 1534735413513635. doi: 10.1177/1534735413513635

Tang, F. Q., Wang, D. S., Duan, C. J., Huang, D. M., Wu, Y., Chen, Y., . . . Cao, Y. (2009). Berberine Inhibits Metastasis of Nasopharyngeal Carcinoma 5-8F Cells by Targeting Rho Kinase-mediated Ezrin Phosphorylation at Threonine 567. Journal of Biological Chemistry, 284(40), 27456-27466. doi: DOI 10.1074/jbc.M109.033795

Tang, J., Feng, Y., Tsao, S., Wang, N., Curtain, R., & Wang, Y. (2009). Berberine and Coptidis rhizoma as novel antineoplastic agents: a review of traditional use and biomedical investigations. J Ethnopharmacol, 126(1), 5-17. doi: 10.1016/j.jep.2009.08.009

Tsang, C. M., Lau, E. P., Di, K., Cheung, P. Y., Hau, P. M., Ching, Y. P., . . . Feng, Y. (2009a). Berberine inhibits Rho GTPases and cell migration at low doses but induces G2 arrest and apoptosis at high doses in human cancer cells. Int J Mol Med, 24(1), 131-138.

Tsang, C. M., Lau, E. P. W., Di, K. J., Cheung, P. Y., Hau, P. M., Ching, Y. P., . . . Feng, Y. B. (2009b). Berberine inhibits Rho GTPases and cell migration at low doses but induces G2 arrest and apoptosis at high doses in human cancer cells. Int J Mol Med, 24(1), 131-138. doi: DOI 10.3892/ijmm_00000216

Uemura, N., Okamoto, S., Yamamoto, S., Matsumura, N., Yamaguchi, S., Yamakido, M., . . . Schlemper, R. J. (2001). Helicobacter pylori infection and the development of gastric cancer. N Engl J Med, 345(11), 784-789. doi: 10.1056/NEJMoa001999

Wang, G. Y., Lv, Q. H., Dong, Q., Xu, R. Z., & Dong, Q. H. (2009). Berbamine induces Fas-mediated apoptosis in human hepatocellular carcinoma HepG2 cells and inhibits its tumor growth in nude mice. Journal of Asian Natural Products Research, 11(3), 219-228. doi: Pii 910840020

Doi 10.1080/10286020802675076

Wang, L., Cao, H., Lu, N., Liu, L., Wang, B., Hu, T., . . . Yan, F. (2013). Berberine inhibits proliferation and down-regulates epidermal growth factor receptor through activation of Cbl in colon tumor cells. Plos One, 8(2), e56666. doi: 10.1371/journal.pone.0056666

Wang, L., Liu, L., Shi, Y., Cao, H., Chaturvedi, R., Calcutt, M. W., . . . Yan, F. (2012). Berberine induces caspase-independent cell death in colon tumor cells through activation of apoptosis-inducing factor. Plos One, 7(5), e36418. doi: 10.1371/journal.pone.0036418

Wang, N., Feng, Y. B., Lau, E. P. W., Tsang, C. M., Ching, Y. P., Man, K., . . . Tsao, S. W. (2010). F-Actin Reorganization and Inactivation of Rho Signaling Pathway Involved in the Inhibitory Effect of Coptidis Rhizoma on Hepatoma Cell Migration. INTEGRATIVE CANCER THERAPIES, 9(4), 354-364. doi: 10.1177/1534735410379121

Wang, N., Feng, Y. B., Zhu, M. F., Tsang, C. M., Man, K., Tong, Y., & Tsao, S. W. (2010). Berberine Induces Autophagic Cell Death and Mitochondrial Apoptosis in Liver Cancer Cells: The Cellular Mechanism. Journal of Cellular Biochemistry, 111(6), 1426-1436. doi: Doi 10.1002/Jcb.22869

Wang, N., Pan, W., Zhu, M., Zhang, M., Hao, X., Liang, G., & Feng, Y. (2011). Fangchinoline induces autophagic cell death via p53/sestrin2/AMPK signaling in human hepatocellular carcinoma cells. 164(2b), 731-742.

Wang, X. N., Han, X., Xu, L. N., Yin, L. H., Xu, Y. W., Qi, Y., & Peng, J. Y. (2008). Enhancement of apoptosis of human hepatocellular carcinoma SMMC-7721 cells through synergy of berberine and evodiamine. Phytomedicine, 15(12), 1062-1068. doi: DOI 10.1016/j.phymed.2008.05.002

Wang, X. Q., Yao, X., Zhu, Z. A., Tang, T. T., Dai, K. R., Sadovskaya, I., . . . Jabbouri, S. (2009). Effect of berberine on Staphylococcus epidermidis biofilm formation. International Journal of Antimicrobial Agents, 34(1), 60-66. doi: DOI 10.1016/j.ijantimicag.2008.10.033

Wartenberg, M., Budde, P., de Marees, M., Grunheck, F., Tsang, S. Y., Huang, Y., . . . Sauer, H. (2003). Inhibition of tumor-induced angiogenesis and matrix-metalloproteinase expression in confrontation cultures of embryoid bodies and tumor spheroids by plant ingredients used in traditional Chinese medicine. Laboratory Investigation, 83(1), 87-98. doi: Doi 10.1097/01.Lab.0000049348.51663.2f

Wu, C. M., Li, T. M., Tan, T. W., Fong, Y. C., & Tang, C. H. (2013). Berberine Reduces the Metastasis of Chondrosarcoma by Modulating the alpha v beta 3 Integrin and the PKC delta , c-Src, and AP-1 Signaling Pathways. Evid Based Complement Alternat Med, 2013, 423164. doi: 10.1155/2013/423164

Wu, K., Yang, Q., Mu, Y., Zhou, L., Liu, Y., Zhou, Q., & He, B. (2012). Berberine inhibits the proliferation of colon cancer cells by inactivating Wnt/beta-catenin signaling. International Journal of Oncology, 41(1), 292-298. doi: 10.3892/ijo.2012.1423

Wu, X. Z., Xie, G. R., & Chen, D. (2007). Hypoxia and hepatocellular carcinoma: The therapeutic target for hepatocellular carcinoma. J Gastroenterol Hepatol, 22(8), 1178-1182. doi: 10.1111/j.1440-1746.2007.04997.x

Xu, Y., Wang, Y., Yan, L., Liang, R. M., Dai, B. D., Tang, R. J., . . . Jiang, Y. Y. (2009). Proteomic analysis reveals a synergistic mechanism of fluconazole and berberine against fluconazole-resistant Candida albicans: endogenous ROS augmentation. J Proteome Res, 8(11), 5296-5304. doi: 10.1021/pr9005074

Yan, K. Q., Zhang, C., Feng, J. B., Hou, L. F., Yan, L., Zhou, Z. L., . . . Xu, Z. H. (2011). Induction of G1 cell cycle arrest and apoptosis by berberine in bladder cancer cells. European Journal of Pharmacology, 661(1-3), 1-7. doi: DOI 10.1016/j.ejphar.2011.04.021

Yan, L., Yan, K., Kun, W., Xu, L., Ma, Q., Tang, Y., . . . Xu, Z. (2013). Berberine inhibits the migration and invasion of T24 bladder cancer cells via reducing the expression of heparanase. Tumour Biol, 34(1), 215-221. doi: 10.1007/s13277-012-0531-z

Yang, X., & Huang, N. (2013). Berberine induces selective apoptosis through the AMPKmediated mitochondrial/caspase pathway in hepatocellular carcinoma. Mol Med Rep, 8(2), 505-510. doi: 10.3892/mmr.2013.1506

Ye, X., Feng, Y., Tong, Y., Ng, K. M., Tsao, S., Lau, G. K., . . . Kobayashi, S. (2009). Hepatoprotective effects of Coptidis rhizoma aqueous extract on carbon tetrachloride-induced acute liver hepatotoxicity in rats. J Ethnopharmacol, 124(1), 130-136.

Yip, N. K., & Ho, W. S. (2013). Berberine induces apoptosis via the mitochondrial pathway in liver cancer cells. Oncol Rep, 30(3), 1107-1112. doi: 10.3892/or.2013.2543

Yu, F. S., Yang, J. S., Lin, H. J., Yu, C. S., Tan, T. W., Lin, Y. T., . . . Chung, J. G. (2007). Berberine inhibits WEHI-3 leukemia cells in vivo. In Vivo, 21(2), 407-412.

Yu, H. H., Kim, K. J., Cha, J. D., Kim, H. K., Lee, Y. E., Choi, N. Y., & You, Y. O. (2005). Antimicrobial activity of berberine alone and in combination with ampicillin or oxacillin against methicillin-resistant Staphylococcus aureus. J Med Food, 8(4), 454-461. doi: 10.1089/jmf.2005.8.454

Zhang, D. Y., & Friedman, S. L. (2012). Fibrosis-dependent mechanisms of hepatocarcinogenesis. Hepatology, 56(2), 769-775. doi: 10.1002/hep.25670

Zhang, L., Yang, L., & Zheng, X. (1997). A study of Helicobacterium pylori and prevention and treatment of chronic atrophic gastritis. J Tradit Chin Med, 17(1), 3-9.

Zhang, X. L., Gu, L. B., Li, J. S., Shah, N., He, J., Yang, L., . . . Zhou, M. X. (2010). Degradation of MDM2 by the Interaction between Berberine and DAXX Leads to Potent Apoptosis in MDM2-Overexpressing Cancer Cells. Cancer Research, 70(23), 9895-9904. doi: Doi 10.1158/0008-5472.Can-10-1546

Zhu, M., Wang, N., Tsao, S. W., Yuen, M. F., Feng, Y., Wan, T. S., . . . Feng, Y. (2011). Up-regulation of microRNAs, miR21 and miR23a in human liver cancer cells treated with Coptidis rhizoma aqueous extract. Exp Ther Med, 2(1), 27-32. doi: 10.3892/etm.2010.164

Role and Metabolism of Heme-derived Iron in Cancer

Mailin Li* and Barbara Wegiel*

1 Introduction

Iron is an essential cofactor for many biological processes including DNA synthesis, oxygen transport, and ATP generation. Iron metabolism, recycling, and transport, is thus controlled at multiple levels. Cells undergoing rapid proliferation, such as cancer cells, are characterized by increased demand for iron and accelerated iron turnover.

Heme degradation provides the major source of iron used in iron recycling. Residential macrophages of the spleen and liver express high levels of heme oxygenase-1 (HO-1), an enzyme that degrades heme to ferrous iron (Fe^{2+}), biliverdin (BV), and carbon monoxide (CO). Tumor associated macrophages (TAM) are present in the tumor microenvironment and, dependent on their polarization phenotypes, contribute to tumor development or regression in part by regulating iron availability. "Classically activated" M1 macrophages are pro-inflammatory, express high intracellular levels of ferritin that sequesters iron, and promote tumor regression. In contrast, M2 macrophages favor tumor growth in part through upregulated HO-1-mediated iron generation and increased iron export. As HO-1 is expressed in residential macrophages and recruited monocytes in the tumor stroma, the role of iron recycling in the tumor microenvironment depends heavily on TAM activity.

In this chapter, we focus on the altered status of iron homeostasis and heme degradation in TAM and how HO-1 expression in both cancer cells and TAM may contribute to carcinogenesis.

2 Heme and Iron Recycling During Homeostasis

The average human body contains three to four grams of iron distributed throughout various organs. Hemoglobin found on circulating and developing erythrocytes binds one to two grams of total iron, while hepatocytes and residential macrophages (Kupffer cells) of the liver store an additional gram (Ganz 2007). A further significant portion of iron is present in myoglobin in muscles and in various other hemoproteins like cytochromes and nitric oxide synthase (Ganz 2007). Heme iron from hemoglobin and myoglobin derived from red meat provides the largest source of external iron and is uptaken by enterocytes via receptor-mediated endocytosis in the small intestine; nonheme iron sources include ferrous and ferric iron derived from plant products, though they are not as readily absorbed (Bastide, Pierre and Corpet 2011). Iron and heme absorption in duodenal enterocytes accounts for 1 to 2 mg of

* Transplant Institute, Department of Surgery, Beth Israel Deaconess Medical Center, Harvard Medical School, Boston, MA, USA

iron intake daily, yet the same amount of iron lost through shedding of intestinal epithelial cells and extravasated red blood cells, making physiological iron levels a constant parameter (Ganz 2007; Walsh, Kaldor, Brading and George 1955). Although there is no system for large scale removal of iron from the body, various organs do contribute to the regulation of iron levels: through reduced iron absorption by duodenal mucosa, reduced iron export by the same epithelial cells through the peptide hormone hepcidin, and sequestration of already circulating iron in the liver and spleen in ferritin and hemosiderin (Ganz 2003; Shoden, Gabrio and Finch 1953).

The relatively small exchange of iron between the body and the environment contrasts with the large amount of iron redistributed between tissues and cells. Monocytes and macrophages of the spleen, liver, lymph nodes and bone marrow form the mononuclear phagocyte system (MNP, the reticuloendothelial system), and are responsible for the degradation of hemoglobin from senescent red blood cells and generation of a systemic iron pool. The majority of recycled iron is then incorporated into nascent erythrocytes of the bone marrow (Pollycove and Mortimer 1961). Iron hemoglobin from red blood cells (RBCs) produces 25 to 30 mg of iron per day, allowing for the production of 200 billion new erythrocytes every day (Munoz, Villar and Garcia-Erce 2009).

Iron is the reactive core of a variety of enzymes necessary in all cell types. It forms the catalytic site in ribonucleotide reductases necessary for DNA synthesis, facilitates the coordination of oxygen and carbon dioxide in hemoglobin and myoglobin, and is additionally involved in ATP generation through the iron sulfur clusters of cytochromes in the mitochondrial oxidative chain (Beinert *et al.*, 1983; Elford, Freese, Passamani and Morris, 1970; Perutz, 1979). Iron chelation has been shown to arrest human lymphocytes at the G1/S phase checkpoint due to inhibition of DNA synthesis (Lederman, Cohen, Lee, Freedman and Gelfand, 1984). Iron metabolism also has been shown to regulate cell cycle activity by affecting expression and activity of cyclins A, D, an E and cyclin dependent kinases in cancer cells. Iron chelation was shown to block cyclin dependent kinase, specifically cdks 2, 4 and 6 activities leading to hypophosphorylation of Rb and blockage of cell cycle progression(Gao and Richardson 2001; Kulp, Green and Vulliet, 1996; Lucas *et al.*, 1995; Mitra *et al.*, 1999; Nurtjahja-Tjendraputra, Fu, Phang and Richardson 2007). As such, iron is often the limiting factor for synthesis of proteins, DNA and cell growth.

Highly proliferative cells, such as cancer cells, have high iron requirements. Early studies on iron metabolism in cancer showed that addition of iron to culture media of hepatoma cells enhanced cell growth via increased iron retention, and this effect was reversed with addition of the iron chelator, desferroxamine (Hann, Stahlhut and Hann, 1990). Similar studies on iron deprivation have been performed in neuroblastoma (Blatt and Stitely, 1987), leukemia (Foa, Maiolo, Lombardi, Villa and Polli, 1986; Kim *et al.*, 2011), breast cancer (Reddel, Hedley and Sutherland, 1985) and hepatocellular carcinoma (Ba *et al.*, 2011) cell lines showing iron deprivation to block cancer growth. Iron deprivation was shown to have minimal or no effect on normal non-transformed cells growth. Moreover, other iron depleting compounds such as deferasirox, tachpyridine, and thiosemicarbazones were also effective in suppressing cancer cell growth *in vivo* and *in vitro*(Kim *et al.*, 2011; Lui *et al.*, 2013; Torti *et al.*, 1998; Turner *et al.*, 2005)

In addition to iron chelation, mechanisms reducing iron uptake—through transferrin—and enhancing iron export—through ferroportin—were also shown to be effective approaches for inhibition of cancer growth. Blockage of transferrin receptors with monoclonal antibody blocked growth of human melanoma xenografts (Trowbridge and Domingo, 1981). Similarly, overexpression of iron exporter ferroportin or alteration of ferroportin expression may also be viable options for cancer therapy (Pinnix *et al.*, 2010; Sow *et al.*, 2009).

The multiple processes in which iron participates are due to its flexible coordination chemistry and redox reactivity allowing oxygen binding and transfer of electrons with ease (Aisen, Enns and Wessling-Resnick 2001). However, the same high energy properties of iron makes it cytotoxic as free iron reacts in Fenton chemistry to generate hydroxyl radicals and reactive oxygen species that damage cellular macromolecules indiscriminately (Graf, Mahoney, Bryant and Eaton, 1984). The most significantly damaged molecules include DNA (double stranded breaks, base shifts, base modifications) and lipids (oxidation) (Chevion, 1988; Lloyd and Phillips, 1999; Mello Filho, Hoffmann and Meneghini, 1984; Meneghini, 1997; Morel *et al.*, 1990). Dietary analyses have linked high fats and heme-iron intake to colon cancer and ovarian cancers, likely due to the generation of lipid peroxyl radicals that have DNA damaging capacities (Sawa *et al.*, 1998; Yamaguchi *et al.*, 2008). Transgenic mice fed a high iron diet were also shown to have increased accumulation of lipid peroxidation products and DNA oxidative damage correlating with increased risk of developing hepatocellular carcinoma (Furutani *et al.*, 2006). Iron is thus capable of accelerating tumor growth as both a limited resource and through the generation of ROS and DNA mutations.

As mentioned previously, various organs participate in regulating iron homeostasis but there is no efficient mechanism for large-scale removal of iron from the body (Ganz 2007; Kohgo, Ikuta, Ohtake, Torimoto and Kato 2008). Iron overloading can occur through abnormalities due to genetic disorders, repeat blood transfusions, chronic inflammation and dietary choices. Iron that exceeds export and sequestering capacities circulates as non-transferrin bound iron which then accumulates in the liver, heart, and pancreas (Andrews, 1999; Brissot, Ropert, Le Lan and Loreal 2012; Cabantchik, Breuer, Zanninelli and Cianciulli 2005). Such free iron causes organ dysfunction through enhanced ROS production and can lead to liver failure, cirrhosis, arrhythmias, heart failure, and diabetes (Brissot *et al.*, 2012; Hirano *et al.*, 2001). Diseases characterized by high iron accumulation like hereditary hemochromatosis, beta-thalassemia and end stage liver disease have been associated with increased risk of hepatocellular carcinoma (Kowdley 2004; Pietrangelo 2010). Similarly to cancer cells, invading pathogens also depend on iron for their exponential growth, resulting in iron withholding by the MNP system as a form of primary immune defense. Continued iron sequestration in these instances however, results in chronic anemia with symptoms of decreased survival of mature red blood cells and poor maturation of erythroid precursors (Rivera *et al.*, 2005). These data suggest that iron is a critical regulator of cell proliferation and therefore imbalance in iron recycling, storage or uptake may result in pro-proliferative disease and/or malignancy.

Heme degradation is mediated by the heme-oxygenase family of enzymes. Although there are two isoforms of the heme oxygenases, HO-1 is the predominant form associated with iron recycling and hemoglobin turnover and is highly expressed in the specialized cells of the MNP system—specifically the macrophages of the spleen and liver. HO-1 is generally considered to be a cytoprotective molecule as it degrades proinflammatory heme and generates biologically active products biliverdin, carbon monoxide gas, and free iron (Maines, 1988; Tenhunen, Marver and Schmid, 1968). Through its importance in macrophages, HO-1 is also a critical mediator of iron recycling. A case study of a 6-year-old boy suffering from HO-1 deficiency reported persistent erythrocyte fragmentation, increased serum iron and heme levels, and iron deposition in distal tissues (Kawashima, Oda, Yachie, Koizumi and Nakanishi 2002; Yachie *et al.,* 1999). Similar MNP system-related abnormalities were made for HO-1 knockout *(Hmox -/-)* mice which are characterized by high oxidative stress, low survival in utero, and exaggerated response to tissue injury (Poss and Tonegawa, 1997). *Hmox -/-* mice, in addition to dysfunctional and mostly absent residential splenic and liver macrophages, showed tissue inflammation due to intravascular erythrocyte hemolysis and iron overload in the kidneys, suggesting difficulties with iron trafficking (Kovtunovych, Eckhaus, Ghosh, Ollivierre-Wilson and Rouault 2010). Furthermore, bone marrow progenitor cells isolated from HO-1 knockout mice were unable to differentiate fully even under favorable macrophage growth conditions, suggesting the importance of HO-1 in the maturation of myeloid cells (Wegiel *et al.,* 2014).

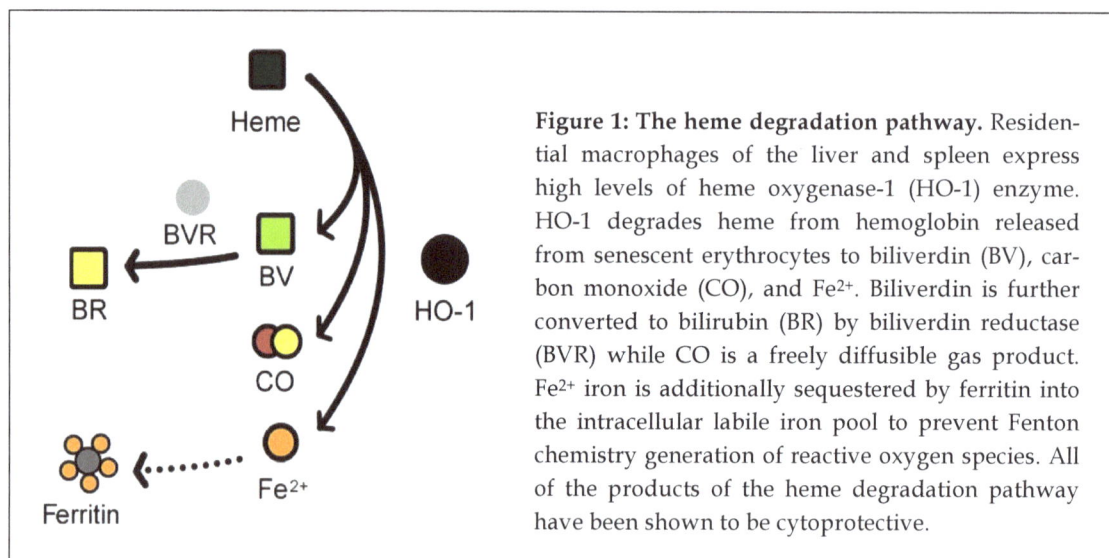

Figure 1: The heme degradation pathway. Residential macrophages of the liver and spleen express high levels of heme oxygenase-1 (HO-1) enzyme. HO-1 degrades heme from hemoglobin released from senescent erythrocytes to biliverdin (BV), carbon monoxide (CO), and Fe^{2+}. Biliverdin is further converted to bilirubin (BR) by biliverdin reductase (BVR) while CO is a freely diffusible gas product. Fe^{2+} iron is additionally sequestered by ferritin into the intracellular labile iron pool to prevent Fenton chemistry generation of reactive oxygen species. All of the products of the heme degradation pathway have been shown to be cytoprotective.

As mentioned previously, the energy potential and flexibility of heme to be incorporated into a variety of hemoproteins is due to the coordination chemistry possible with the iron center of the heme porphyrin. Biological iron is rarely found unaccompanied, likely due to its insolubility and reactivity. Generation of intracellular iron in the heme degradation pathway leads to induction of heavy chain of ferritin, a sequestration molecule considered to possess protective properties. Ferritins have been shown to not only play a role in iron storage and detoxification but also mediate cytoprotective effects in several models of the diseases mimicking and mediating in part the effects observed with induction of HO-1 (Harrison and Arosio, 1996). Overexpression of ferritin was shown to inhibit tumor human H1299 xenografts growth (Nie, Chen, Sheftel, Pantopoulos and Ponka 2006). Deficiency in light chain of ferritin in human leads to reduced cellular iron availability, diminished levels of cytosolic catalase superoxide dismutase 1 (SOD1) protein levels, enhanced reactive oxygen species (ROS) production and higher levels of oxidized proteins (Cozzi *et al.,* 2013). Expression of ferritin is induced by acute inflammatory cytokines such as IFNγ, IL-6, and TNF-α that increase iron sequestration in macrophages (Feelders *et al.,* 1998).

3   Iron Degradation in Macrophages of the Mononuclear Phagocyte (MNP) System

Iron regulation by macrophages of the mononuclear phagocyte system (MNP) is facilitated through two pathways: uptake of circulating iron complexes or uptake of heme/hemoglobin. Circulating heme complexes include transferrin (Tf)-bound iron (Fe_2-Tf) at physiological iron concentrations, and non-transferrin-bound iron (NTBI) under iron overload conditions (Trinder, Fox, Vautier and Olynyk 2002). NTBI is biologically more toxic than Tf-bound iron. Among the NTBI fractions, labile plasma iron (LPI) is the most toxic because unlike Tf-bound iron, the cellular uptake of NTBI is not dependent on the presence of transferrin receptors (TfR), and therefore the resulting iron is diffusely distributed throughout the organs (Breuer, Hershko and Cabantchik 2000; Cabantchik *et al.*, 2005).

Ferric iron Fe^{3+} bound to transferrin (Fe_2-Tf) is the primary form of physiological iron found circulating in the blood. Transport of iron between organs and uptake of iron is facilitated by Tf and transferrin receptor (TfR1). The Fe_2-Tf complex binds to transferrin receptor 1 (TfR1) on the cell surface and is endocytosed. Once internalized, the endosome is acidified, uncoupling ferric iron from transferrin (Dautry-Varsat, Ciechanover and Lodish, 1983). STEAP3 reductase catalyzes the conversion of ferric (Fe3+) iron to ferrous (Fe2+) iron which binds to the divalent metal transporter 1 (DMT1; also known as natural resistance associated macrophage protein (NRAMP2)) (Ohgami *et al.*, 2005). DMT1 then transports the ferrous ion across the endosomal compartment to the cytoplasm (Fleming *et al.*, 1997; Gunshin *et al.*, 1997). In the cytoplasm, ferrous iron is either directly utilized by mitochondria for synthesis of heme and iron-sulfur complexes or stored by ferritin into the intracellular labile iron pool (Napier, Ponka and Richardson 2005). Apo-transferrin bound to its receptor is recycled to the cell surface where they uncouple at neutral pH, and both participate in additional cycles of iron transport and intake (Figure 2).

Ferroportin is thus far the only iron export channel discovered in mammalian cells (Donovan *et al.*, 2005). Iron for delivery to systemic tissues is first exported by ferroportin, oxidized to ferric iron by multicopper ferroxidase cerruloplasmin and then scavenged by transferrin which maintains Fe^{3+} in a redox inert state for delivery (Harris, Durley, Man and Gitlin, 1999). Iron export is negatively regulated by hepcidin, a circulating peptide hormone that binds to ferroportin, leading to its internalization and degradation (Nemeth *et al.*, 2004). Hepcidin is produced by the liver in the state of high iron intake and under inflammatory conditions, resulting in reduced iron absorption by duodenal enterocytes and iron retention in macrophages (Feelders *et al.*, 1998).

Iron transport is controlled at the post-transcriptional level via two iron regulatory proteins (IRP1 and IRP2) and iron responsive elements (IREs). IREs are found within both the 5′ and 3′ UTRs of various target mRNAs encoding proteins involved in iron trafficking: ferritin and ferroportin mRNAs contain IREs in their 5′ UTRs, and transferrin receptor and DMT1 contain IREs in their 3′ UTR (Hubert and Hentze 2002; Torti and Torti 2013). Binding of IRPs to IREs occurs only in conditions of low iron and serves to increase levels of intracellular iron. Binding of IRPs to 5′ UTRs blocks mRNA translation, reducing expression of proteins involved in iron storage and efflux, while binding of IRPs to 3′ UTRs inhibits mRNA degradation, stabilizing expression of iron importers. In conditions of high intracellular iron IRP1 acquires an iron sulfur cluster and is converted to a cytoplasmic acontinase, IRP2 is degraded,

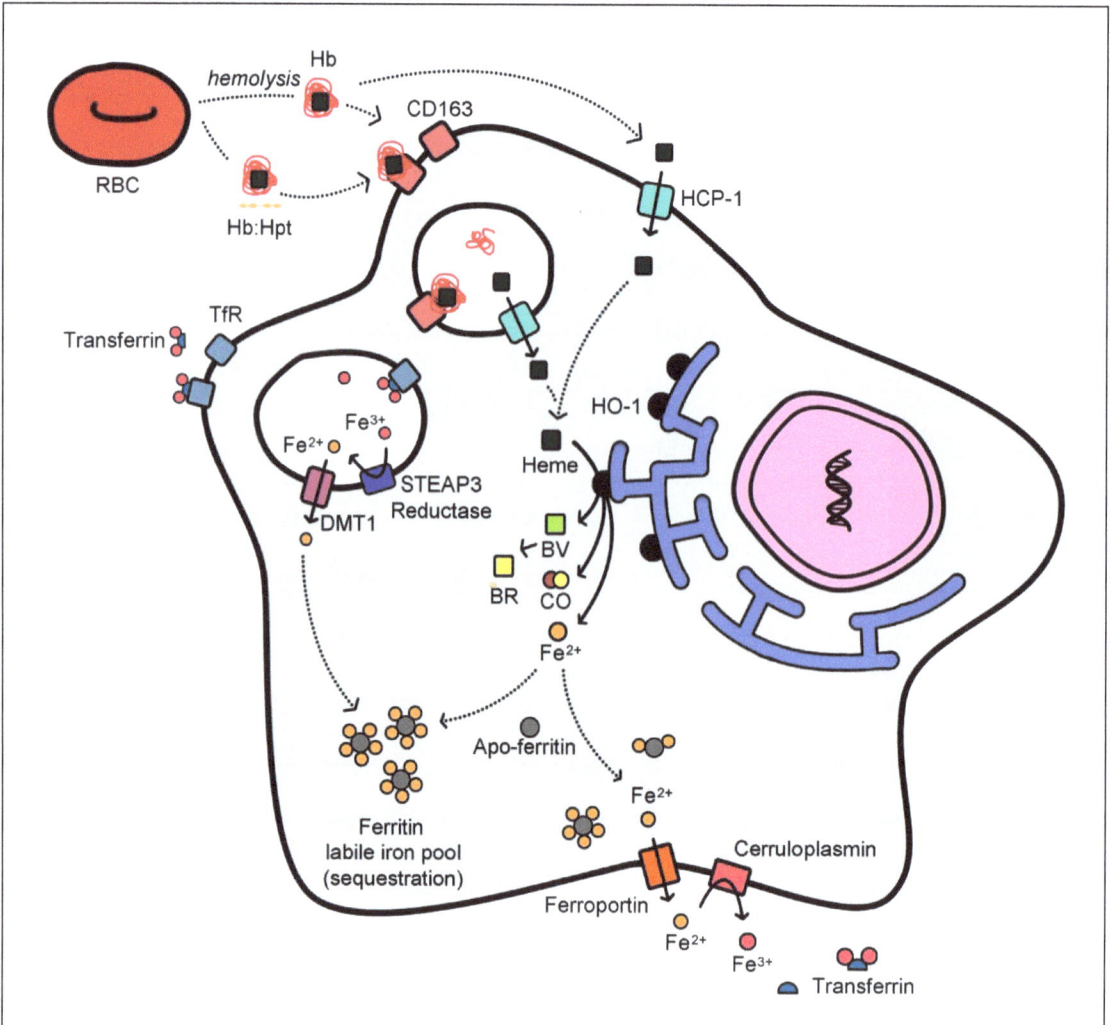

Figure 2: Scheme of iron recycling in macrophages. Iron is derived from two primary pathways: intake of transferrin bound iron and degradation of hemoglobin (Hb). Circulating iron is bound to transferrin. Macrophages uptake diferric-bound transferrin through endocytosis via the transferrin receptor (TfR). Acidification of the endosome releases iron from transferrin, which is then reduced by Steap3 metalloreductase before transport to the cytosol via divalent metal transporter (DMT1). Additionally, hemolysis of RBCs released hemoglobin, which could be bound by circulating hapto-globin (Hb:Hpt). Macrophage specific CD163 scavenge both hemoglobin and hemoglo-bin:haptoglobin complexes and allows for endocytic heme degradation. Acidification of the endo-somal compartment uncouples heme from its globin component. Heme is then transported to the cytosol by heme transporter heme carrier protein 1 (HCP-1). Heme degradation through ER-anchored heme oxygenase-1 (HO-1) produces biliverdin (BV), which is then reduced to bilirubin (BR) by biliverdin reductase (BVR), carbon monoxide (CO), and Fe^{2+} iron. Heavy and light chains of ferritin sequester free iron generated from both heme degradation and iron import into the labile iron pool until utilization by mitochondria or export. Release of iron from macrophages is facilitated through ferroportin followed by oxidation by membrane bound ceruloplasmin and is finally bound to transporter transferrin.

and ferritin and ferroportin mRNA is translated (Thomson, Rogers and Leedman, 1999). In addition to iron levels, IREs are sensitive to factors such as nitric oxide, reactive oxygen species, and hypoxia (Pantopoulos, Gray and Hentze, 1995; Pantopoulos *et al.*, 1997; Tacchini, Recalcati, Bernelli-Zazzera and Cairo, 1997) suggesting their function during oxidative stress or injury associated with ischemia-reperfusion.

Macrophages have the capacity to not only endocytose senescent erythrocytes but also scavenge hemoglobin and free heme released from hemolysis of red blood cells. Endocytosis of free heme and hemoglobin by the monocytes/macrophage is mediated by scavenger receptor CD163. CD163 is currently the only known pathway for intake of free circulating hemoglobin and hemoglobin:haptoglobin complexes (Kristiansen *et al.*, 2001; Moller, Peterslund, Graversen and Moestrup 2002; Schaer *et al.*, 2006). Following ingestion of the receptor:ligand complexes, increased acidification of the endosomal compartment uncouples both hemoglobin:CD163 and subsequently heme from its globin component as well. Free heme is exported to the cytoplasm by the heme transporters HCP-1 and then degraded by ER-bound heme oxygenase-1 (HO-1) while globins are digested in the maturing lysosome, and the receptor is eventually recycled back to the cell surface (Schaer, Vallelian, Imhof, Schoedon and Schaer 2008). Schaer et al showed colocalization of iron transporter DMT1 within the late endosome/lysososome suggesting heme breakdown and release of iron occurring in the lysosome (Schaer *et al.*, 2008). Although he attributed this to nonenzymatic heme degradation due to the various peroxides or at low pH in the presence of proteases, Gagnon et al provided evidence that phagosomal membrane is derived from the endoplasmic reticulum, suggesting ER associated HO-1 could catalyse heme degradation and iron recycling within the phagolysosome as well (Gagnon *et al.*, 2002).

4   Cancer and Reprogramming of Iron Homeostasis: Role of Tumor-associated Macrophages (TAM)

Because iron is key in the regulation of cell growth, cancer cells reprogram their iron metabolism and transport to facilitate enhanced iron acquisition. Studies on the role of iron in tumorigenesis have shown that iron accumulates in the tumor stroma (Alkhateeb, Han and Connor 2013). Tumor stroma consists of a mixture of cell types including endothelial cells, fibroblasts, and various other cells such as lymphocytes, myeloid cells and smooth muscle cells. Accumulation of iron in the stroma suggests that iron-dependent effects may be mediated by cells in the tumor microenvironment rather than tumor cells themselves.

Among the cells in tumor stroma, macrophages have the highest iron storage capabilities. Increased infiltration of ferritin-rich CD68 positive macrophages was detected in more advanced breast cancer tumors characterized by high histological grade (Alkhateeb *et al.*, 2013). Tumor associated macrophages (TAM) and infiltrating monocytes and polarized macrophages express different profiles of iron receptors, iron transporters and exporters. TAM in the tumor stroma is present in close proximity to cancer cells and therefore can facilitate their growth and metastasis. There are two distinct polarization statuses of tumor-associated macrophages: "classically activated" M1s and "alternatively activated" M2s (Figure 3). M1 macrophages are generated *in vitro* by stimulation with lipopolysaccharide (LPS) and IFNγ while M2 macrophages are typically polarized under Th2 stimulatory conditions including IL4 and

A. M1 "Classically Activated"

IL-1β
IFN-γ
LPS
TLR ligands
CSF/GMCSF

TLR IFN-γR
CD86
MHC II
ferritin

IL6, IL-12, IL-13
ROS, RNI
TNFα
MCP-1

Proinflammatory
Anti-tumoral
Efficient APC capacity
Immune Response Promotion
Iron Sequestration

B. M2 "Alternatively Activated"

IL4
IL13
MCSF
IL33

CD163
TfR
Mannose Receptor
DMT-1
HO-1
HCP-1
Ferroportin

IL-10, IL-1Ra
TGF-β
MMP9
VEGF, EGF

Antiinflammatory
Supports Tumor Growth
Angiogenic Support/Tissue Remodeling and Repair
Immune Inhibition
Enhanced Heme Degradation and Iron Export

Figure 3: Iron metabolism during macrophage polarization. M1 macrophages display an anti-tumoral phenotype by activating immune responses, generation of reactive oxygen species (ROS) and reactive nitrogen intermediates (RNI), and iron sequestration via increased ferritin synthesis. M2 macrophages promote tumor growth through induction of angiogenesis, immunosuppression, and enhanced iron generation and export. IFNγ, interferon-gamma; CSF, colony stimulating factor; GMCSF, granulocyte stimulating factor; TLRs, toll like receptors; TNFα, tumor necrosis factor; MCP-1, monocyte chemoattractant protein 1; MCSF, macrophage colony stimulating factor; TfR transferrin receptor; DMT-1, Divalent Metal Transporter; HCP-1, Heme Carrier Protein; TGF-β, Transforming Growth Factor; MMP, Metalloproteinase; VEGF, Vascular Endothelial Growth Factor; EGF, Epithelial Growth Factor.

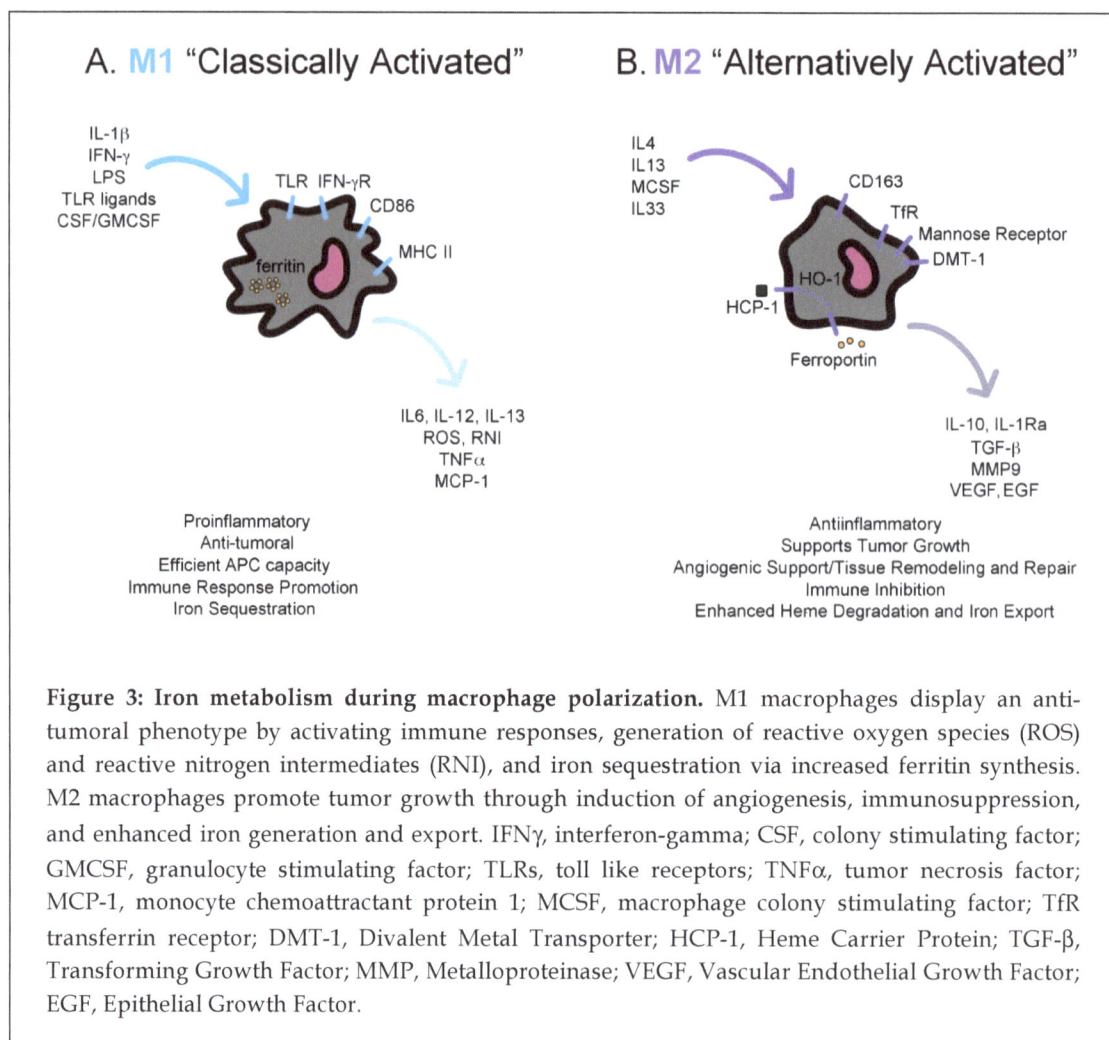

IL13 (Mantovani and Locati 2013). The M1 phenotype is proinflammatory and is characterized by the release of inflammatory cytokines, reactive nitrogen intermediates, reactive oxygen species, and anti-tumoral activities (Mantovani, Sozzani, Locati, Allavena and Sica 2002). In contrast, M2 macrophages are involved in tissue remodeling and repair with immunosuppressive and anti-inflammatory functions that promote tumor growth (Mantovani *et al.*, 2002; Sica and Mantovani 2012). M2 macrophages show low IL12 expression, high IL10 expression, high scavenging potential, and ability to support angiogenesis, tissue remodeling and repair (Biswas, Sica and Lewis 2008). It is prudent to mention now that while dividing the macrophage population under the properties mentioned above is tempting, such classifications are general observed characteristics, and that macrophages display remarkable plasticity with some expressing none or all M1/M2 markers, and these even subject to change depending on the local environment. Recently, vascular cell adhesion molecule 1 (VCAM-1) positive and CD11b low population with intermittent expression of mannose receptor (MMR, CD206) was shown to influence mammary tumor growth in transgenic model (Franklin *et al.*, 2014).

High levels of iron released within the tumor microenvironment provide a source of iron for cancer proliferation. Since M2 macrophages exhibit a gene expression profile consistent with iron efflux — an increase in ferroportin and decreased ferritin accumulation — M2 macrophages may represent a mechanism behind promotion of cancer growth (Corna *et al.*, 2010; Recalcati *et al.*, 2010). Measurements of iron release into the culture medium showed that after 4 hours, M2 macrophages released approximately four times more iron as M1 (Recalcati *et al.*, 2010). Supernatants from M2 macrophage cultures were shown to promote tumor cell proliferation, an effect inhibited by iron chelation, suggesting that M2 macrophages may promote tumor growth at least partly by supplementing tumor cells with iron (Corna *et al.*, 2010; Recalcati *et al.*, 2010). In a model of urethane-induced lung carcinogenesis, cancer growth was associated with a phenotypic switch from M1 (early initiation) to M2 (late promotion and progression). However, depletion of alveolar macrophages during both early and late stages impaired tumor growth suggesting a tumor-promoting role for M1 macrophages as well, though dependent on the tumor progression stage (Zaynagetdinov *et al.*, 2011).

Although ferritin is most commonly found as an intracellular iron storage protein, ferritin has also been found in circulation. Increased levels of serum ferritin correlated with poor clinical outcome in breast cancer patients (Alkhateeb *et al.*, 2013). Macrophages, but not breast cancer cells, were able to actively secrete L ferritin *in vitro* in an nonclassical secretion pathway following N-glycolyslation and ER/golgi processing, an effect enhanced in response to pro-inflammatory cytokines (Cohen *et al.*, 2010). Macrophages are known to extensively infiltrate breast tumors and are often rich in ferritin (Simson and Spicer, 1972). Staining of ferritin in tissue stroma showed high density of ferritin rich CD68+ TAM in the stroma of invasive ductal carcinomas (Alkhateeb *et al.*, 2013). Ferritin was shown to increase proliferation of T47D and MCF7 epithelial breast cancer cells lines however with little intracellular iron level changes (Alkhateeb *et al.*, 2013). Release of ferritin by M2 macrophages within the stroma in breast tumors may represent a mechanism by which ferritin stimulates tumor growth and progression. The role of iron in cancer progression is summarized in Table 1.

Tumors regulate their own iron metabolism in ways to favor net iron influx and retention. TfR1 is highly expressed in breast cancer (Hogemann-Savellano *et al.*, 2003; Shindelman *et al.*, 1981), leukemia (Sutherland *et al.*, 1981), lymphoma (Habeshaw *et al.*, 1983), prostate cancer (Keer *et al.*, 1990), and lung cancer (Kukulj *et al.*, 2010). Analysis of squamous cell carcinomas showed that expression of TfR1 is a marker of poor prognosis and outcome. Small interfering RNA against TfR used in culture resulted in reduced proliferation and cell cycle arrest (Chan *et al.*, 2014; Schaar, Medina, Moore, Strair and Ting 2009). High TfR1 expression has additionally been associated with poor response to tamoxifen treatment and short breast cancer-specific survival (Habashy *et al.*, 2010). Heme transporter heme carrier protein 1 (HCP-1) was shown to be highly expressed in Caco-2 and HeLa cancer cell lines and moderately expressed in Hep2G and HEK293 cells suggesting the higher demands for heme uptake by cancer cells (Latunde-Dada, Takeuchi, Simpson and McKie 2006). A study on small lung cancer cell and a variety of human lung cancer tumors additionally showed upregulated heme transporters HCP-1 and heme responsive gene 1 (HRG-1) expression in combination with enhanced ALAS1 expression (the rate limiting enzyme involved in heme synthesis) and increased production of hemoproteins like cytochromes and cytoglobins (Hooda *et al.*, 2013). These data, in addition to evidence regarding altered localization of HO-1 and potential altered function suggest perhaps cancer cells in part utilize heme and iron independent of HO-1 involvement. Though one might ex pect intracellular ferritin to diminish with accelerated iron-containing macromolecle synthesis, intracellular iron has been shown to be upregulated

	Cancer	M1	M2
Uptake	⇑ TfR1 expression in breast cancer (Hogemann-Savellano *et al.*, 2003; Shindelman, Ortmeyer and Sussman, 1981), leukemic cells (Sutherland *et al.*, 1981), non-Hodgekin lymphoma (Habeshaw, Lister, Stansfeld and Greaves, 1983), prostate cancer (Keer *et al.*, 1990), colorectal carcinoma (Brookes *et al.*, 2006; Prutki *et al.*, 2006) and tumors from non small cell lung cancer patients (Kukulj *et al.*, 2010). ⇑ Iron importer DMT1(Brookes *et al.*, 2006). ⇑ STEAP family (1,2,3) metalloreductases (Ohgami *et al.*, 2005; Torti and Torti 2011)	⇓ TfR1 (Corna *et al.*, 2010). ⇓ HCP-1 expression following stimulation with TLR1-9 agonists (Schaer *et al.*, 2008). ⇓ STEAP3 (Corna *et al.*, 2010). ⇓ STEAP3 in LPS-stimulated macrophages (Zhang *et al.*, 2012). ⇑ NRAMP1(Corna *et al.*, 2010)	⇑ CD163 scavenger receptor (Sierra-Filardi, Vega, Sanchez-Mateos, Corbi and Puig-Kroger 2010). ⇔ HCP-1 heme transporter found to colocalize with endocytosed hemoglobin:haptoglobin processes following CD163-mediated uptake (Schaer *et al.*, 2008). ⇑ TfR1 (Corna *et al.*, 2010) (Mantovani *et al.*, 2002). ⇑ DMT1 expression levels though may be of different splice variants based on maturation of endosome (Corna *et al.*, 2010; Schaer *et al.*, 2008)
Utilization	⇑ Ferritin expression in breast cancer associated with worse clinical outcome (Alkhateeb *et al.*, 2013). ⇑ H ferritin following continual heme treatment in Caco-2 and BT-20 tumor cells (Cermak *et al.*, 1993). ⇔ Intracellular iron levels following ferritin stimulation in MC7 and T47D breast cancer cell lines (Alkhateeb *et al.*, 2013). ⇑ Ribonucleotide reductase correlated with increased growth rate (Elford *et al.*, 1970).	⇓ IRP1 and 2 binding activity (Corna *et al.*, 2010; Recalcati *et al.*, 2010) ⇑ H ferritin (Corna *et al.*, 2010; Recalcati *et al.*, 2010) ⇓ HO-1 (Corna *et al.*, 2010; Recalcati *et al.*, 2010)	⇑ HO-1 (Corna *et al.*, 2010; Recalcati *et al.*, 2010; Sierra-Filardi *et al.*, 2010) ⇓ H ferritin (Corna *et al.*, 2010; Recalcati *et al.*, 2010) ⇑ IRP binding activity (Corna *et al.*, 2010; Recalcati *et al.*, 2010) ⇑ IRP protein levels (Corna *et al.*, 2010; Recalcati *et al.*, 2010)
Transport	⇓ Ferroportin in colorectal carcinoma (Brookes *et al.*, 2006), breast cancer cell lines(Jiang, Elliott and Head 2010) and breast cancer patients(Miller *et al.*, 2011; Pinnix *et al.*, 2010)	⇓ Ferroportin(Recalcati *et al.*, 2010) ⇓ Ferroportin following treatment with TLR1-9 agonists(Schaer *et al.*, 2008)	⇑ Ferroportin (Corna *et al.*, 2010; Recalcati *et al.*, 2010; Vallelian *et al.*, 2010)

Table 1: Altered Iron Homeostasis in Cancer Cells and Macrophages of the Tumor Microenvironment.

in a variety of cancers (Alkhateeb *et al.*, 2013). Treatment with hemin and FeSO₄ was shown to induce H-ferritin in breast cancer cells but not colon cancer cells, allowing for protection against subsequent oxidants; Cermak et al hypothesized this as due to the differences between basal ferritin amounts and that while acute exposure of tumors to heme-derived iron allowed for oxidant-mediated sensitivity and lysis, chronic exposure to oxidants may result in resistance to oxidant stressors, especially due to increased intracellular iron storage capacity (Cermak *et al.*, 1993). These two observations suggest that cancer cells have a high rate of iron import and utilization with little export.

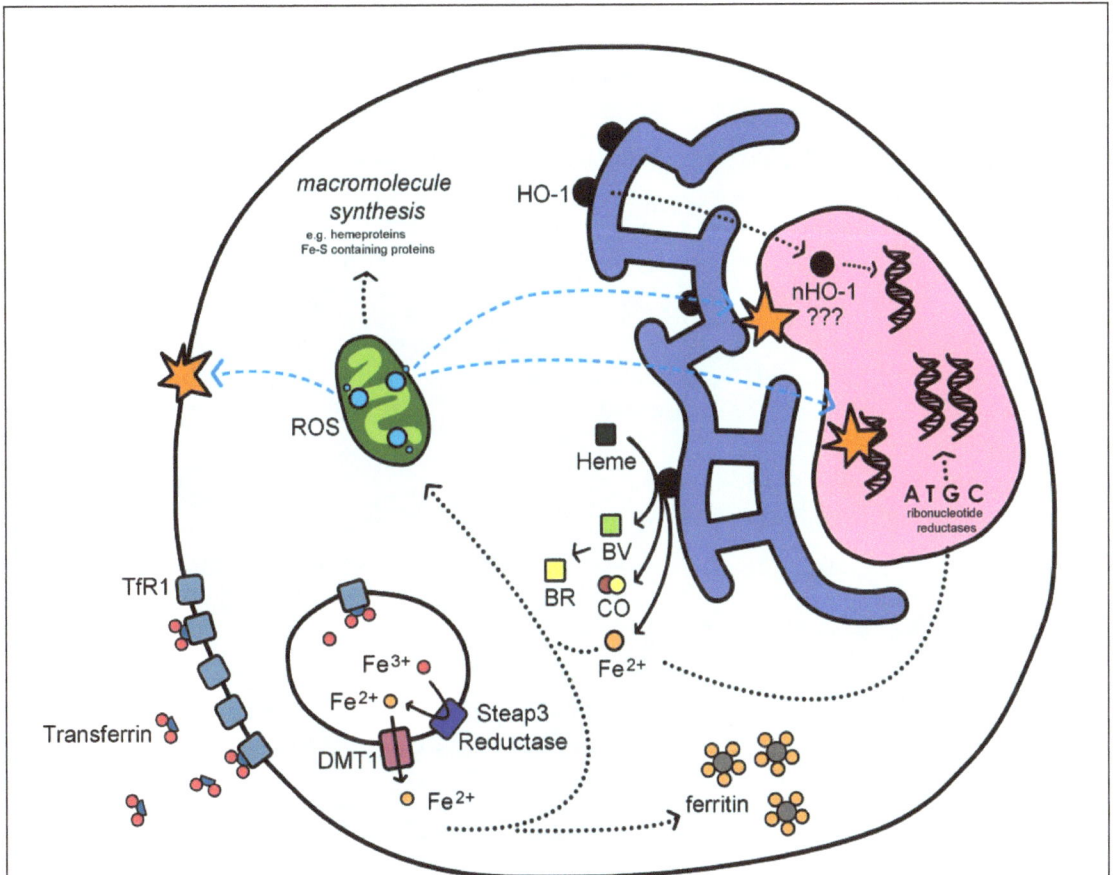

Figure 4: Scheme of iron import and utilization by cancer cells. Cancer cells maintain high level of total iron import through increased expression of transferrin receptors and minimal ferroportin expression. Low ferritin measurements and high aminolevulinic acid synthase (ALAS1) activity in cancer cells indicate low sequestration and high iron utilization by mitochondria. Iron is essential for macromolecule synthesis such as various hemoproteins, iron-sulfur (Fe-S) containing proteins, and ribonucleotide reductases that synthesize deoxyribonucleotides that are utilized by cancer cells for their abnormal and accelerated growth. Free iron further contributes to carcinogenesis by Fenton chemistry through catalysis of mitochondrial and lipid mediated ROS formation that causes DNA mutations. Nuclear translocation of HO-1 has also been reported for various cancers, though its function in the nucleus is currently unknown.

The role of HO-1 in cancer has been either linked to more advanced disease in the presence of dysfunctional HO-1 in the nucleus in prostate cancer (Sacca *et al.*, 2007; Wegiel *et al.*, 2013) or to the better prognosis if present in the cytoplasm in breast cancer (Lin, Shen, Hou, Yang and Chen 2008). Recent data suggests an alternative utilization of HO-1 protective properties in assisting in the progression of malignant cells (Jozkowicz, Was and Dulak 2007). The protective properties of HO-1 can also be considered as a hallmarks of carcinogenesis, and elevated HO-1 expression have been reported in various tumor tissues. In renal cell carcinoma, elevated HO-1 in tumor tissues was suggested to contribute to neoplastic development by reducing oxidative damage caused by cytochrome P450 metabolites (Goodman, Choudhury, da Silva, Schwartzman and Abraham, 1997). Overexpression of HO-1 accelerated tumor growth through the promotion of angiogenesis in prostate cancer (Birrane, Li, Yang, Tachado and Seng, 2013). HO-1 is also implicated as BCR-ABL-mediated antiapoptotic survival signal in chronic myeloid leukemia (Tibullo *et al.*, 2013). Importantly, HO-1 expression is also potently increased in response to chemotherapy, radiation, and photodynamic therapy (Jozkowicz *et al.*, 2007).

While HO-1 normally carries out catabolism of heme on the endoplasmic reticulum, membrane-bound caveaole, or in mitochondria, recently the truncated isoform has been described in the nucleus of cancer cells. While HO-1 has also been located in endothelial cell calveolae to modulate carbon monoxide (CO) and nitric oxide (NO) production (Kim, Wang, Galbiati, Ryter and Choi, 2004) and in mitochondria to protect against mitochondrial oxidative stress (Bindu *et al.*, 2011), nuclear translocation is atypical in that the HO-1 enzyme is both modified—nuclear translocation is dependent on proteolytic cleavage of a c-terminal tail—and has abrogated enzymatic activity (Lin *et al.*, 2007; Wegiel *et al.*, 2013). Nuclear HO-1 showed protective and progressive effects in prostate cancer (Sacca *et al.*, 2007), head and neck squamous cell carcinoma (Gandini *et al.*, 2012), and oral epithelial dysplasia (Lee *et al.*, 2008). Nuclear localization has also been correlated to higher VEGF production (Birrane *et al.*, 2013) and resistance to chemotherapy (Tibullo *et al.*, 2013). Interestingly, unlike BVR, HO-1 does not have DNA binding motifs and thus cannot act as a transcription factor, although many have speculated on the role of HO-1 mediated chromatin modifications and transactivation of transcription factors including AP-1 or NFκB (Lin *et al.*, 2007). The specifics of how nuclear translocation of HO-1 affects tumor growth have yet to be elucidated.

5   Heme Degradation-derived Iron in Tissue Homeostasis and Cancer

Information about the role and expression of HO-1 in TAMs is limited. HO-1 was identified as a key gene out of 54 genes associated with iron recycling that distinguished the polarization status between M1 and M2 macrophages.(Recalcati *et al.*, 2010) During the early stages of cancer, myeloid cells are recruited from the blood into the tissues and in the presence of pathogen or sterile inflammation differentiate and are polarized towards M1 "classically activated" macrophages that activate an immune response, promote inflammation, sequester iron, promote cancer cell regression, and inhibit development of tumours (Sica, Schioppa, Mantovani and Allavena, 2006). However, in the later stages of cancer progression, recruited and resident macrophages in the tumor microenvironment become polarized towards an "alternatively activated" M2 phenotype with anti-inflammatory, immunosuppressive, pro-angiogenic, and favour iron intake and iron export characteristics. Since HO-1 is expressed in both M1 and M2 macrophages, being more pronounced in M2 macrophages, we speculate that HO-1 may have a significant role in shaping the tumor microenvironment. The switch between M1 and M2 macrophages is important for responses against the tumor as well as tumor maintenance.

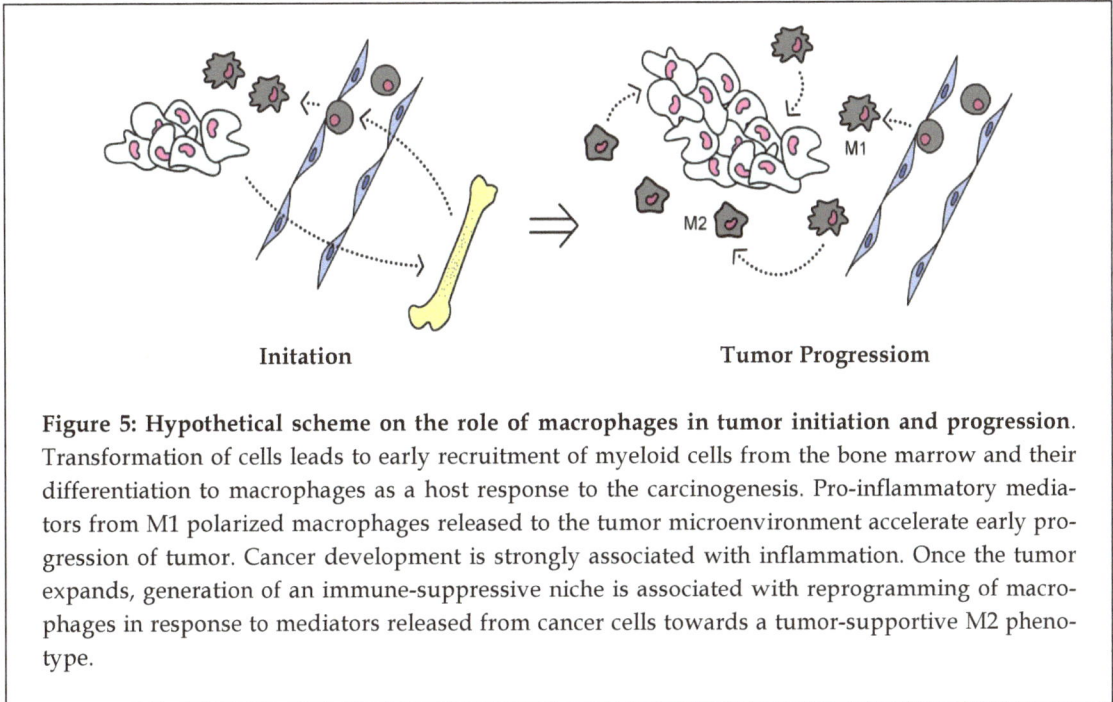

Initation   Tumor Progressiom

Figure 5: Hypothetical scheme on the role of macrophages in tumor initiation and progression. Transformation of cells leads to early recruitment of myeloid cells from the bone marrow and their differentiation to macrophages as a host response to the carcinogenesis. Pro-inflammatory mediators from M1 polarized macrophages released to the tumor microenvironment accelerate early progression of tumor. Cancer development is strongly associated with inflammation. Once the tumor expands, generation of an immune-suppressive niche is associated with reprogramming of macrophages in response to mediators released from cancer cells towards a tumor-supportive M2 phenotype.

In metastatic melanoma, HO-1 expression was primarily detected in CD163-positive TAM, typically associated with M2 polarization (Sierra-Filardi *et al.*, 2010). Administration of cobalt protoporphyrin, a potent inducer of HO-1, resulted in increased IL-10 release from M2 macrophages, suggesting that HO-1 is important for the anti-inflammatory activities of MCSF M2 polarized macrophages (Sierra-Filardi *et al.*, 2010). M1-polarizing cytokines (GM-CSF, IFNγ) inhibited, while IL-4 enhanced, M-CSF-driven HO-1 expression (Sierra-Filardi *et al.*, 2010). MCSF-stimulated macrophages showed high levels of HO-1 and their functional status depends on the generation of carbon monoxide (Wegiel *et al.*, 2014). Furthermore, binding of hemoglobin-haptoglobin to CD163 cells elicited IL10 secretion and resulted in HO-1 induction (Philippidis *et al.*, 2004). Surprisingly, stable overexpression of HO-1 cells resulted in lower ferritin concentrations while the labile iron was not shown to increase significantly (Li *et al.*, 2012).

6   Concluding Remarks

In summary, iron metabolism, recycling and storage are critical determinants of cancer development and progression. All above processes are controlled by macrophages and therefore

TAM with altered iron homeostasis may contribute to cancer growth and promotion. The heme degradation pathway and HO-1 are important regulator of iron recycling and utilization and as such dictate cancer growth and metastases. Cancer cells are characterized by increased iron intake and use, and M2 macrophages are uniquely positioned in the tumor microenvironment to facilitate enhanced heme degradation and iron export that contributes to cancer progression to more advance disease.

References

Aisen, P., C. Enns and M. Wessling-Resnick (2001). Chemistry and biology of eukaryotic iron metabolism. Int J Biochem Cell Biol 33(10), 940-959.

Alkhateeb, A. A., B. Han and J. R. Connor (2013). Ferritin stimulates breast cancer cells through an iron-independent mechanism and is localized within tumor-associated macrophages. Breast Cancer Res Treat 137(3), 733-744.

Andrews, N. C. (1999). Disorders of iron metabolism. N Engl J Med 341(26), 1986-1995.

Ba, Q., M. Hao, H. Huang, J. Hou, S. Ge, Z. Zhang, J. Yin, R. Chu, H. Jiang, F. Wang, K. Chen, H. Liu and H. Wang (2011). Iron deprivation suppresses hepatocellular carcinoma growth in experimental studies. Clin Cancer Res 17(24), 7625-7633.

Bastide, N. M., F. H. Pierre and D. E. Corpet (2011). Heme iron from meat and risk of colorectal cancer: a meta-analysis and a review of the mechanisms involved. Cancer Prev Res (Phila) 4(2), 177-184.

Beinert, H., M. H. Emptage, J. L. Dreyer, R. A. Scott, J. E. Hahn, K. O. Hodgson and A. J. Thomson (1983). Iron-sulfur stoichiometry and structure of iron-sulfur clusters in three-iron proteins: evidence for [3Fe-4S] clusters. Proc Natl Acad Sci U S A 80(2), 393-396.

Bindu, S., C. Pal, S. Dey, M. Goyal, A. Alam, M. S. Iqbal, S. Dutta, S. Sarkar, R. Kumar, P. Maity and U. Bandyopadhyay (2011). Translocation of heme oxygenase-1 to mitochondria is a novel cytoprotective mechanism against non-steroidal anti-inflammatory drug-induced mitochondrial oxidative stress, apoptosis, and gastric mucosal injury. J Biol Chem 286(45), 39387-39402.

Birrane, G., H. Li, S. Yang, S. D. Tachado and S. Seng (2013). Cigarette smoke induces nuclear translocation of heme oxygenase 1 (HO-1) in prostate cancer cells: nuclear HO-1 promotes vascular endothelial growth factor secretion. Int J Oncol 42(6), 1919-1928.

Biswas, S. K., A. Sica and C. E. Lewis (2008). Plasticity of macrophage function during tumor progression: regulation by distinct molecular mechanisms. J Immunol 180(4), 2011-2017.

Blatt, J. and S. Stitely (1987). Antineuroblastoma activity of desferoxamine in human cell lines. Cancer Res 47(7), 1749-1750.

Breuer, W., C. Hershko and Z. I. Cabantchik (2000). The importance of non-transferrin bound iron in disorders of iron metabolism. Transfus Sci 23(3), 185-192.

Brissot, P., M. Ropert, C. Le Lan and O. Loreal (2012). Non-transferrin bound iron: a key role in iron overload and iron toxicity. Biochim Biophys Acta 1820(3), 403-410.

Brookes, M. J., S. Hughes, F. E. Turner, G. Reynolds, N. Sharma, T. Ismail, G. Berx, A. T. McKie, N. Hotchin, G. J. Anderson, T. Iqbal and C. Tselepis (2006). Modulation of iron transport proteins in human colorectal carcinogenesis. Gut 55(10), 1449-1460.

Cabantchik, Z. I., W. Breuer, G. Zanninelli and P. Cianciulli (2005). LPI-labile plasma iron in iron overload. Best Pract Res Clin Haematol 18(2), 277-287.

Cermak, J., J. Balla, H. S. Jacob, G. Balla, H. Enright, K. Nath and G. M. Vercellotti (1993). Tumor cell heme uptake induces ferritin synthesis resulting in altered oxidant sensitivity: possible role in chemotherapy efficacy. Cancer Res 53(21), 5308-5313.

Chan, K. T., M. Y. Choi, K. K. Lai, W. Tan, L. N. Tung, H. Y. Lam, D. K. Tong, N. P. Lee and S. Law (2014). Overexpression of transferrin receptor CD71 and its tumorigenic properties in esophageal squamous cell carcinoma. Oncol Rep 31(3), 1296-1304.

Chevion, M. (1988). A site-specific mechanism for free radical induced biological damage: the essential role of redox-active transition metals. Free Radic Biol Med 5(1), 27-37.

Cohen, L. A., L. Gutierrez, A. Weiss, Y. Leichtmann-Bardoogo, D. L. Zhang, D. R. Crooks, R. Sougrat, A. Morgenstern, B. Galy, M. W. Hentze, F. J. Lazaro, T. A. Rouault and E. G. Meyron-Holtz (2010). Serum ferritin is derived primarily from macrophages through a nonclassical secretory pathway. Blood 116(9), 1574-1584.

Corna, G., L. Campana, E. Pignatti, A. Castiglioni, E. Tagliafico, L. Bosurgi, A. Campanella, S. Brunelli, A. A. Manfredi, P. Apostoli, L. Silvestri, C. Camaschella and P. Rovere-Querini (2010). Polarization dictates iron handling by inflammatory and alternatively activated macrophages. Haematologica 95(11), 1814-1822.

Cozzi, A., P. Santambrogio, D. Privitera, V. Broccoli, L. I. Rotundo, B. Garavaglia, R. Benz, S. Altamura, J. S. Goede, M. U. Muckenthaler and S. Levi (2013). Human L-ferritin deficiency is characterized by idiopathic generalized seizures and atypical restless leg syndrome. J Exp Med 210(9), 1779-1791.

Dautry-Varsat, A., A. Ciechanover and H. F. Lodish (1983). pH and the recycling of transferrin during receptor-mediated endocytosis. Proc Natl Acad Sci U S A 80(8), 2258-2262.

Donovan, A., C. A. Lima, J. L. Pinkus, G. S. Pinkus, L. I. Zon, S. Robine and N. C. Andrews (2005). The iron exporter ferroportin/Slc40a1 is essential for iron homeostasis. Cell Metab 1(3), 191-200.

Elford, H. L., M. Freese, E. Passamani and H. P. Morris (1970). Ribonucleotide reductase and cell proliferation. I. Variations of ribonucleotide reductase activity with tumor growth rate in a series of rat hepatomas. J Biol Chem 245(20), 5228-5233.

Feelders, R. A., G. Vreugdenhil, A. M. Eggermont, P. A. Kuiper-Kramer, H. G. van Eijk and A. J. Swaak (1998). Regulation of iron metabolism in the acute-phase response: interferon gamma and tumour necrosis factor alpha induce hypoferraemia, ferritin production and a decrease in circulating transferrin receptors in cancer patients. Eur J Clin Invest 28(7), 520-527.

Fleming, M. D., C. C. Trenor, 3rd, M. A. Su, D. Foernzler, D. R. Beier, W. F. Dietrich and N. C. Andrews (1997). Microcytic anaemia mice have a mutation in Nramp2, a candidate iron transporter gene. Nat Genet 16(4), 383-386.

Foa, P., A. T. Maiolo, L. Lombardi, L. Villa and E. E. Polli (1986). Inhibition of proliferation of human leukaemic cell populations by deferoxamine. Scand J Haematol 36(1), 107-110.

Franklin, R. A., W. Liao, A. Sarkar, M. V. Kim, M. R. Bivona, K. Liu, E. G. Pamer and M. O. Li (2014). The cellular and molecular origin of tumor-associated macrophages. Science 344(6186), 921-925.

Furutani, T., K. Hino, M. Okuda, T. Gondo, S. Nishina, A. Kitase, M. Korenaga, S. Y. Xiao, S. A. Weinman, S. M. Lemon, I. Sakaida and K. Okita (2006). Hepatic iron overload induces hepatocellular carcinoma in transgenic mice expressing the hepatitis C virus polyprotein. Gastroenterology 130(7), 2087-2098.

Gagnon, E., S. Duclos, C. Rondeau, E. Chevet, P. H. Cameron, O. Steele-Mortimer, J. Paiement, J. J. Bergeron and M. Desjardins (2002). Endoplasmic reticulum-mediated phagocytosis is a mechanism of entry into macrophages. Cell 110(1), 119-131.

Gandini, N. A., M. E. Fermento, D. G. Salomon, J. Blasco, V. Patel, J. S. Gutkind, A. A. Molinolo, M. M. Facchinetti and A. C. Curino (2012). Nuclear localization of heme oxygenase-1 is associated with tumor progression of head and neck squamous cell carcinomas. Exp Mol Pathol 93(2), 237-245.

Ganz, T. (2003). Hepcidin, a key regulator of iron metabolism and mediator of anemia of inflammation. Blood 102(3), 783-788.

Ganz, T. (2007). Molecular control of iron transport. J Am Soc Nephrol 18(2), 394-400.

Gao, J. and D. R. Richardson (2001). The potential of iron chelators of the pyridoxal isonicotinoyl hydrazone class as effective antiproliferative agents, IV: The mechanisms involved in inhibiting cell-cycle progression. Blood 98(3), 842-850.

Goodman, A. I., M. Choudhury, J. L. da Silva, M. L. Schwartzman and N. G. Abraham (1997). Overexpression of the heme oxygenase gene in renal cell carcinoma. Proc Soc Exp Biol Med 214(1), 54-61.

Graf, E., J. R. Mahoney, R. G. Bryant and J. W. Eaton (1984). Iron-catalyzed hydroxyl radical formation. Stringent requirement for free iron coordination site. J Biol Chem 259(6), 3620-3624.

Gunshin, H., B. Mackenzie, U. V. Berger, Y. Gunshin, M. F. Romero, W. F. Boron, S. Nussberger, J. L. Gollan and M. A. Hediger (1997). Cloning and characterization of a mammalian proton-coupled metal-ion transporter. Nature 388(6641), 482-488.

Habashy, H. O., D. G. Powe, C. M. Staka, E. A. Rakha, G. Ball, A. R. Green, M. Aleskandarany, E. C. Paish, R. Douglas Macmillan, R. I. Nicholson, I. O. Ellis and J. M. Gee (2010). Transferrin receptor (CD71) is a marker of poor prognosis in breast cancer and can predict response to tamoxifen. Breast Cancer Res Treat 119(2), 283-293.

Habeshaw, J. A., T. A. Lister, A. G. Stansfeld and M. F. Greaves (1983). Correlation of transferrin receptor expression with histological class and outcome in non-Hodgkin lymphoma. Lancet 1(8323), 498-501.

Hann, H. W., M. W. Stahlhut and C. L. Hann (1990). Effect of iron and desferoxamine on cell growth and in vitro ferritin synthesis in human hepatoma cell lines. Hepatology 11(4), 566-569.

Harris, Z. L., A. P. Durley, T. K. Man and J. D. Gitlin (1999). Targeted gene disruption reveals an essential role for ceruloplasmin in cellular iron efflux. Proc Natl Acad Sci U S A 96(19), 10812-10817.

Harrison, P. M. and P. Arosio (1996). The ferritins: molecular properties, iron storage function and cellular regulation. Biochim Biophys Acta 1275(3), 161-203.

Hirano, K., T. Morinobu, H. Kim, M. Hiroi, R. Ban, S. Ogawa, H. Ogihara, H. Tamai and T. Ogihara (2001). Blood transfusion increases radical promoting non-transferrin bound iron in preterm infants. Arch Dis Child Fetal Neonatal Ed 84(3), F188-193.

Hogemann-Savellano, D., E. Bos, C. Blondet, F. Sato, T. Abe, L. Josephson, R. Weissleder, J. Gaudet, D. Sgroi, P. J. Peters and J. P. Basilion (2003). The transferrin receptor: a potential molecular imaging marker for human cancer. Neoplasia 5(6), 495-506.

Hooda, J., D. Cadinu, M. M. Alam, A. Shah, T. M. Cao, L. A. Sullivan, R. Brekken and L. Zhang (2013). Enhanced heme function and mitochondrial respiration promote the progression of lung cancer cells. PLoS One 8(5), e63402.

Hubert, N. and M. W. Hentze (2002). Previously uncharacterized isoforms of divalent metal transporter (DMT)-1: implications for regulation and cellular function. Proc Natl Acad Sci U S A 99(19), 12345-12350.

Jiang, X. P., R. L. Elliott and J. F. Head (2010). Manipulation of iron transporter genes results in the suppression of human and mouse mammary adenocarcinomas. Anticancer Res 30(3), 759-765.

Jozkowicz, A., H. Was and J. Dulak (2007). Heme oxygenase-1 in tumors: is it a false friend? Antioxid Redox Signal 9(12), 2099-2117.

Kawashima, A., Y. Oda, A. Yachie, S. Koizumi and I. Nakanishi (2002). Heme oxygenase-1 deficiency: the first autopsy case. Hum Pathol 33(1), 125-130.

Keer, H. N., J. M. Kozlowski, Y. C. Tsai, C. Lee, R. N. McEwan and J. T. Grayhack (1990). Elevated transferrin receptor content in human prostate cancer cell lines assessed in vitro and in vivo. J Urol 143(2), 381-385.

Kim, H. P., X. Wang, F. Galbiati, S. W. Ryter and A. M. Choi (2004). Caveolae compartmentalization of heme oxygenase-1 in endothelial cells. FASEB J 18(10), 1080-1089.

Kim, J. L., H. N. Kang, M. H. Kang, Y. A. Yoo, J. S. Kim and C. W. Choi (2011). The oral iron chelator deferasirox induces apoptosis in myeloid leukemia cells by targeting caspase. Acta Haematol 126(4), 241-245.

Kohgo, Y., K. Ikuta, T. Ohtake, Y. Torimoto and J. Kato (2008). Body iron metabolism and pathophysiology of iron overload. Int J Hematol 88(1), 7-15.

Kovtunovych, G., M. A. Eckhaus, M. C. Ghosh, H. Ollivierre-Wilson and T. A. Rouault (2010). Dysfunction of the heme recycling system in heme oxygenase 1-deficient mice: effects on macrophage viability and tissue iron distribution. Blood 116(26), 6054-6062.

Kowdley, K. V. (2004). Iron, hemochromatosis, and hepatocellular carcinoma. Gastroenterology 127(5 Suppl 1), S79-86.

Kristiansen, M., J. H. Graversen, C. Jacobsen, O. Sonne, H. J. Hoffman, S. K. Law and S. K. Moestrup (2001). Identification of the haemoglobin scavenger receptor. Nature 409(6817), 198-201.

Kukulj, S., M. Jaganjac, M. Boranic, S. Krizanac, Z. Santic and M. Poljak-Blazi (2010). Altered iron metabolism, inflammation, transferrin receptors, and ferritin expression in non-small-cell lung cancer. Med Oncol 27(2), 268-277.

Kulp, K. S., S. L. Green and P. R. Vulliet (1996). Iron deprivation inhibits cyclin-dependent kinase activity and decreases cyclin D/CDK4 protein levels in asynchronous MDA-MB-453 human breast cancer cells. Exp Cell Res 229(1), 60-68.

Latunde-Dada, G. O., K. Takeuchi, R. J. Simpson and A. T. McKie (2006). Haem carrier protein 1 (HCP1): Expression and functional studies in cultured cells. FEBS Lett 580(30), 6865-6870.

Lederman, H. M., A. Cohen, J. W. Lee, M. H. Freedman and E. W. Gelfand (1984). Deferoxamine: a reversible S-phase inhibitor of human lymphocyte proliferation. Blood 64(3), 748-753.

Lee, J., S. K. Lee, B. U. Lee, H. J. Lee, N. P. Cho, J. H. Yoon, H. R. Choi, S. K. Lee and E. C. Kim (2008). Upregulation of heme oxygenase-1 in oral epithelial dysplasias. Int J Oral Maxillofac Surg 37(3), 287-292.

Li, C., M. E. Lonn, X. Xu, G. J. Maghzal, D. M. Frazer, S. R. Thomas, B. Halliwell, D. R. Richardson, G. J. Anderson and R. Stocker (2012). Sustained expression of heme oxygenase-1 alters iron homeostasis in nonerythroid cells. Free Radic Biol Med 53(2), 366-374.

Lin, C. W., S. C. Shen, W. C. Hou, L. Y. Yang and Y. C. Chen (2008). Heme oxygenase-1 inhibits breast cancer invasion via suppressing the expression of matrix metalloproteinase-9. Mol Cancer Ther 7(5), 1195-1206.

Lin, Q., S. Weis, G. Yang, Y. H. Weng, R. Helston, K. Rish, A. Smith, J. Bordner, T. Polte, F. Gaunitz and P. A. Dennery (2007). Heme oxygenase-1 protein localizes to the nucleus and activates transcription factors important in oxidative stress. J Biol Chem 282(28), 20621-20633.

Lloyd, D. R. and D. H. Phillips (1999). Oxidative DNA damage mediated by copper(II), iron(II) and nickel(II) fenton reactions: evidence for site-specific mechanisms in the formation of double-strand breaks, 8-hydroxydeoxyguanosine and putative intrastrand cross-links. Mutat Res 424(1-2), 23-36.

Lucas, J. J., A. Szepesi, J. Domenico, K. Takase, A. Tordai, N. Terada and E. W. Gelfand (1995). Effects of iron-depletion on cell cycle progression in normal human T lymphocytes: selective inhibition of the appearance of the cyclin A-associated component of the p33cdk2 kinase. Blood 86(6), 2268-2280.

Lui, G. Y., P. Obeidy, S. J. Ford, C. Tselepis, D. M. Sharp, P. J. Jansson, D. S. Kalinowski, Z. Kovacevic, D. B. Lovejoy and D. R. Richardson (2013). The iron chelator, deferasirox, as a novel strategy for cancer treatment: oral activity against human lung tumor xenografts and molecular mechanism of action. Mol Pharmacol 83(1), 179-190.

Maines, M. D. (1988). Heme oxygenase: function, multiplicity, regulatory mechanisms, and clinical applications. FASEB J 2(10), 2557-2568.

Mantovani, A. and M. Locati (2013). Tumor-associated macrophages as a paradigm of macrophage plasticity, diversity, and polarization: lessons and open questions. Arterioscler Thromb Vasc Biol 33(7), 1478-1483.

Mantovani, A., S. Sozzani, M. Locati, P. Allavena and A. Sica (2002). Macrophage polarization: tumor-associated macrophages as a paradigm for polarized M2 mononuclear phagocytes. Trends Immunol 23(11), 549-555.

Mello Filho, A. C., M. E. Hoffmann and R. Meneghini (1984). Cell killing and DNA damage by hydrogen peroxide are mediated by intracellular iron. Biochem J 218(1), 273-275.

Meneghini, R. (1997). Iron homeostasis, oxidative stress, and DNA damage. Free Radic Biol Med 23(5), 783-792.

Miller, L. D., L. G. Coffman, J. W. Chou, M. A. Black, J. Bergh, R. D'Agostino, Jr., S. V. Torti and F. M. Torti (2011). An iron regulatory gene signature predicts outcome in breast cancer. Cancer Res 71(21), 6728-6737.

Mitra, J., C. Y. Dai, K. Somasundaram, W. S. El-Deiry, K. Satyamoorthy, M. Herlyn and G. H. Enders (1999). Induction of p21(WAF1/CIP1) and inhibition of Cdk2 mediated by the tumor suppressor p16(INK4a). Mol Cell Biol 19(5), 3916-3928.

Moller, H. J., N. A. Peterslund, J. H. Graversen and S. K. Moestrup (2002). Identification of the hemoglobin scavenger receptor/CD163 as a natural soluble protein in plasma. Blood 99(1), 378-380.

Morel, I., G. Lescoat, J. Cillard, N. Pasdeloup, P. Brissot and P. Cillard (1990). Kinetic evaluation of free malondialdehyde and enzyme leakage as indices of iron damage in rat hepatocyte cultures. Involvement of free radicals. Biochem Pharmacol 39(11), 1647-1655.

Munoz, M., I. Villar and J. A. Garcia-Erce (2009). An update on iron physiology. World J Gastroenterol 15(37), 4617-4626.

Napier, I., P. Ponka and D. R. Richardson (2005). Iron trafficking in the mitochondrion: novel pathways revealed by disease. Blood 105(5), 1867-1874.

Nemeth, E., M. S. Tuttle, J. Powelson, M. B. Vaughn, A. Donovan, D. M. Ward, T. Ganz and J. Kaplan (2004). Hepcidin regulates cellular iron efflux by binding to ferroportin and inducing its internalization. Science 306(5704), 2090-2093.

Nie, G., G. Chen, A. D. Sheftel, K. Pantopoulos and P. Ponka (2006). In vivo tumor growth is inhibited by cytosolic iron deprivation caused by the expression of mitochondrial ferritin. Blood 108(7), 2428-2434.

Nurtjahja-Tjendraputra, E., D. Fu, J. M. Phang and D. R. Richardson (2007). Iron chelation regulates cyclin D1 expression via the proteasome: a link to iron deficiency-mediated growth suppression. Blood 109(9), 4045-4054.

Ohgami, R. S., D. R. Campagna, E. L. Greer, B. Antiochos, A. McDonald, J. Chen, J. J. Sharp, Y. Fujiwara, J. E. Barker and M. D. Fleming (2005). Identification of a ferrireductase required for efficient transferrin-dependent iron uptake in erythroid cells. Nat Genet 37(11), 1264-1269.

Pantopoulos, K., N. K. Gray and M. W. Hentze (1995). Differential regulation of two related RNA-binding proteins, iron regulatory protein (IRP) and IRPB. RNA 1(2), 155-163.

Pantopoulos, K., S. Mueller, A. Atzberger, W. Ansorge, W. Stremmel and M. W. Hentze (1997). Differences in the regulation of iron regulatory protein-1 (IRP-1) by extra- and intracellular oxidative stress. J Biol Chem 272(15), 9802-9808.

Perutz, M. F. (1979). Regulation of oxygen affinity of hemoglobin: influence of structure of the globin on the heme iron. Annu Rev Biochem 48, 327-386.

Philippidis, P., J. C. Mason, B. J. Evans, I. Nadra, K. M. Taylor, D. O. Haskard and R. C. Landis (2004). Hemoglobin scavenger receptor CD163 mediates interleukin-10 release and heme oxygenase-1 synthesis: antiinflammatory monocyte-macrophage responses in vitro, in resolving skin blisters in vivo, and after cardiopulmonary bypass surgery. Circ Res 94(1), 119-126.

Pietrangelo, A. (2010). Hereditary hemochromatosis: pathogenesis, diagnosis, and treatment. Gastroenterology 139(2), 393-408, 408 e391-392.

Pinnix, Z. K., L. D. Miller, W. Wang, R. D'Agostino, Jr., T. Kute, M. C. Willingham, H. Hatcher, L. Tesfay, G. Sui, X. Di, S. V. Torti and F. M. Torti (2010). Ferroportin and iron regulation in breast cancer progression and prognosis. Sci Transl Med 2(43), 43ra56.

Pollycove, M. and R. Mortimer (1961). The quantitative determination of iron kinetics and hemoglobin synthesis in human subjects. J Clin Invest 40, 753-782.

Poss, K. D. and S. Tonegawa (1997). Heme oxygenase 1 is required for mammalian iron reutilization. Proc Natl Acad Sci U S A 94(20), 10919-10924.

Prutki, M., M. Poljak-Blazi, M. Jakopovic, D. Tomas, I. Stipancic and N. Zarkovic (2006). Altered iron metabolism, transferrin receptor 1 and ferritin in patients with colon cancer. Cancer Lett 238(2), 188-196.

Recalcati, S., M. Locati, A. Marini, P. Santambrogio, F. Zaninotto, M. De Pizzol, L. Zammataro, D. Girelli and G. Cairo (2010). Differential regulation of iron homeostasis during human macrophage polarized activation. Eur J Immunol 40(3), 824-835.

Reddel, R. R., D. W. Hedley and R. L. Sutherland (1985). Cell cycle effects of iron depletion on T-47D human breast cancer cells. Exp Cell Res 161(2), 277-284.

Rivera, S., L. Liu, E. Nemeth, V. Gabayan, O. E. Sorensen and T. Ganz (2005). Hepcidin excess induces the sequestration of iron and exacerbates tumor-associated anemia. Blood 105(4), 1797-1802.

Sacca, P., R. Meiss, G. Casas, O. Mazza, J. C. Calvo, N. Navone and E. Vazquez (2007). Nuclear translocation of haeme oxygenase-1 is associated to prostate cancer. Br J Cancer 97(12), 1683-1689.

Sawa, T., T. Akaike, K. Kida, Y. Fukushima, K. Takagi and H. Maeda (1998). Lipid peroxyl radicals from oxidized oils and heme-iron: implication of a high-fat diet in colon carcinogenesis. Cancer Epidemiol Biomarkers Prev 7(11), 1007-1012.

Schaar, D. G., D. J. Medina, D. F. Moore, R. K. Strair and Y. Ting (2009). miR-320 targets transferrin receptor 1 (CD71) and inhibits cell proliferation. Exp Hematol 37(2), 245-255.

Schaer, C. A., F. Vallelian, A. Imhof, G. Schoedon and D. J. Schaer (2008). Heme carrier protein (HCP-1) spatially interacts with the CD163 hemoglobin uptake pathway and is a target of inflammatory macrophage activation. J Leukoc Biol 83(2), 325-333.

Schaer, D. J., C. A. Schaer, P. W. Buehler, R. A. Boykins, G. Schoedon, A. I. Alayash and A. Schaffner (2006). CD163 is the macrophage scavenger receptor for native and chemically modified hemoglobins in the absence of haptoglobin. Blood 107(1), 373-380.

Shindelman, J. E., A. E. Ortmeyer and H. H. Sussman (1981). Demonstration of the transferrin receptor in human breast cancer tissue. Potential marker for identifying dividing cells. Int J Cancer 27(3), 329-334.

Shoden, A., B. W. Gabrio and C. A. Finch (1953). The relationship between ferritin and hemosiderin in rabbits and man. J Biol Chem 204(2), 823-830.

Sica, A. and A. Mantovani (2012). Macrophage plasticity and polarization: in vivo veritas. J Clin Invest 122(3), 787-795.

Sica, A., T. Schioppa, A. Mantovani and P. Allavena (2006). Tumour-associated macrophages are a distinct M2 polarised population promoting tumour progression: potential targets of anti-cancer therapy. Eur J Cancer 42(6), 717-727.

Sierra-Filardi, E., M. A. Vega, P. Sanchez-Mateos, A. L. Corbi and A. Puig-Kroger (2010). Heme Oxygenase-1 expression in M-CSF-polarized M2 macrophages contributes to LPS-induced IL-10 release. Immunobiology 215(9-10), 788-795.

Simson, J. V. and S. S. Spicer (1972). Ferritin particles in macrophages and in associated mast cells. J Cell Biol 52(3), 536-541.

Sow, F. B., G. R. Alvarez, R. P. Gross, A. R. Satoskar, L. S. Schlesinger, B. S. Zwilling and W. P. Lafuse (2009). Role of STAT1, NF-kappaB, and C/EBPbeta in the macrophage transcriptional regulation of hepcidin by mycobacterial infection and IFN-gamma. J Leukoc Biol 86(5), 1247-1258.

Sutherland, R., D. Delia, C. Schneider, R. Newman, J. Kemshead and M. Greaves (1981). Ubiquitous cell-surface glycoprotein on tumor cells is proliferation-associated receptor for transferrin. Proc Natl Acad Sci U S A 78(7), 4515-4519.

Tacchini, L., S. Recalcati, A. Bernelli-Zazzera and G. Cairo (1997). Induction of ferritin synthesis in ischemic-reperfused rat liver: analysis of the molecular mechanisms. Gastroenterology 113(3), 946-953.

Tenhunen, R., H. S. Marver and R. Schmid (1968). The enzymatic conversion of heme to bilirubin by microsomal heme oxygenase. Proc Natl Acad Sci U S A 61(2), 748-755.

Thomson, A. M., J. T. Rogers and P. J. Leedman (1999). Iron-regulatory proteins, iron-responsive elements and ferritin mRNA translation. Int J Biochem Cell Biol 31(10), 1139-1152.

Tibullo, D., I. Barbagallo, C. Giallongo, P. La Cava, N. Parrinello, L. Vanella, F. Stagno, G. A. Palumbo, G. Li Volti and F. Di Raimondo (2013). Nuclear translocation of heme oxygenase-1 confers resistance to imatinib in chronic myeloid leukemia cells. Curr Pharm Des 19(15), 2765-2770.

Torti, S. V. and F. M. Torti (2011). Ironing out cancer. Cancer Res 71(5), 1511-1514.

Torti, S. V. and F. M. Torti (2013). Iron and cancer: more ore to be mined. Nat Rev Cancer 13(5), 342-355.

Torti, S. V., F. M. Torti, S. P. Whitman, M. W. Brechbiel, G. Park and R. P. Planalp (1998). Tumor cell cytotoxicity of a novel metal chelator. Blood 92(4), 1384-1389.

Trinder, D., C. Fox, G. Vautier and J. K. Olynyk (2002). Molecular pathogenesis of iron overload. Gut 51(2), 290-295.

Trowbridge, I. S. and D. L. Domingo (1981). Anti-transferrin receptor monoclonal antibody and toxin-antibody conjugates affect growth of human tumour cells. Nature 294(5837), 171-173.

Turner, J., C. Koumenis, T. E. Kute, R. P. Planalp, M. W. Brechbiel, D. Beardsley, B. Cody, K. D. Brown, F. M. Torti and S. V. Torti (2005). Tachpyridine, a metal chelator, induces G2 cell-cycle arrest, activates checkpoint kinases, and sensitizes cells to ionizing radiation. Blood 106(9), 3191-3199.

Vallelian, F., C. A. Schaer, T. Kaempfer, P. Gehrig, E. Duerst, G. Schoedon and D. J. Schaer (2010). Glucocorticoid treatment skews human monocyte differentiation into a hemoglobin-clearance phenotype with enhanced heme-iron recycling and antioxidant capacity. Blood 116(24), 5347-5356.

Walsh, R. J., I. Kaldor, I. Brading and E. P. George (1955). The availability of iron in meat: some experiments with radioactive iron. Australas Ann Med 4(4), 272-276.

Wegiel, B., D. Gallo, E. Csizmadia, C. Harris, J. Belcher, G. M. Vercellotti, N. Penacho, P. Seth, V. Sukhatme, A. Ahmed, P. P. Pandolfi, L. Helczynski, A. Bjartell, J. L. Persson and L. E. Otterbein (2013). Carbon monoxide expedites metabolic exhaustion to inhibit tumor growth. Cancer Res 73(23), 7009-7021.

Wegiel, B., A. Hedblom, M. Li, D. Gallo, E. Csizmadia, C. Harris, Z. Nemeth, B. S. Zuckerbraun, M. Soares, J. L. Persson and L. E. Otterbein (2014). Heme oxygenase-1 derived carbon monoxide permits maturation of myeloid cells. Cell Death Dis 5, e1139.

Yachie, A., Y. Niida, T. Wada, N. Igarashi, H. Kaneda, T. Toma, K. Ohta, Y. Kasahara and S. Koizumi (1999). Oxidative stress causes enhanced endothelial cell injury in human heme oxygenase-1 deficiency. J Clin Invest 103(1), 129-135.

Yamaguchi, K., M. Mandai, S. Toyokuni, J. Hamanishi, T. Higuchi, K. Takakura and S. Fujii (2008). Contents of endometriotic cysts, especially the high concentration of free iron, are a possible cause of carcinogenesis in the cysts through the iron-induced persistent oxidative stress. Clin Cancer Res 14(1), 32-40.

Zaynagetdinov, R., T. P. Sherrill, V. V. Polosukhin, W. Han, J. A. Ausborn, A. G. McLoed, F. B. McMahon, L. A. Gleaves, A. L. Degryse, G. T. Stathopoulos, F. E. Yull and T. S. Blackwell (2011). A critical role for macrophages in promotion of urethane-induced lung carcinogenesis. J Immunol 187(11), 5703-5711.

Zhang, F., Y. Tao, Z. Zhang, X. Guo, P. An, Y. Shen, Q. Wu, Y. Yu and F. Wang (2012). Metalloreductase Steap3 coordinates the regulation of iron homeostasis and inflammatory responses. Haematologica 97(12), 1826-1835.

NER Pathway and Wild-Type p53 in Platinum-Drug Resistance and Inhibition of Chemoresistance with PCK3145, a PSP94 Peptide Derivative

Jing Jie Yu[*][†]

1 Introduction

This chapter is devoted to investigations of DNA repair gene ERCC1 and mechanistic studies of chemoresistance focusing on p53, Chk2, and MZF1. It proposes a new hypothetic chemo-sensitizer, PSP94, and its peptide derivative, PCK3145, to reverse chemoresistance and im-prove clinical outcomes for treatment of some cancers.

The rate of cancer death has declined in the United States from a peak of 215.1 in 1991 to 171.8 in 2010. This 20% decline translates to the prevention of more than a million cancer deaths. Still, a total of 1,665,540 new cancer cases and 585,720 cancer deaths are projected to occur in the US in 2014 (Greenlee *et al.*, 2001; Siegel *et al.*, 2014).

Chemotherapy is a standard treatment for human cancers. Platinum compounds (DNA-targeting drugs) and other anticancer agents are effective and have been widely used in clinical settings. However, adverse effects and especially tumor resistance to chemotherapy are major treatment obstacles affecting the life-quality of patients and therapeutic outcomes, often leading to treatment failure (Kelland *et al.*, 2007; Cossa *et al.*, 2009; Reed, 1998; Figg *et al.*, 2013; Curt, 2000; Curt *et al.*, 2000).

Drug-resistance is multifactorial in nature. Its mechanisms involve a complex network of cellular pathways and molecular changes with numerous cross-interactions at different stages (Gottesman *et al.*, 2002; Fojo & Bates, 2003; Annunziata & Kohn, 2013; Bates *et al.*, 1999; Lage, 2008). Resistance to platinum-compounds may occur due to alterations of drug influx and efflux; altered activation or metabolism; modified drug-induced damage or drug-targets; evasion of apoptosis (Longley & Johnston, 2005; Redmond *et al.*, 2008); and dynamic chroma-tin modification (Sharma *et al.*, 2010). Multi-drug resistance (MDR) proteins, RPN2, β-catenin and PI3K, have been reported as promising molecular targets for the reversal of drug-resistance (Berns *et al.*, 2007; Chen, 2010; Honma *et al.*, 2008; Yeung *et al.*, 2010). To date, how-ever, no successful chemosensitizers or diagnostic/prognostic assays for the prediction of therapy response have been developed.

[*] WVU Cancer Institute and Molecular Medicine Core
[†] Department of Biochemistry, School of Medicine; Department of Basic Pharmaceutical Sciences, School of Pharmacy; Robert C. Byrd Health Sciences Center, West Virginia University, Morgantown, WV, USA

Transcription factor p53, a DNA-binding protein containing DNA-binding, oligomerization, and transcriptional activation domains (Lamb & Crawford, 1986; Matlashewski *et al.*, 1984; Jeffery *et al.*, 1995; Cho *et al.*, 1994), plays a key role in DNA damage response to genotoxic stress by binding directly to the promoters of target genes and altering the rate at which they are transcribed (Lakin & Jackson, 1999; Vogelstein *et al.*, 2000). Embryo cells lacking p53 are resistant to anticancer drugs; these cells become sensitive to those drugs and die via apoptosis when p53 is restored (Brown & Wouters, 1999). Wild-type p53 protein has a role in the inhibition of DNA synthesis following DNA damage, suggesting a mechanism for how the loss of wild-type p53 may contribute to tumorigenesis (Fojo, 2002; Kastan *et al.*, 1991). Mutations of p53 have been associated with resistance to platinum-based chemotherapy and shortened survival in ovarian cancer (Reles *et al.*, 2001).

Checkpoint kinase 2 (*Chk2*), a serine/threonine kinase and encoded protein, contains a forkhead-associated protein interaction domain. It resides at the heart of the DNA damage/repair pathway and is responsible for the maintenance of mammalian genomic integrity. Studies suggest that Chk2 inhibition in combination with genotoxic agents might have therapeutic value (Hirao *et al.*, 2002; Yu *et al.*, 2001; Liang *et al.*, 2011). Inhibition of Chk2 expression reduces DNA-damage-induced cell cycle checkpoints and enhances apoptosis in p53-defective HEK-293 cells (Antoni *et al.*, 2007; Liang *et al.*, 2011). Molecular or genetic targeting of Chk2 prevents the release of survivin from mitochondria and enhances DNA-damage-induced tumor cell apoptosis, thus inhibiting *in vivo* growth of resistant tumors, providing a rational approach for treatment (Ghosh *et al.*, 2006).

Myeloid zinc finger 1 (*MZF1*), located on chromosome 19q, band 13.3, encodes a transcription factor protein (Morris, 1994). MZF1 is involved in growth, differentiation and apoptosis of myeloid progenitors and plays a key role in regulating transcription during differentiation along the myeloid lineage (Morris *et al.*, 1995; Perrotti *et al.*, 1995; Hromas *et al.*, 1996). MZF1 overexpression inhibits hematopoiesis (Hromas *et al.*, 1996), raising the possibility that it functions as a transcriptional repressor. We hypothesized that MZF1 may be involved in the function of ERCC1 (a marker for chemoresistance to platinum therapy) promoter and investigated MZF1 effects on ERCC1 transcription and expression (Yan *et al.*, 2006).

Prostatic secretory protein 94 (*PSP94*), also known as β-microsemino-protein or the long isoform of MSMB, is found in a variety of human tissues (Baijal-Gupta *et al.*, 2000; Lilja & Abrahamsson, 1988; Weiber *et al.*, 1990). Studies indicate that PSP94 expression decreases with the progression of prostate cancer; thus, it is a promising mechanism for cancer treatment and a biomarker for early detection (Whitaker *et al.*, 2010). Recently, we found decreased levels of PSP94 in chemoresistant ovarian cancer patients. Functional analysis indicated a critical role of PSP94 in chemoresistance, apparently by regulating downstream signaling of the Lin28b/Let-7 pathway. More importantly, PSP94 peptide derivative PCK3145 selectively suppressed growth of resistant cancer cells (*in vitro*) and tumor-bearing animals (*in vivo*) (Yan *et al.*, 2014).

On the treatment horizon, we are currently investigating the molecular mechanisms of dicycloplatin (DCP), a novel platinum analog developed in China (Yang *et al.*, 2010), approved by the Chinese State Food and Drug Administration (SFDA) in 2012. The molecular mechanisms appear to be similar to cisplatin and carboplatin but with fewer side-effects and broader therapeutic application (Yu *et al.*, 2014). We are exploring the possibility of a clinical trial with DCP in the United States.

2 Platinum Compounds and Nucleotide Excision Repair (NER) Pathway

Platinum-based chemotherapeutic agents such as cisplatin and carboplatin are the mainstream drugs for treating advanced cancers. Studies show that cells treated with genotoxic agents swiftly respond by activating DNA-damage checkpoint response. This prompts repair of DNA lesions, slowing replication or eliciting apoptosis in the case of massive or irreparable lesions to the DNA. Platinum drugs cause cell death by forming covalent crosslinks in DNA (DNA-adduct) that interfere with DNA replication and transcription, which leads to cell death (Johnson *et al.*, 1994; Kelland, 2007; Reed, 1998; Behrens *et al.*, 1987).

In response to DNA damage, cells evoke signal transduction pathways at G1/S, S or G2/M checkpoints to delay the cell cycle progression, allowing time to correct errors before moving on to the next phase. Two primary pathways are initiated in response to DNA damage. One is mediated by the ATM-Chk2 axis, the other by the ATR-Chk1 axis (Bartek & Lukas, 2003; Pommier *et al.*, 2006). DNA damage activates ATM (ataxia telangiectasia-mutated) and ATR (ATM-Rad3-related) kinases, the two apical protein kinases of the DNA damage response pathways (Abraham, 2001). ATM and ATR, in turn, activate Chk1 and Chk2, two key kinases, leading to initiation of DNA damage response pathways and cell cycle arrest. Generally, ATM- and ATR-initiated pathways function separately, but crosstalk between them occurs. Studies suggest that the ATM pathway mainly responds to ionizing radiation (IR)-induced DNA damage signal (Pandita *et al.*, 2000), while ATR pathway responds to UV and genotoxic drugs (Wright *et al.*, 1998; Hannan *et al.*, 2002; Zhang *et al.*, 2003). Platinum-therapeutic agents have a broad range of antitumor activity and are employed to treat many types of cancer. Unfortunately, many patients relapse following treatment and become refractory to those agents due to development of acquired resistance.

2.1 Mechanism of Action of Platinum Compounds

There are four drug-action steps in platinum chemotherapy: 1) **Uptake** (Cell Entry), which is not a matter of simple diffusion but involves plasma membrane proteins or transporter proteins, such as the copper transporter CTR1 (Lee *et al.*, 2002; Gottesman *et al.*, 2002). Studies suggest that about 50% of the initial rate of uptake occurs via passive diffusion and the rest is facilitated by transporters (active transport). Research findings indicate that reduced transport of platinum drugs is associated with decreased drug accumulation, which leads to drug resistance, and transporter CTR1-deficient cells seem to be cisplatin-resistant phenotype (Köberle *et al.*, 2010; Ishida *et al.*, 2002); 2) **Activation**, by which the parental drug is converted to active species that bind to the target or meant to attack the cancer cell DNA, usually achieved by hydrolysis inside the cell due to a much lower concentration of chloride ion. In other words, platinum is most effective at low intracellular and extracellular pH (Kuin *et al.*, 1999), and pH value was significantly increased in cisplatin-resistant cells with reduced DNA binding activity (Chau & Stewart, 1999; Murakami *et al.*, 2001); 3) **DNA Binding,** when the active species bind with the DNA and cause DNA crosslinks, the potency of the drug directly related to ability to form bi-functional interstrand and/or intrastrand crosslinks on DNA, thus disrupting cellular processes such as transcription and replication, leading to apoptosis; and 4) **Cellular Response**. With regard to the last step, platinum drugs provoke a complex series of cellular reactions. Lethal drug doses kill cells primarily by forming DNA adducts, causing cell-cycle arrest at the G2 phase. Platinum-DNA adducts are recognized by cellular proteins, including some that enhance the survival of cancer cells through the DNA repair system; others hasten death by conferring sensitivity to the drug and triggering apoptosis. Each step of drug-action is important in successful platinum chemotherapy. Defects or altera-tions of involved kinases/enzymes within the process can cause reduced drug efficacy and treatment failure (Mueller, 2008; Yu, 2009; Johnson *et al.*, 1994).

2.2 Increased DNA Repair is a Primary Mechanism of Acquired Resistance to Platinum Drugs

Clinical resistance to platinum therapy is positively associated with expression of human DNA repair gene ERCC1 (Dabholkar *et al.*, 1994) and is effected through the platinum-induced DNA adduct repair pathway (Behrens *et al.*, 1987; Eastman, 1983). Enhanced DNA repair of platinum-DNA adducts or removal of cisplatin-induced interstrand and intrastrand crosslinks has been observed in cisplatin-resistant cell models, and DNA repair inhibitors in some models can potentiate cisplatin cytotoxicity (Masuda *et al.*, 1988; Parker *et al.*, 1991; Johnson *et al.*, 1994). *In vitro* studies of platinum-resistant ovarian cancer A2780/CP70 cells showed a 6-fold increase in ERCC1 mRNA level in response to cisplatin exposure, caused by increased transcription and by prolonged mRNA half-life (Li *et al.*, 1998).

2.3 Nucleotide Excision Repair is Associated with Cellular and Clinical Resistance to Platinum Chemotherapy

Nucleotide excision repair (NER) is the critical DNA repair pathway. It appears to be the ma-jor mechanism for removal of platinum-induced DNA adducts, resulting in resistance to plat-inum drug therapy. NER enzyme-complexes remove bulky, transcription-blocking lesions caused by endogenous and environmental insults to DNA, including platinum-induced ad-ducts (Huang *et al.*, 1992; Moggs *et al.*, 1996; Furuta *et al.*, 2002). NER-defective cells are hyper-sensitive to platinum drugs, and enhanced DNA repair has been implicated in the cisplatin-resistant phenotype (Lee *et al.*, 1993; Zhen *et al.*, 1992; Sood & Buller, 1996). The major steps in the NER process are shown in Figure 1: damage recognition, dual-incision of DNA (on 5' and 3' sides of the lesion), removal of incised nucleotides and deoxyribose, and gap fill-in synthe-sis (Sancar & Tang, 1993; Matsunaga *et al.*, 1995; Reardon & Sancar, 2002; Hoeijmakers, 1993; Wood, 1997; Petit & Sancar, 1999).

NER is accomplished by a large multi-protein complex composed of nearly two-dozen enzymes (Wakasugi & Sancar, 1999). It is suggested that low levels of NER factors render tu-mors more susceptible to platinum drugs (Welsh *et al.*, 2004; Chang *et al.*, 2005). Among the NER enzymes, excision repair cross-complementing 1 (ERCC1) plays a pivotal role in the re-moval of bulky platinum-lesions (Olaussen *et al.*, 2007; Reed, 2005; Shirota *et al.*, 2001). ERCC1/XPF heterodimer with XPG are responsible for the dual-incision process (Sancar, 1994; Matsunaga *et al.*, 1995; Hoeijmakers, 1993).

2.4 DNA-Damage Repair Signaling Pathway Activated by Platinum Drugs

In an investigation of cisplatin-induced molecular signature in ovarian cancer A2780 (cispla-tin-sensitive) cells, we found that several kinases of the DNA-damage repair pathway were

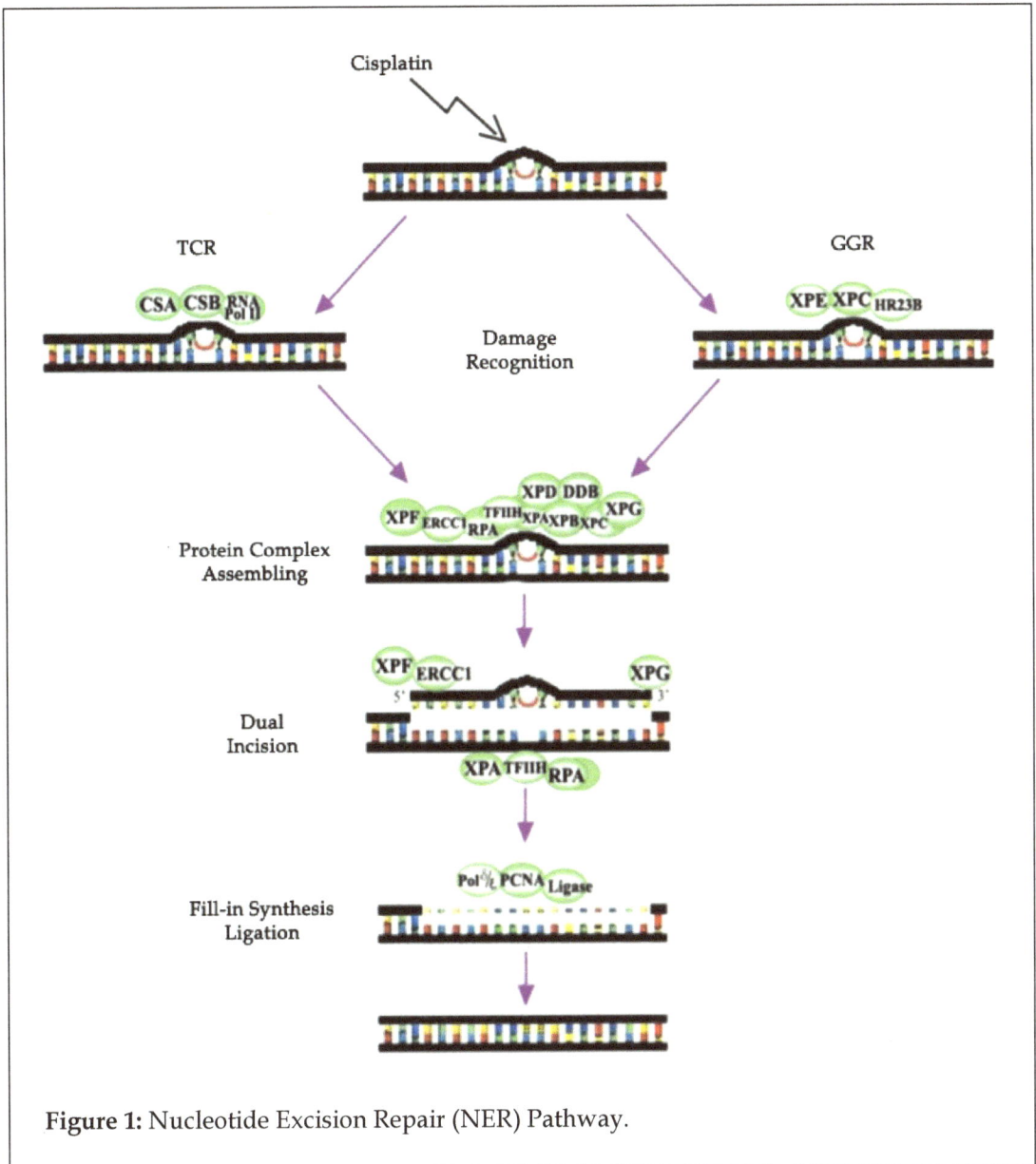

Figure 1: Nucleotide Excision Repair (NER) Pathway.

activated 1-h after drug exposure. As shown in Figure 2A, we observed phosphorylation of p53 at serine 15, p53 at serine 20, and Chk2 at threonine 68; we also found increased proteins of p53, p48 and p21 (Liang *et al.*, 2011). Among the activated signals, Chk2 is particularly interesting. We observed that Chk2 is activated and regulated by p53 in a wild-type p53 cell model (see section 5 for additional comments).

In another investigation of dicycloplatin-activated DNA-damage response pathway in the same cells, two major factors - p53 and Chk2 - were activated in a manner similar to cisplatin-induction (Figure 2B), suggesting that the molecular mechanism of dicycloplatin anti-cancer activity may be similar to cisplatin (Yu *et al.*, 2014).

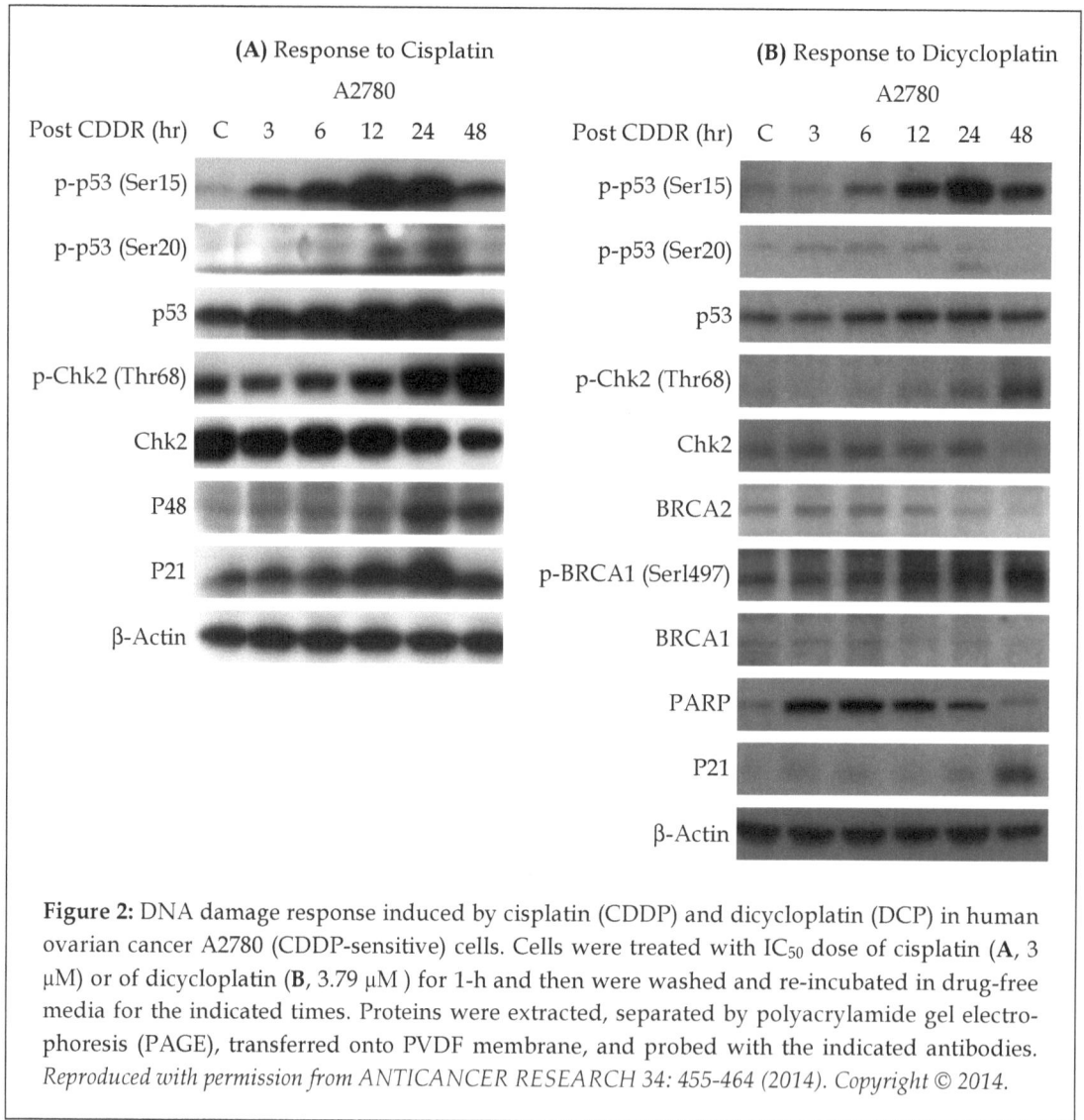

Figure 2: DNA damage response induced by cisplatin (CDDP) and dicycloplatin (DCP) in human ovarian cancer A2780 (CDDP-sensitive) cells. Cells were treated with IC_{50} dose of cisplatin (**A**, 3 μM) or of dicycloplatin (**B**, 3.79 μM) for 1-h and then were washed and re-incubated in drug-free media for the indicated times. Proteins were extracted, separated by polyacrylamide gel electro-phoresis (PAGE), transferred onto PVDF membrane, and probed with the indicated antibodies. *Reproduced with permission from ANTICANCER RESEARCH 34: 455-464 (2014). Copyright © 2014.*

3   ERCC1 Predicts Chemosensitivity and Serves as a Prognostic Marker

ERCC1 is an essential component of the NER pathway, which is the only known mechanism for the removal of intrastrand/interstrand bulky DNA-adducts. ERCC1-defective mice show elevated p53 levels and liver-cell nuclear abnormalities with death before weaning (McWhir *et al.*, 1993). Studies indicate that high levels of ERCC1 expression reflect elevated DNA repair capacity and are associated with clinical resistance to platinum-based chemotherapy (Lee *et al.*, 1993; Zhen *et al.*, 1992; Reed, 2006) and, theoretically, to other chemotherapeutic agents that involve the DNA-damage repair mechanism. In addition, an SNP of ERCC1 gene pre-dicts chemosensitivity to platinum drug and overall survival (Yu *et al.*, 1997; Ryu *et al.*, 2004). Thus, ERCC1 is a useful marker in platinum chemotherapy.

3.1 Overexpression of ERCC1 is Associated with Enhanced DNA Repair Activity and Clinical Resistance to Platinum Chemotherapy

In vitro studies suggest that ERCC1 expression in cisplatin-hypersensitive, repair-deficient cells is 50- to 30-fold lower than in platinum-resistant cells (Taverna *et al.*, 1994). Overexpression of ERCC1 and other NER genes is associated with increased DNA repair activity and clinical resistance to cisplatin treatment (Parker *et al.*, 1991; Johnson *et al.*, 1994; Dabholkar *et al.*, 1992; Dabholkar *et al.*, 1994; Yu *et al.*, 1996). NER genes such as ERCC1 and XPA in human ovarian cancer tissues are at low levels in platinum-sensitive tumors (responders), and the same genes are expressed at high levels in platinum-resistant patients (non-responders) (Dabholkar *et al.*, 1994). Data from *in vitro* systems have shown that suppressed ERCC1 expression by siRNA enhances or restores sensitivity of human cancer cells to cisplatin (Chang *et al.*, 2005). These findings have significant therapeutic implications.

3.2 SNP of the ERCC1 Gene Serves as an Important Biomarker for Platinum Sensitivity and Overall Survival

The author discovered a significant single nucleotide polymorphism (SNP) in the ERCC1 gene (GenBank Acc # AF001925). This SNP converts a common codon usage to an infrequent codon usage, reducing frequency of use 2-fold, prompting the prediction that this SNP would be associated with reduced ERCC1 translation and improved response to platinum chemotherapy (Yu *et al.*, 1997). The discovery of this ERCC1 SNP has been shown by other researchers to be an important biomarker associated with platinum sensitivity and predicts better overall survival of cancer patients with colorectal, testicular and non-small-cell lung cancers treated with platinum-combination therapy (Figg *et al.*, 2013; Stoehlmacher *et al.*, 2004; Mendoza *et al.*, 2013; Olaussen *et al.*, 2007). Ryu and colleagues investigated 109 patients with non-small-cell lung cancer (NSCLC) treated with cisplatin combination chemotherapy and compared survival rate of patients with and without ERCC1 SNP, Asn118Asn (C→T). The median survival time in patients showing C/C genotype was 480 days, which was significantly more than the 281 days of patients with the variant genotype (T/T or C/T) (P = 0.0058). Genotype effect on patient survival and hazard ratios adjusted for age, sex and other confounders was determined using Cox-proportional hazards model (a survival model). The ERCC1 SNP, response to chemotherapy, weight loss and performance status were significantly associated with overall survival (P=0.0001, 0.0001, 0.0028, and 0.0184, respectively), suggesting that the C/C genotype in codon 118 of ERCC1 is a surrogate marker for predicting better survival in NSCLC patients treated with cisplatin combination chemotherapy (Ryu *et al.*, 2004). Other studies also report that patients homozygous for the ERCC1 118 C allele demonstrated significantly better survival, indicating that ERCC1 SNP assessment could be an important component of tailored chemotherapy trials (Isla *et al.*, 2004; Kang, *et al.*, 2006).

3.3 Advances and Translational Implications of ERCC1

Of interest, the Eddie Reed team investigated the relationship between mRNA expression of ERCC1 and XPB, two key genes in the NER pathway, and clinical resistance to platinum chemotherapy in histological subtypes of human epithelial ovarian cancer. We observed that mRNA levels of ERCC1 and XPB tend to be higher in clear cell tumors, as opposed to other types of epithelial ovarian cancer. This finding is consistent with the long-standing observation that clear cell tumors are more likely to show *de novo* drug resistance against DNA-damaging agents in the clinic (Reed *et al.*, 2003).

Olaussen and colleagues retrospectively evaluated 761 tumor samples from patients with metastatic lung cancer who participated in the International Adjuvant Lung Cancer Trial. The results showed a statistically significant survival benefit in patients with low levels of ERCC1 who had received platinum chemotherapy, compared to patients with low levels of ERCC1 who did not receive chemotherapy and patients with high levels of ERCC1 who received cisplatin chemotherapy (Olaussen *et al.*, 2006).

Cobo *et al.* (2007) reported the results of a prospective trial using ERCC1 mRNA levels to assign patients with NSCLC to chemotherapy. In this trial, 444 patients with stage IIIB or stage IV diseases were randomly assigned into two arms. In the control arm, patients received the well-established docetaxel/cisplatin combination therapy. In the genotypic arm, patients with high levels of ERCC1 received a non-platinum-containing regimen of gemcitabine/docetaxel, and patients with low levels of ERCC1 received cisplatin/docetaxel. The study met its primary end-point: response rates were significantly higher in the genotypic arm (50.3%), compared to the control arm (39.3%).

4   MZF1 Repressively Regulates ERCC1 Expression

MZF1 expresses predominantly in myeloid progenitor cells and totipotent hemopoietic cells. This gene has been reported as a bi-functional transcriptional regulator, repressing transcription in non-hematopoietic cells and activating transcription in cells of hematopoietic origin. Consensus MZF1 binding sites were found in the promoters of several hematopoietic cell-specific genes, including CD34, c-myc, lactoferrin and myeloperoxidase (Hromas *et al.*, 1991; Morris *et al.*, 1995; Perrotti *et al.*, 1995; Hromas *et al.*, 1996). We hypothesized that MZF1 plays a role in the *ERCC1* promoter. Using constitutive and drug-induced strategies in cell models, we found that MZF1 and AP1 coordinately regulate ERCC1 transcription in response to cisplatin-induced DNA damage/repair (Yan *et al.*, 2006; Li *et al.*, 1998).

4.1   Increased AP1 and Suppressed MZF1 Binding Activities are Induced by Cisplatin

To determine how the *ERCC1* gene is regulated after cisplatin treatment, Li and Yan examined the effect of cisplatin on the expression of AP1 (*c-jun* and *c-fos*) and MZF1 in human ovarian cancer A2780/CP70 (cisplatin-resistant) cells and observed that cisplatin exposure increased mRNA expression of *c-fos* and *c-jun,* and decreased MZF1 mRNA expression by nearly 75% at 48-h. Li and Yan also identified functional cis-elements corresponding transfactors AP1 and MZF1 through analysis of ERCC1 promoter region by Electrophoresis Mobility Shift Assay (EMSA). In response to cisplatin exposure, the AP1 site and the MZF1 site within *ERCC1* promoter formed DNA-protein complexes; binding activities of AP1 increased and binding activities of MZF1 decreased during time course (Li *et al.*, 1998; Yan *et al.*, 2006).

4.2   Within the ERCC1 Promoter Region, AP1 And MZF1 Coordinately Regulate ERCC1 in Response to Cisplatin Treatment

Our investigations confirmed that the region -220 to -110 of *ERCC1* promoter is essential to constitutive ERCC1 expression. A more forward upstream region containing AP1 and MZF1 binding sites is responsible for cisplatin-induced ERCC1 up-regulation. Specifically, the induction of ERCC1 expression in A2780/CP70 cells exposed to cisplatin results from increases in the expression of transactivation factors that bind the AP1 site in the 5'-flanking region of *ERCC1* promoter and in the level of *c-jun* phosphorylation, which enhances transactivation. This increases transactivation of ERCC1 expression in cisplatin-treated A2780/CP70 cells (Li *et al.*, 1998). Moreover, overexpression of MZF1 repressed ERCC1 transcription in cisplatin-treated cells, suggesting that MZF1 acts as repressor of ERCC1 transcription upon cisplatin exposure (Yan *et al.*, 2006). Put together, these findings suggest that within the *ERCC1* promoter region AP1 and MZF1 are the cis-elements reacting to cisplatin treatment. During cellular response to cisplatin stimulation, higher ERCC1 expression contributes to an increase in cisplatin-induced DNA-adduct repair, resulting in drug resistance. Thus, the transcriptional factors AP1 and MZF1, particularly the latter, may be targeted as modulators of ERCC1 expression.

5   Wild-Type p53 Plays a Role in the Upstream Regulation of Chk2 Activation

Under normal conditions, wild-type p53 is maintained at a low expression level due to the extremely short half-life of the polypeptide and its largely-inactive state that is inefficient for its function (Lakin & Jackson, 1999; Vogelstein *et al.*, 2000; Selivanova, 2001). In response to genotoxic stress, wild-type p53 proteins form a tetramer that binds DNA, preventing its transactivation function (Cho *et al.*, 1994; Blagosklonny, 2002). This leads to activation of numerous genes that cause growth arrest and apoptosis (Mirza *et al.*, 2002; Vogelstein *et al.*, 2000; Fojo, 2002). In response to DNA damage, post-translational modifications of p53 increase protein levels by dramatically extending the half-life of the protein (Maltzman & Czyzyk, 1984; Price & Calderwood, 1993; Maki & Howley, 1997); the control of p53 mRNA translation plays a key role in the p53-induction response (Kastan *et al.*, 1991). In this regard, both the 5' and 3' untranslated regions of p53 mRNA have been implicated in regulating p53 mRNA translation (Mosner *et al.*, 1995; Fu & Benchimol, 1997). Elevated p53 is seen in massive DNA injury, indicating its role as monitor of DNA damage (Lakin & Jackson, 1999).

After exposure to ionizing radiation, Chk2 is rapidly activated by ATM and DNA-PK (DNA-dependent protein kinase) via phosphorylation at Thr68, causing homodimerization and subsequent trans-activating auto-phosphorylations at Thr383 and Thr387, and cis-phosphorylation at Ser516. Activated Chk2, in turn, phosphorylates downstream substrates, including Cdc25A at serine123 and Cdc25C at Ser215, and inhibits Cdc25C phosphatase, preventing mitosis and leading to cell-cycle arrest at G1 phase. This protein also interacts with and phosphorylates BRCA1, allowing it to recover after DNA damage (Bartek & Lukas, 2003; Pommier *et al.*, 2006; Antoni *et al.*, 2007; Falck *et al.*, 2001; Ahn & Prives, 2002). Chk2 inhibition also increases the level of mitotic catastrophe and sensitizes proliferating cells to doxorubicin-induced apoptosis (Castedo *et al.*, 2004). In addition to augmenting the effect of cytotoxic drugs, Chk2 inhibitors may elicit radioprotection or chemoprotection of normal tissue via abrogation of p53-dependent apoptosis (Jobson *et al.*, 2009).

5.1   Cisplatin Induces Phosphorylation of p53 and Chk2

Liang and colleagues investigated platinum-induced activation and regulation of Chk2, which further defined the relationship between two central mediators, p53 and Chk2. Human ovarian cancer A2780 (cisplatin-sensitive) cells (analyzed and classified as p53 wild-type) were exposed to cisplatin at IC$_{50}$ dose for 1-h, followed by western blotting to analyze the levels of selected proteins of the DNA damage response pathway. As shown in Figure 2 (A), at 12-h after cisplatin exposure, the p53 level is highly accumulated, accompanied by p53 phosphorylation at Ser-15 and Ser-20, Chk2 phosphorylation at Thr-68. Of note, the greatest increase in p53 phosphorylation induced by cisplatin occurred 12 hours before the primary increase in Chk2 phosphorylation, hinting that p53, as an upstream regulator, modulates Chk2, resulting in activation of downstream proteins P48 and P21 (Liang *et al.*, 2011).

Damia *et al.* (2001) reported that cisplatin and taxol induce different patterns of p53 phosphorylation. Both cisplatin and taxol induced p53 phosphorylation at serine 20, but only cisplatin induced p53 phosphorylation at serine 15. This finding is similar to the report by Liang *et al.* (2011).

5.2   Overexpression of p53 Increases Chk2 Phosphorylation in Wild-Type p53 Cells but Not in p53-Null Cells

To investigate our hypothesis that only wild-type p53 phenotype possesses the p53 function, cDNA-transfection was performed in wild-type p53 A2780 cells and in p53-null SKOV3 cells. Twenty-four hours after transfection, cells were treated with cisplatin. Figure 3 shows that cisplatin-induced Chk2 phosphorylation is increased after p53 cDNA transfection in only the wild-type p53 cell model. Overexpression of p53 doubled the amount of Chk2 phosphorylation in wild-type p53 A2780 cells (Figure 3A). In contrast, western analysis showed no effect on Chk2 phosphorylation by p53 transfection in p53-null SKOV3 cells (Figure 3B). In other words, transfection of p53 in p53-null cells failed to alter Chk2 activation (Liang *et al.*, 2011).

5.3   Inhibition of p53 by Specific siRNA Inhibits Chk2 Phosphorylation

To confirm the above observations, we performed p53 knock-off siRNA assays using small interfering RNA (siRNA) to silence the p53, and then measured Chk2 expression. As shown in Figure 4, in cells not treated with cisplatin, the siRNA to human p53 produced a decrease of phosphorylated Chk2, compared to the nonspecific siRNA-treated control. This decreased level may reflect a constitutive level of activated Chk2 68-phosphothreonine that is normally regulated by p53. Cells transfected by specific siRNA to p53 and treated with cisplatin showed a great reduction of phosphorylated Chk2 at Thr-68, suggesting that p53 modulates 68-threonine phosphorylation of Chk2 (Liang *et al.*, 2011).

These results indicate that in specific conditions Chk2 activation at Thr-68 phosphorylation is regulated by p53 in response to cisplatin treatment in wild-type p53 cells but not in p53-deficient cells. Cells without wild-type p53 could survive, conceivably, via an alternative pathway in response to cisplatin treatment. *Therefore, we strongly suggest that p53 mutational status be included in any p53-related studies due to the functional differentiation of wt-p53 and p53-mutant.*

Moreover, Pabla and colleagues studied ATR-Chk2 signaling in p53 activation and DNA-damage response during cisplatin-induced apoptosis and demonstrated a critical role for ATR. They observed the following: ATR was activated during cisplatin treatment and co-localized with H2AX, forming nuclear foci at the site of DNA damage; blocking ATR inhibited cisplatin-induced p53 activation and renal cell apoptosis; cisplatin-induced p53 activation and apoptosis were suppressed in ATR-deficient fibroblasts; downstream of ATR, both Chk1

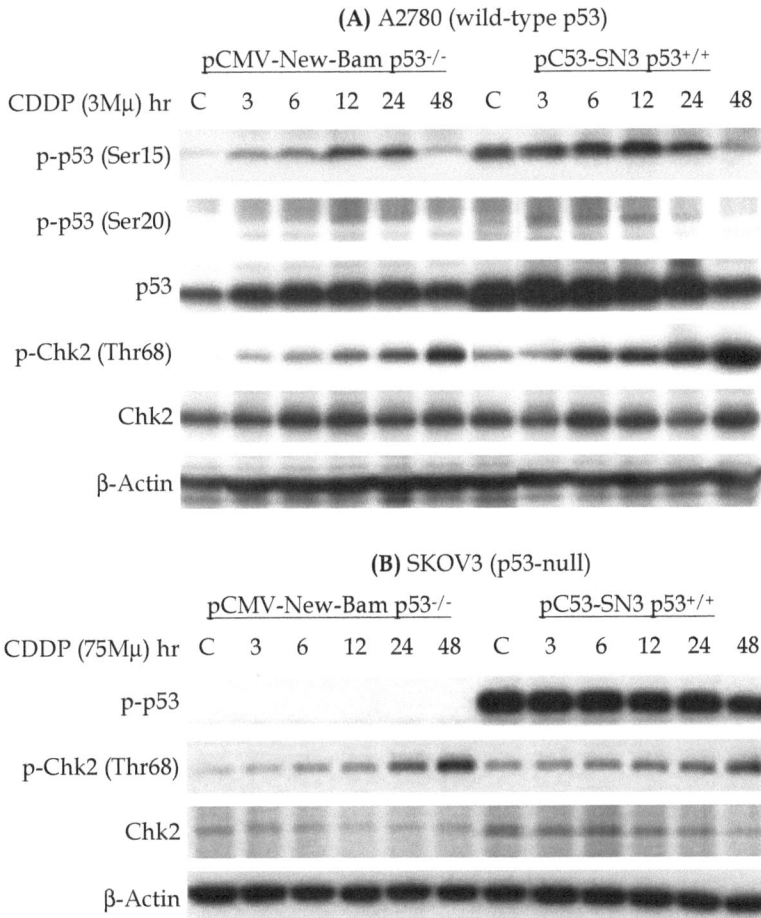

Figure 3: Overexpression of p53 by cDNA transfection in wild-type p53 and cisplatin-sensitive A2780 cells (**Panel A**) and p53-null SKOV3 cells (**Panel B**). Cells were transfected with the plasmid pC53-SN3 (which expresses wild-type human p53) or pCMV-Neo-Bam (empty vector) for overexpression of wild-type human p53. Twenty-four hours after transfection, cells were treated with cisplatin at IC_{50} doses (3 μM for A2780 and 75 μM for SKOV3) for 1-h and then were continuously incubated with fresh media (drug free) for indicated hours. Cell lysate was obtained by lysing the cells in lysate buffer and used for Western blot analysis with antibodies (for A2780 cells) of anti-p-p53(Ser15), anti-p-p53(Ser20), anti-p53, anti-p-Chk2(Thr68), anti-Chk2, or anti-β-Actin, respectively. For p53-null SKOV3 cells, the last 4 antibodies were applied. *Reprinted with permission from Chemotherapy Research and Practice, 1-8 (2011). Copyright © 2011.*

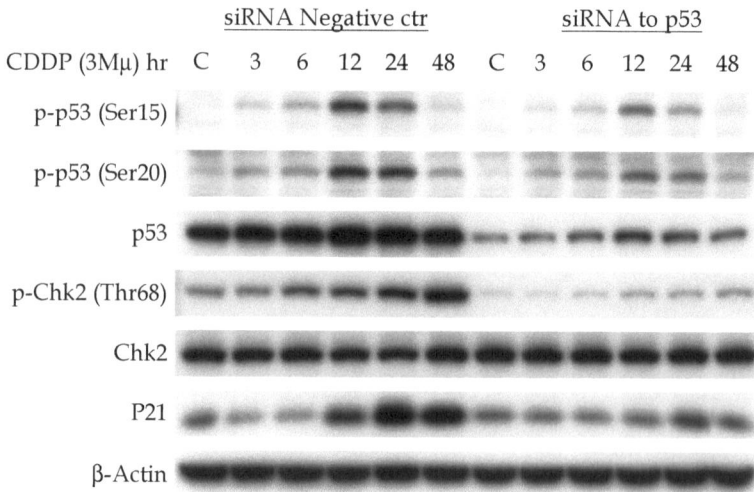

Figure 4: Inhibition of p53 by specific siRNA to p53 in CDDP-sensitive A2780 cells. siRNA against p53 (SMARTpool p53) were transfected into A2780 cells using Lipofectamine 2000. A negative nonspecific siRNA was used as control. Twenty-four hours after transfection, cells were treated with cisplatin for 1-h at 3 μM concentration. At the end of 1-h exposure to cisplatin, cells were washed and incubated with fresh media. The protein level of p-p53(Ser15), p-p53(Ser20), p53, p-Chk2 (Thr68), Chk2, p21, and β-Actin were determined by Western blotting. *Reprinted with permission from Chemotherapy Research and Practice, 1-8 (2011). Copyright © 2011.*

and Chk2 were phosphorylated during cisplatin treatment in an ATR-dependent manner; and inhibition of Chk2 repressed cisplatin-induced p53 activation and apoptosis (Pabla *et al.*, 2008).

6 Decreased PSP94 Expression Contributes to Drug Resistance and Restoration of PSP94 Sensitizes Drug-Resistant Tumors to Anticancer Agents

Studies indicate that expression of prostatic secretory protein 94 (*PSP94*), the long isoform of *MSMB*, decreases with the progression of prostate cancer, and that the PSP94 pathway is a promising target for improved cancer treatment and a biomarker for early detection (Whitaker *et al.*, 2010). In a preliminary study, we found that PSP94 is altered in ovarian cancer patients, suggesting that this gene may play an important role in human ovarian cancer (Guo *et al.*, 2012.). We hypothesized that PSP94 might be involved in ovarian tumor development and chemoresistance. Recently, Yan and colleagues launched several PSP94 investigations. The findings are reported in this section.

6.1 PSP94 Expression is Decreased in Patients with Chemoresistant Ovarian Cancer

PSP94 mRNA expression was measured by real-time quantitative PCR in 49 ovarian tumor samples (18 ERCC1 high expression; 31 ERCC1 low expression). As shown in Figure 5, PSP94 mean expression was significantly reduced in the ERCC1-high tumor samples, the chemoresistant phenotype, compared to ERCC1-low samples, the chemosensitive phenotype (1.54 vs. 0.44, respectively; p=0.004). These data indicate a possible role of PSP94 in the development of chemoresistance (Yan *et al.*, 2014).

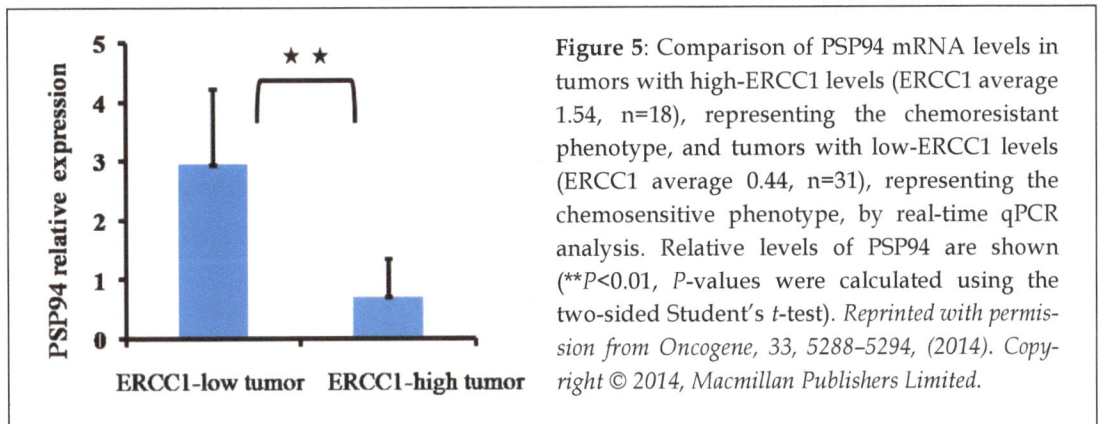

Figure 5: Comparison of PSP94 mRNA levels in tumors with high-ERCC1 levels (ERCC1 average 1.54, n=18), representing the chemoresistant phenotype, and tumors with low-ERCC1 levels (ERCC1 average 0.44, n=31), representing the chemosensitive phenotype, by real-time qPCR analysis. Relative levels of PSP94 are shown (**$P<0.01$, *P*-values were calculated using the two-sided Student's *t*-test). *Reprinted with permission from Oncogene, 33, 5288–5294, (2014). Copyright © 2014, Macmillan Publishers Limited.*

6.2 PSP94 Plays an Important Role in Acquired Drug Resistance

Our hypothesis was that PSP94 may sensitize paclitaxel-resistant cells but not sensitive cells by a mechanism of apoptosis or pre-apoptosis though a Caspase signaling pathway, such as PAK2-p34. To better understand the role of PSP94 in the development of chemoresistance, we generated the drug-resistant ovarian cancer cell line O432-RP by *in vitro* chronic exposure to increased concentrations of paclitaxel for 4 to 6 cycles. Each cycle included a 24-h exposure to the drug and subsequent recovery with normal medium. In the end, the IC_{50} dose of paclitaxel in the drug-resistant O432-RP cells was 100-fold higher than in the parental O432 cells. The *in vitro* data in Figure 6 demonstrate that PSP94 contributes to drug resistance in ovarian cancer. As seen in Fig. 6a, PSP94 protein levels were significantly reduced in drug-resistant O432-RP cells, in contrast to the drug-sensitive O432 cells (Western blot analysis).

Overexpression of PSP94 in drug-resistant O432-RP cells by cDNA transfection (O432-RP-psp-O) resulted in higher PSP94 proteins, compared to O432-RP-C control cells (Fig. 6b left-panel). These stable-expression cells were treated with increasing concentrations of paclitaxel and evaluated with cell survival assays. The survival rate of O432-RP-psp-O cells was significantly reduced, compared to control cells (Fig. 6b right-panel), suggesting a reversal of resistance.

Knockdown of PSP94 expression by siRNA in drug-sensitive O432 cells (O432-psp-D) led to substantially reduced PSP94 protein level (Fig. 6c left-panel). Survival of O432-psp-D cells was substantially enhanced with increasing doses of paclitaxel, compared to control O432 cells (Fig. 6c right-panel), suggesting that downregulation of PSP94 is sufficient to increase drug resistance. These findings indicate an important role of PSP94 in the development of resistance during chemotherapy (Yan *et al.*, 2014).

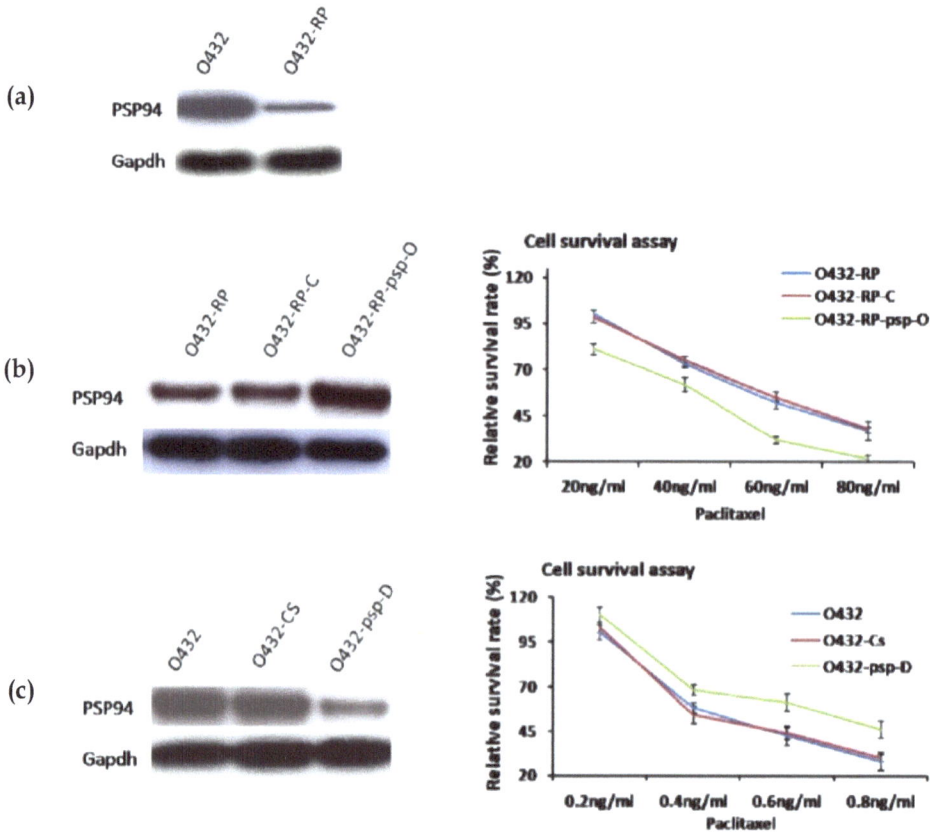

Figure 6: (a) *PSP94 expression decreases in acquired paclitaxel-resistant cells.* O432: ovarian cancer sensitive cells; O432-RP: paclitaxel-resistant cells. The PSP94 protein levels are shown in immunoblots with specific antibodies. (b) *Overexpression of PSP94 in O432-RP cells re-sensitizes drug-resistant cells.* O432-RP-psp-O cells (stably transfected with PSP94 cDNA) express higher levels of PSP94 than control cells O432-RP (transfected with reagent only) and O432-RP-C (stably transfected with control pCI-neo vector). Cells were plated at 10–20% confluence and treated with paclitaxel at different concentrations for 24-h, then in fresh medium for 7–10 days and assayed for cell survival. (c) *Downregulation of PSP94 in O432 cells results in increased drug resistance.* O432-psp-D cells (transfected with PSP94 siRNA) express lower levels of PSP94 compared to control cells of O432 (mock-transfected with reagent only) and O432-Cs (transfected with no-targeting siRNA). Cells were treated with paclitaxel at different concentrations for 24-h (starting 48-h after siRNAs transfection) and cultured with fresh medium for 7–10 days for relative cell survival rates. *Reprinted with permission from Oncogene, 33, 5288–5294, (2014). Copyright © 2014, Macmillan Publishers Limited.*

To determine if PSP94 might be an effective therapeutic target in the treatment of drug-resistant ovarian tumors, xenografts of the resistant O432-RP line (O432-RP-psp-O) and control (O432-RP-C) were generated in mice. O432-RP-psp-O cells or control O432-RP-C cells were injected into the flanks of mice. When tumor volume reached 100 mm³ +/- 10%, the tumor-bearing animals were treated with paclitaxel once a week for 2-3 weeks. At the end of treatment, tumors of O432-RP-psp-O shrank significantly in size, compared to O432-RP-C control tumors (p=0.001). These data demonstrate that restoration of PSP94 protein can sensitize drug-resistant tumors to chemotherapeutic agents, repressing tumor growth (Yan *et al.*, 2014).

7   PCK3145, a PSP94 Peptide Derivative, Reverses Chemoresistance

Recombinant PSP94 protein and its peptide derivative PCK3145 repress prostate cancer cell growth (Shukeir *et al.*, 2003; Shukeir *et al.*, 2004). Lin28a and Lin28b, the RNA binding proteins and direct upstream regulators and inhibitors of the Let-7 family, negatively control Let-7 biosynthesis (Piskounova *et al.*, 2011; Viswanathan *et al.*, 2008). The miRNAs of the Let-7 family consists of more than ten members with conserved functions across diverse species, from worms to humans (Pasquinelli *et al.*, 2000). Deregulation of Let-7 has been linked to many types of cancer and other diseases (Boyerinas *et al.*, 2010; Pasquinelli *et al.*, 2000). Lin28b, an RNA binding protein, was recently identified as a direct upstream target and inhibitor of the Let-7 family (Piskounova *et al.*, 2011; Viswanathan *et al.*, 2008) with important functions in embryonic stem cells and embryonal carcinoma (Guo *et al.*, 2006; Hagan *et al.*, 2009; King *et al.*, 2011; Viswanathan *et al.*, 2009). Signaling of Lin28b to Let-7 is crucial in the development and the deregulation of the balance between these two genes in various diseases (Ji & Wang, 2010).

7.1   PCK3145 Selectively Represses Drug-Resistant Cancer Cells and Tumor Growth

After treatment with PCK3145, *in vitro* cell survival in O432-RP, O432-RP-C and O432-PSP-D cell lines (3 drug-resistant phenotypes with low PSP94 levels) was significantly reduced, compared to vehicle PBS treatment, indicating that growth of resistant cells was selectively inhibited in these models (p=0.003, 0.004 & 0.026, respectively) (Yan *et al.*, 2014). In addition, as shown in Figure 7, O432-RP cells treated with PCK3145 alone and in combination with paclitaxel demonstrated that the latter is more effective than PCK3145 alone (Fig. 7A, p=0.034), hinting that PCK3145 can re-sensitize cells to drug treatment.

In vivo, O432-RP tumor-bearing animals treated with PCK3145 alone and in combination with paclitaxel showed that tumor volume was significantly smaller at the end of treatment, compared to control for both treatments (Figs. 7B & 7C, p=0.036 for PCK3145 alone and P = 0.002 for PCK3145 plus paclitaxel). This indicates that PCK3145 is a potential target to reverse resistance or to treat drug-resistant tumors (Yan *et al.*, 2014).

7.2   PSP94 Confers Chemoresistance via Modulation of Lin28b and miRNAs of Let-7 Pathway

PSP94 and microRNAs play important roles in the development of drug resistance (Bitarte *et al.*, 2011; Garofalo *et al.*, 2012). To identify potential mechanisms of PSP94 and miRNA function in the PSP94-directed signaling pathway in the development of drug resistance, gene expression profiles for O432-RP-psp-O and O432-RP-C cells were recently investigated using microRNA qPCR Array. MicroRNA levels of the Let-7 family were significantly decreased in O432-RP-psp-O cells (PSP94 overexpressed), compared to control O432-RP-C cells. We also

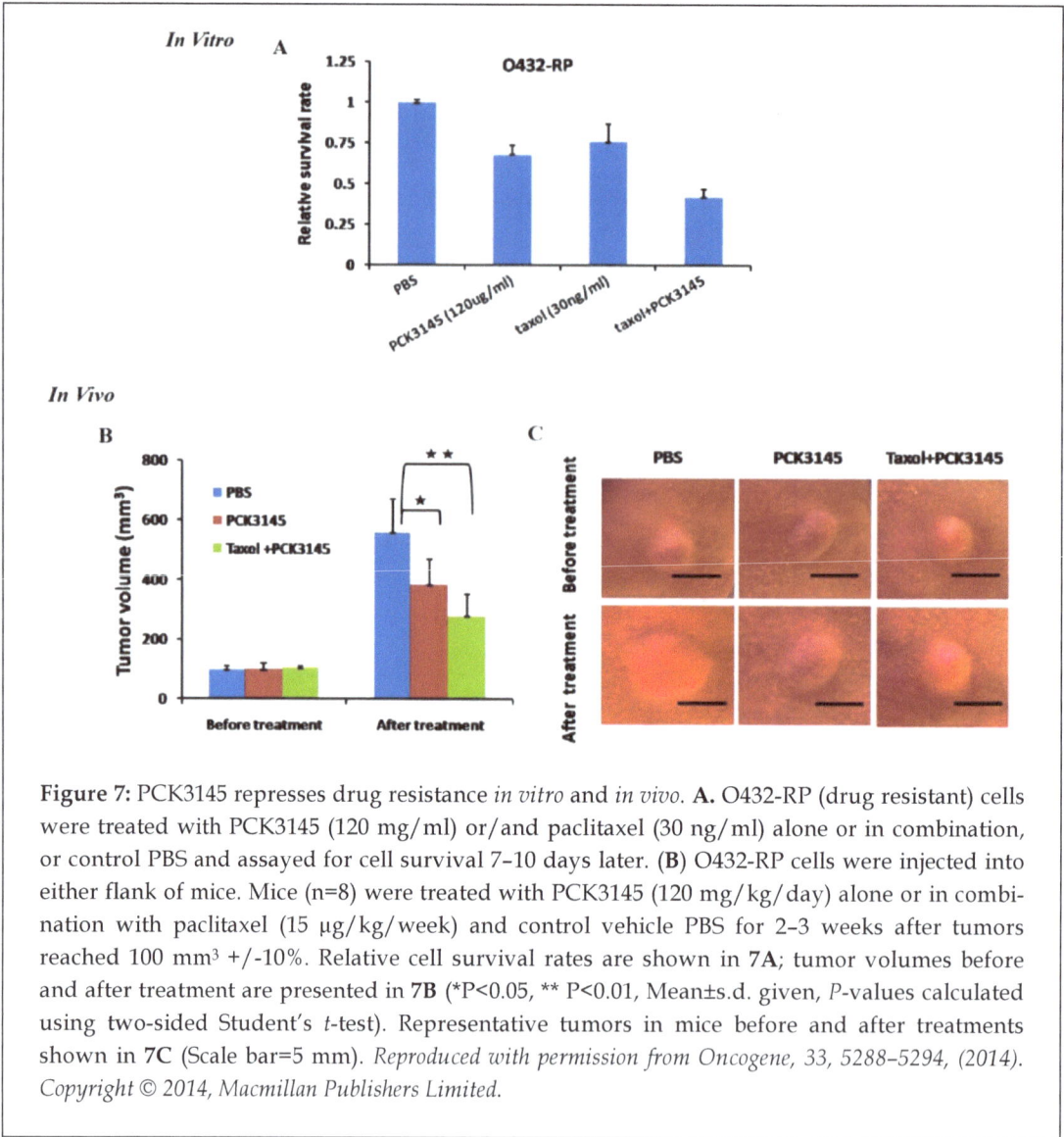

Figure 7: PCK3145 represses drug resistance *in vitro* and *in vivo*. **A.** O432-RP (drug resistant) cells were treated with PCK3145 (120 mg/ml) or/and paclitaxel (30 ng/ml) alone or in combination, or control PBS and assayed for cell survival 7–10 days later. **(B)** O432-RP cells were injected into either flank of mice. Mice (n=8) were treated with PCK3145 (120 mg/kg/day) alone or in combination with paclitaxel (15 μg/kg/week) and control vehicle PBS for 2–3 weeks after tumors reached 100 mm^3 +/-10%. Relative cell survival rates are shown in **7A**; tumor volumes before and after treatment are presented in **7B** (*P<0.05, ** P<0.01, Mean±s.d. given, *P*-values calculated using two-sided Student's *t*-test). Representative tumors in mice before and after treatments shown in **7C** (Scale bar=5 mm). *Reproduced with permission from Oncogene, 33, 5288–5294, (2014). Copyright © 2014, Macmillan Publishers Limited.*

evaluated protein expressions of Lin28a and Lin28b and found significantly increased Lin28b (but not Lin28a) levels in O432-RP-psp-O cells. In PSP94 knockdown O432-psp-D cells, Lin28b decreased, whereas Let-7 miRNA levels increased in O432-psp-D cells, compared to control cells (data not shown). Furthermore, overexpressed Lin28b in drug-resistant O432-PR cells resulted in less resistance to drug treatment, indicating that Lin28b is involved in the molecular network of chemoresistance. These preliminary findings suggest that PSP94 may mediate chemoresistance by regulating the Lin28b→Let-7 signaling pathway (Yan *et al.*, 2014).

8   Conclusion

In conclusion, our long-term investigations found the following: (1) elevated ERCC1 expression represents increased DNA repair activity (the clinical resistant phenotype), and the

ERCC1 SNP is an important biomarker that associates with platinum sensitivity and predicts better overall survival of cancer patients; (2) wild-type p53, a monitor of DNA damage, plays a critical role in drug resistance, and any research involving the p53 gene should determine its mutational status due to functional differentiation of wt-p53 and p53-mutant; (3) Chk2, an upstream regulator of the DNA repair pathway, and MZF1, the negative mediator of the ERCC1 gene, appear to have regulatory functions and are possible targets to control ERCC1 expression; (4) PSP94 plays an important role in the development of acquired resistance, and it reverses resistance in the mouse model; and (5) improved clinical outcomes for cancer patients might be achieved by applying PSP94 or its peptide derivative PCK3145 to re-sensitize drug-resistant tumors.

Dedication

This chapter is dedicated to the memory of Eddie Reed, MD. Dr. Reed mentored many of the researchers who conducted studies discussed in this chapter. His leadership and support in the investigation of ERCC1 expression in clinical samples provided valuable insights for improving the management of cancer.

Acknowledgements

My personal involvement in research presented in this chapter spans a period of 25 years. I would like to thank the following colleagues for their significant contributions to our research and for other valuable support: Eddie Reed and Meenakshi (Dabholkar) Reed, National Institute on Minority Health and Health Disparities, NIH; Scot C. Remick, Laura F. Gibson, William P. Petros, Bingxue Yan, Xiaobing Liang, and Yi Guo, Mary Babb Randolph Cancer Center, and Michael D. Schaller, Department of Biochemistry, West Virginia University; John E. Prescott, Association of American Medical Colleges; Qingdi Quentin Li, Intramural Research Program, NCI, NIH; Qing-Wu Yan, HNRCA, Tufts University; Daniel C. Flynn, College of Health Sciences, University of Delaware; Gregory A. Curt, AstraZeneca; Michael M. Gottesman, Susan Bates, Antonio Tito Fojo, Elise C. Kohn, and William Douglas Figg, Center for Cancer Research, NCI, NIH; Ricardo Parker, School of Health and Human Services, National University; Kang Bo Lee, Obstetric and Gynecologic Clinics, Seoul, Korea. Xuqing Yang and Qinhua Song, Sopo-Xingda Pharmaceutical, Inc., P.R. China. Special thanks to Michael D. Mueller and Yi Guo for editorial assistance.

References

Abraham, R. T. (2001). Cell cycle checkpoint signaling through the ATM and ATR kinases. Genes & Development, 15(17), 2177-2196.

Ahn, J. & Prives, C. (2002). Checkpoint kinase 2 (Chk2) monomers or dimers phosphorylate Cdc25C after DNA damage regardless of threonine 68 phosphorylation. Journal of Biological Chemistry, 277(50), 48418-48426.

Annunziata, C. M. & Kohn, E. C. (2013). Novel Facts About FAK: New Connections to Drug Resistance. Journal of the National Cancer Institute, 105(19), 1430-1431.

Antoni, L., Sodha, N., Collins, I., & Garrett, M. D. (2007). CHK2 kinase: cancer susceptibility and cancer therapy - two sides of the same coin? Nature Reviews Cancer, 7(12), 925-936.

Bates, S. E., Zhan, Z. R., Regis J., & Gamelin E. (1999). Measuring MDR-1 by Quantitative RT-PCR. In Cytotoxic Drug Resistance Mechanisms, Pp.63-77.

Baijal-Gupta, M., Clarke, M. W., Finkelman, M. A., McLachlin, C. M., & Han, V. K. (2000). Prostatic secretory protein (PSP94) expression in human female reproductive tissues, breast and in endometrial cancer cell lines. Journal of Endocrinology, 165(2), 425-433.

Bartek, J. & Lukas, J. (2003). Chk1 and Chk2 kinases in checkpoint control and cancer. Cancer Cell, 3(5), 421-429.

Behrens, B. C., Hamilton, T. C., Masuda, H., Grotzinger, K. R., Whang-Peng, J, Louie, K. G., & Ozols, R. F. (1987). Characterization of a cis-diamminedichloroplatinum(II)-resistant human ovarian cancer cell line and its use in evaluation of platinum analogues. Cancer Research, 47(2), 414-418.

Berns, K., Horlings, H. M., Hennessy, B. T., Madiredjo, M., Hijmans, E. M., Beelen, K., ... Bernards, R. (2007). A functional genetic approach identifies the PI3K pathway as a major determinant of trastuzumab resistance in breast cancer. Cancer Cell, 12(4), 395-402.

Bitarte, N., Bandres, E., Boni, V., Zarate, R., Rodriguez, J., Gonzalez-Huarriz, M., ... Garcia-Foncillas, J. (2011). MicroRNA-451 is involved in the self-renewal, tumorigenicity, and chemoresistance of colorectal cancer stem cells. Stem Cells, 29(11), 1661-1671.

Blagosklonny, M. V. (2002). p53: an ubiquitous target of anticancer drugs. International Journal of Cancer, 98(2), 161-166.

Boyerinas, B., Park, S. M., Hau, A., Murmann, A. E., Peter, M. E. (2010). The role of let-7 in cell differentiation and cancer. Endocrine-Related Cancer, 17(1), F19-F36.

Brown, M. J., Wouters, B. G. (1999). Apoptosis, p53, and tumor cell sensitivity to anticancer agents. Cancer Research 59(7), 1391-1399.

Castedo, M., Perfettini, J. L., Roumier, T., Yakushijin, K., Horne, D., Medema, R., & Kroemer, G. (2004). The cell cycle checkpoint kinase Chk2 is a negative regulator of mitotic catastrophe. Oncogene, 23(25), 4353-4361.

Chang, I. Y., Kim, M. H., Kim, H. B., Lee, D. Y., Kim, S. H., Kim, H. Y., & You, H. J. (2005). Small interfering RNA induced suppression of ERCC1 enhances sensitivity of human cancer cells to cisplatin. Biochemical and Biophysical Research Communications, 327(1), 225-233.

Chau, Q., & Stewart, D. J. (1999). Cisplatin efflux, binding and intracellular pH in the HTB56 human lung adenocarcinoma cell line and the E-8/0.7 cisplatin-resistant variant. Cancer Chemotherapy Pharmacology, 44(3), 193-202.

Chen, T. (2010). Overcoming drug resistance by regulating nuclear receptors. Advanced Drug Delivery Reviews, 62(13), 1257-1264.

Cho, Y., Gorina, S., Jeffrey, P. D., & Pavletich, N. P. (1994). Crystal structure of a p53 tumor suppressor-DNA complex: understanding tumorigenic mutations. Science, 265(5170), 346-355.

Clump, D. A., Yu, J. J., Cho, Y. J., Gao, R., Jett, J., Zot, H., ... Flynn, D. C. (2010). A polymorphic variant of AFAP-110 enhances cSrc activity. Translational Oncology, 3(4), 276-285.

Cobo, M., Isla, D., Massuti, B., Montes, A., Sanchez, J. M., Provencio, M., ... Rosell, R. (2007). Customizing cisplatin based on quantitative excision repair cross complementing 1 mRNA expression: a phase III trial in non-small-cell lung cancer. Journal of Clinical Oncology, 25(19), 2747-2754.

Cossa, G., Gatti, L., Zunino, F., & Perego, P. (2009). Strategies to Improve the Efficacy of Platinum Compounds. Current Medicinal Chemistry, 16(19), 2355-2365.

Curt, G. A. (2000). The Impact of Fatigue on Patients with Cancer: Overview of FATIGUE 1 and 2. The Oncologist, 5 (suppl. 2), 9-12.

Curt, G. A., Breitbart, W., Cella, D. F., Groopman, J. E., Horning, S. J., Itri, L. M., ... Vogelzang, N. J. (2000). Impact of cancer-related fatigue on the lives of patients: New Findings from the Fatigue Coalition. The Oncologist, 5(5), 353-360.

Dabholkar, M., Bostick-Bruton, F., Weber, C., Bohr, V. A., Egwuagu, C., & Reed, E. (1992). ERCC1 and ERCC2 expression in malignant tissues from ovarian cancer patients. Journal of the National Cancer Institute, 84(19), 1512-1517.

Dabholkar, M., Vionnet, J., Bostick-Bruton, F., Yu, J. J., & Reed, E. (1994). Messenger RNA levels of XPAC and ERCC1 in ovarian cancer tissue correlate with response to platinum-based chemotherapy. Journal of Clinical Investigation, 94(2), 703-708.

Damia, G., Filiberti, L., Vikhanskaya, F., Carrassa, L., Taya, Y. (2001). Cisplatinum and Taxol Induce Different Patterns of p53 Phosphorylation. Neoplasia, 3(1), 10-16.

Eastman, A. (1983). Characterization of the adducts produced in DNA by cis-diamminedichloroplatinum(II) and cis-dichloro(ethylenediamine)platinum(II). Biochemistry, 22(16), 3927-3933.

Falck, J., Mailand, N., Syljuasen, R. G., Bartek, J., & Lukas, J. (2001). The ATM-Chk2-Cdc25A checkpoint pathway guards against radioresistant DNA synthesis. Nature, 410(6830), 842-847.

Figg, W. D., Chau, C. H., Madan, R. A., Gulley, J. L., Gao, R., Sissung, T. M., … Dahut, W. L. (2013). Phase II study of satraplatin and prednisone in patients with metastatic castration-resistant prostate cancer: a pharmacogenetic assessment of outcome and toxicity. Clinical Genitourinary Cancer, 11(3), 229-237.

Flynn, D. C., Koay, T. C., Humphries, C. G. & Guappone, A. C. (1995). AFAP-120 a variant form of the src sh2/sh3-binding partner afap-110 is detected in brain and contains a novel internal sequence which binds to a 67-kda protein. Journal of Biological Chemistry, 270(8), 3894-3899.

Fojo, T. (2002). p53 as a therapeutic target: unresolved issues on the road to cancer therapy targeting mutant p53. Drug Resistance Updates, 5(5), 209-216.

Fojo, T. & Bates, S. (2003). Strategies for reversing drug resistance. Oncogene, 22(47), 7512-7523.

Fu, L. & Benchimol, S. (1997). Participation of the human p53 3′UTR in translational repression and activation following gamma-irradiation. The EMBO Journal, 16(13), 4117-4125.

Furuta, T., Ueda, T., Aune, G., Sarasin, A., Kraemer, K. H., & Pommier, Y. (2002). Transcription-coupled nucleotide excision repair as a determinant of cisplatin sensitivity of human cells. Cancer Research, 62(17), 4899-4902.

Garofalo, M., Romano, G., Di Leva, G., Nuovo, G., Jeon, Y. J., Ngankeu, A., … Croce, C. M. (2012). EGFR and MET receptor tyrosine kinase-altered microRNA expression induces tumorigenesis and gefitinib resistance in lung cancers. Nature Medicine, 18(1), 74-82.

Ghosh, J. C., Dohi, T., Raskett, C. M., Kowalik, T. F., & Altieri, D. C. (2006). Activated Checkpoint Kinase 2 Provides a Survival Signal for Tumor Cells. Cancer Research, 66(24), 11576-11579.

Gottesman, M. M., Fojo, T., & Bates, S. E. (2002). Multidrug resistance in cancer: role of ATP-dependent transporters. Nature Reviews Cancer, 2(1), 48-58.

Greenlee, R. T., Hill-Harmon, M. B., Murray, T., & Thun, M. (2001). Cancer Statistics, 2001. CA: A Cancer Journal for Clinicians, 51(1), 15-36.

Guo, Y., Chen, Y., Ito, H., Watanabe, A., Ge, X., Kodama, T., & Aburatani, H. (2006). Identification and characterization of lin-28 homolog B (LIN28B) in human hepatocellular carcinoma. Gene, 384, 51-61.

Guo, Y., Yan, B. X., Mueller, M. D., & Yu, J. J. (2012). The PSP94→Prostasin Pathway and Early Detection of Ovarian Cancer. American Association for Cancer Research Annual Meeting, 53, abst # 3644.

Hagan, J. P., Piskounova, E., & Gregory, R. I. (2009). Lin28 recruits the TUTase Zcchc11 to inhibit let-7 maturation in mouse embryonic stem cells. Nature Structural & Molecular Biology, 16(10), 1021-1025.

Hannan, M. A., Hellani, A., Al-Khodairy, F. M., Kunhi, M., Siddiqui, Y., Al-Yussef, N., Pangue-Cruz, N., Siewertsen, M., Al-Ahdal, M. N., & Aboussekhra, A. (2002). Deficiency in the repair of UV-induced DNA damage in human skin fibroblasts compromised for the ATM gene. Carcinogenesis, 23(10), 1617-1624.

Hirao, A., Cheung, A., Duncan, G., Girard, P. M., Elia, A. J., Wakeham, A., … Mak, T. W. (2002). Chk2 is a tumor suppressor that regulates apoptosis in both an ataxia telangiectasia mutated (ATM)-dependent and an ATM-independent manner. Molecular and Cellular Biology, 22(18), 6521-6532.

Hoeijmakers, J. H. (1993). Nucleotide excision repair I: from E. coli to yeast. Trends in Genetics, 9(5), 173-177.

Honma, K., Iwao-Koizumi, K., Takeshita, F., Yamamoto, Y., Yoshida, T., Nishio, K., … Ochiya, T. (2008). RPN2 gene confers docetaxel resistance in breast cancer. Nature Medicine, 14(9), 939-948.

Hromas, R., Boswell, S., Shen, R. N., Burgess, G., Davidson, A., Cornetta, K., … Robertson, K. (1996). *Forced overexpression of the myeloid zinc finger gene MZF-1 inhibits apoptosis and promotes oncogenesis in interleukin-3-dependent FDCP1 cells. Leukemia, 10(6), 1049-1050.*

Hromas, R., Collins, S. J., Hickstein, D., Raskind, W., Deaven, L. L., O'Hara, P., … Kaushanshy, K. (1991). *A retinoic acid-responsive human zinc finger gene, MZF-1, preferentially expressed in myeloid cells. Journal of Biological Chemistry, 266(22), 14183-14187.*

Hromas, R., Davis, B., Rauscher, F. J., Klemsz, M., Tenen, D., Hoffman, S., … Morris, J. F. (1996). *Hematopoietic transcriptional regulation by the myeloid zinc finger gene, MZF-1. Current Topics in Microbiology and Immunology, 211, 159-164.*

Huang, J. C., Svoboda, D. L., Reardon, J. T., & Sancar, A. (1992). *Human nucleotide excision nuclease removes thymine dimers from DNA by incising the 22nd phosphodiester bond 5' and the 6th phosphodiester bond 3' to the photodimer. Proceedings of the National Academy of Science of the United States of America, 89(8), 3664-3668.*

Ishida, S., Lee, J., Thiele, D.J., & Herskowitz, I. (2002). *Uptake of the anticancer drug cisplatin mediated by the copper transporter Ctr1 in yeast and mammals. Proceedings of the National Academy of Science of the United States of America, 99(22), 14298-14302.*

Isla, D., Sarries, C., Rosell, R., Alonso, G., Domine, M., Taron, M., … Lianes, P. (2004). *Single nucleotide polymorphisms and outcome in docetaxel–cisplatin-treated advanced non-small-cell lung cancer. Annals of Oncology, 15(8), 1194-1203.*

Jeffrey, P. D., Gorina, S., & Pavletich, N. P. (1995). *Crystal structure of the tetramerization domain of the p53 tumor suppressor at 1.7 angstroms. Science, 267(5203), 1498-1502.*

Ji, J. & Wang, X. W. (2010). *A Yin-Yang balancing act of the lin28/let-7 link in tumorigenesis. Journal of Hepatology, 53(5), 974-975.*

Jobson, A. G., Lountos, G. T., Lorenzi, P. L., Llamas, J., Connelly, J., Cerna, D., … Pommier, Y. (2009). *Cellular inhibition of checkpoint kinase 2 (Chk2) and potentiation of camptothecins and radiation by the novel Chk2 inhibitor PV1019 [7-nitro-1H-indole-2-carboxylic acid {4-[1-(guanidinohydrazone)-ethyl]-phenyl}-amide]. Journal of Pharmacology and Experimental Therapeutics, 331(3), 816-826.*

Johnson, S. W., Perez, R. P., Godwin, A. K., Yeung, A. T., Handel, L. M., Ozols, R. F., & Hamilton, T. C. (1994). *Role of platinum–DNA adduct formation and removal in cisplatin resistance in human ovarian cancer cell lines. Biochemical Pharmacology, 47(4), 689-697.*

Johnson, S. W., Shen, D., Pastan, I., Gottesman, M. M., & Hamilton, T. C. (1996). *Cross-resistance, cisplatin accumulation, and platinum–DNA adduct formation and removal in cisplatin-sensitive and -resistant human hepatoma cell lines. Experimental Cell Research, 226(1), 133-139.*

Kang, S., Ju, W., Kim, J. W., Park, N. H., Song, Y. S., Kim, S. C., … Lee, H. P. (2006). *Association between excision repair cross-complementation group 1 polymorphism and clinical outcome of platinum-based chemotherapy in patients with epithelial ovarian cancer. Experimental & Molecular Medicine, 38(3), 320-324.*

Kastan, M. B., Onyekwere, O., Sidransky, D., Vogelstein, B. & Craig, R. W. (1991). *Participation of p53 protein in the cellular response to DNA damage. Cancer Research, 51(23 Pt 1), 6304-6311.*

Kelland, L. (2007). *The resurgence of platinum-based cancer chemotherapy. Nature Reviews Cancer, 7(8), 573-584.*

King, C. E., Wang, L., Winograd, R., Madison, B. B., Mongroo, P. S., Johnstone, C. N., & Rustgi, A. K. (2011). *LIN28B fosters colon cancer migration, invasion and transformation through let-7-dependent and -independent mechanisms. Oncogene, 30(40), 4185-4193.*

Köberle, B., Tomicic, M. T., Usanova, S., Kaina, B. (2010). *Cisplatin resistance: preclinical findings and clinical implications. Biochimica et Biophysica Acta, 1806(2), 172-182.*

Kuin, A., Aalders, M. , Lamfers, M., Zuidam, D. J. van., Essers, M., Beijnen, J. H., & Smets, L. A. (1999). *Potentiation of anticancer drug activity at lowintratumoral pH induced by the mitochondrial inhibitor m-iodobenzylguanidine (MIBG) and its analogue benzylguanidine (BG). British Journal of Cancer, 79(5-6), 793-801.*

Lage, H. (2008). *An overview of cancer multidrug resistance: a still unsolved problem. Cellular and Molecular Life Sciences, 65(20), 3145-3167.*

Lakin, N. D. & Jackson, S. P. (1999). *Regulation of p53 in response to DNA damage. Oncogene, 18(53), 7644-7655.*

Lamb, P. & Crawford, L. (1986). Characterization of the human p53 gene. Molecular and Cellular Biology, 6(5), 1379-1385.

Lee, J., Peña, M. M. O., Nose Y., & Thiele, D. J. (2002). Biochemical Characterization of the Human Copper Transporter Ctr1. Journal of Biological Chemistry, 277(6), 4380-4387.

Lee, K. B., Parker, R. J., Bohr, V. A., Cornelison, T. C., & Reed, E. (1993). Cisplatin sensitivity/resistance in UV-repair deficient Chinese hamster ovary cells of complementation groups 1 and 3. Carcinogenesis, 14(10), 2177-2180.

Li, Q., Gardner, K.., Zhang, L., Tsang, B., Bostick-Bruton F., & Reed E. (1998). Cisplatin induction of ERCC1 mRNA expression in A2780/CP70 human ovarian cancer cells. Journal of Biological Chemistry, 273(36), 23419-23425.

Liang, X. B., Guo, Y., Figg, W. D., Fojo, A. T., Mueller, M. D., & Yu, J. J. (2011). The Role of Wild-Type p53 in Cisplatin-Induced Chk2 Phosphorylation and the Inhibition of Platinum Resistance with a Chk2 Inhibitor. Chemotherapy Research and Practice, 2011, 1-8.

Lilja, H. & Abrahamsson, P. A. (1988). Three predominant proteins secreted by the human prostate gland. Prostate, 12(1), 29-38.

Longley, D. B. & Johnston, P. G. (2005). Molecular mechanisms of drug resistance. Journal of Pathology, 205(2), 275-292.

Maki, C. G. & Howley, P. M. (1997). Ubiquitination of p53 and p21 is differentially affected by ionizing and UV radiation. Molecular and Cellular Biology, 17(1), 355-363.

Maltzman, W. & Czyzyk, L. (1984). UV irradiation stimulates levels of p53 cellular tumor antigen in nontransformed mouse cells. Molecular and Cellular Biology, 4(9), 1689-1694.

Martin, L. P., Hamilton, T. C. & Schilder, R. J. (2008). Platinum Resistance: The Role of DNA Repair Pathways. Clinical Cancer Research, 14(5), 1291-1295.

Masuda, H., Ozols, R. F., Lai, G. M., Fojo, A., Rothenberg, M., & Hamilton, T. C. (1988). Increased DNA repair as a mechanism of acquired resistance to cis-diamminedichloroplatinum (II) in human ovarian cancer cell lines. Cancer Research, 48(20), 5713-5716.

Matlashewski, G., Lamb, P., Pim, D., Peacock, J., Crawford, L., & Benchimol, S. (1984). Isolation and characterization of a human p53 cDNA clone: expression of the human p53 gene. The EMBO Journal, 3(13), 3257-3262.

Matsunaga, T., Mu, D., Park, C. H., Reardon, J. T., & Sancar, A. (1995). Human DNA repair excision nuclease. Analysis of the roles of the subunits involved in dual incisions by using anti-XPG and anti-ERCC1 antibodies. Journal of Biological Chemistry, 270(35), 20862-20869.

McWhir, J., Selfridge, J., Harrison, D. J., Squires, S., & Melton, D. W. (1993). Mice with DNA repair gene (ERCC-1) deficiency have elevated levels of p53, liver nuclear abnormalities and die before weaning. Nature Genetics, 5(3), 217-224.

Mendoza, J., Martínez, J., Hernández, C., Pérez-Montiel, D., Castro, C., Fabián-Morales, E., … Herrera, L. A. (2013). Association between ERCC1 and XPA expression and polymorphisms and the response to cisplatin in testicular germ cell tumours. British Journal of Cancer, 109(1), 68-75.

Mirza, A., McGuirk, M., Hockenberry, T. N., Wu, Q., Ashar, H., Black, S., … Liu S. (2002). Human survivin is negatively regulated by wild-type p53 and participates in p53-dependent apoptotic pathway. Oncogene, 21(17), 2613-2622.

Moggs, J. G., Yarema, K. J., Essigmann, J. M., & Wood, R. D. (1996). Analysis of incision sites produced by human cell extracts and purified proteins during nucleotide excision repair of a 1,3-intrastrand d(GpTpG)- cisplatin adduct. Journal of Biological Chemistry, 271(12), 7177-7186.

Morris, J. F., Hromas, R., & Rauscher, F. J. (1994). Characterization of the DNA-binding properties of the myeloid zinc finger protein MZF1: two independent DNA-binding domains recognize two DNA consensus sequences with a common G-rich core. Molecular and Cellular Biology, 14(3), 1786-1795.

Morris, J. F., Rauscher, F. J., Davis, B., Klemsz, M., Xu, D., Tenen, D., & Hromas, R. (1995). The myeloid zinc finger gene, MZF-1, regulates the CD34 promoter in vitro. Blood, 86(10), 3640-7.

Mosner, J., Mummenbrauer, T., Bauer, C., Sczakiel, G., Grosse, F., & Deppert, W. (1995). Negative feedback regulation of wild-type p53 biosynthesis. The EMBO Journal, 14(18), 4442-4449.

Mueller, M. D. (2008). Report on platinum drug symposium. The West Virginia Medical Journal, 104(4), 8-9.

Murakami, T., Shibuya, I., Ise, T., Chen, Z. S., Akiyama, S. i., Nakagawa, M., … Kohno, K. (2001). Elevated expression of vacuolar proton pump genes and cellular pH in cisplatin resistance. International Journal of Cancer, 93(6), 869-874.

Olaussen, K. A., Dunant, A., Fouret, P., Brambilla, E., André, F., Haddad, V., … Soria, J. C. (2006). DNA repair by ERCC1 in non-small-cell lung cancer and cisplatin-based adjuvant chemotherapy. New England Journal of Medicine, 355(10), 983-9 91.

Olaussen, K. A., Mountzios, G., & Soria, J. C. (2007). ERCC1 as a risk stratifier in platinum-based chemotherapy for non-small-cell lung cancer. Current Opinion in Pulmonary Medicine, 13(4), 284-289.

Pabla, N., Huang, S., Mi, Q. S., Daniel, R., & Dong, Z. (2008). ATR-Chk2 Signaling in p53 Activation and DNA Damage Response during Cisplatin-induced Apoptosis. Journal of Biological Chemistry, 283(10), 6572-6583.

Pandita, T. K., Lieberman, H. B., Lim, D. S., Dhar, S., Zheng, W., Taya, Y., & Kastan, M. B. (2000). Ionizing radiation activates the ATM kinase throughout the cell cycle. Oncogene, 19(11), 1386-1391.

Parker, R. J., Eastman, A., Bostick-Bruton, F., & Reed, E. (1991). Acquired cisplatin resistance in human ovarian cancer cells is associated with enhanced repair of cisplatin-DNA lesions and reduced drug accumulation. Journal of Clinical Investigation, 87(3), 772-777.

Pasquinelli, A. E., Reinhart, B. J., Slack, F., Martindale, M. Q., Kuroda, M. I., Maller, B., … Ruvkun, G. (2000). Conservation of the sequence and temporal expression of let-7 heterochronic regulatory RNA. Nature, 408(6808), 86-89.

Perrotti, D., Melotti, P., Skorski, T., Casella, I., Peschle, C., & Calabretta, B. (1995). Overexpression of the zinc finger protein MZF1 inhibits hematopoietic development from embryonic stem cells: correlation with negative regulation of CD34 and c-Myc promoter activity. Molecular and Cellular Biology, 15(11), 6075-6087.

Petit, C. & Sancar, A. (1999). Nucleotide excision repair: From E. coli to man. Biochimie, 81(1-2), 15-25.

Piskounova, E., Polytarchou, C., Thornton, J. E., LaPierre, R. J., Pothoulakis, C., Hagan, J. P., … Gregory, R. I. (2011). Lin28A and Lin28B inhibit let-7 microRNA biogenesis by distinct mechanisms. Cell, 147(5), 1066-1079.

Pommier, Y., Weinstein, J. N., Aladjem, M. I., & Kohn, K. W. (2006). Chk2 molecular interaction map and rationale for Chk2 inhibitors. Clinical Cancer Research, 12(9), 2657-2661.

Price, B. D. & Calderwood, S. K. (1993). Increased sequence-specific p53-DNA binding activity after DNA damage is attenuated by phorbol esters. Oncogene, 8(11), 3055-3062.

Reardon, J. T. & Sancar, A. (2002). Molecular anatomy of the human excision nuclease assembled at sites of DNA damage. Molecular and Cellular Biology, 22(16), 5938-5945.

Redmond, K. M., Wilson, T. R., Johnston, P. G., & Longley, D. B. (2008). Resistance mechanisms to cancer chemotherapy. Frontiers in Bioscience, 13, 5138-5154.

Reed, E. (1998). Platinum-DNA adduct, nucleotide excision repair and platinum based anti-cancer chemotherapy. Cancer Treatment Reviews, 24(5), 331-344.

Reed, E., Yu, J. J., Davies, A., Gannon, J., Armentrout, S. L. (2003). Clear cell tumors have higher mRNA levels of ERCC1 and XPB than other histological types of epithelial ovarian cancer. Clinical Cancer Research, 9(14), 5299-5305.

Reed, E. (2005). ERCC1 and clinical resistance to platinum-based therapy. Clinical Cancer Research, 11(17), 6100-6102.

Reed, E. (2006). ERCC1 measurements in clinical oncology. New England Journal of Medicine, 355(10), 1054-1055.

Reles, A., Wen, W. H., Schmider, A., Gee, C., Runnebaum, I. B., Kilian, U., … Press, M. F. (2001). Correlation of p53 Mutations with Resistance to Platinum-based Chemotherapy and Shortened Survival in Ovarian Cancer. Clinical Cancer Research, 7(10), 2984-2997.

Ryu, J. S., Hong, Y. C., Han, H. S., Lee, J. E., Kim, S., Park, Y. M., … Hwang, T. S. (2004). Association between polymorphisms of ERCC1 and XPD and survival in non-small-cell lung cancer patients treated with cisplatin combination chemotherapy. Lung Cancer, 44(3), 311-316.

Sancar, A. (1994). Mechanisms of DNA excision repair. Science, 266(5193), 1954-1956.

Sancar, A. & Tang, M. S. (1993). Nucleotide excision repair. Photochemistry and Photobiology, 57(5), 905-921.

Selivanova, G. (2001). Mutant p53: the loaded gun. Current Opinion in Investigational Drugs, 2(8), 1136-1141.

Sharma, S. V., Lee, D. Y., Li, B., Quinlan, M. P., Takahashi, F., Maheswaran, S., … Settleman, J. (2010). A chromatin-mediated reversible drug-tolerant state in cancer cell subpopulations. Cell, 141(1), 69-80.

Shirota, Y., Stoehlmacher, J., Brabender, J., Xiong, Y. P., Uetake, H., Danenberg, K. D., … Lenz, H. J. (2001). ERCC1 and thymidylate synthase mRNA levels predict survival for colorectal cancer patients receiving combination oxaliplatin and fluorouracil chemotherapy. Journal of Clinical Oncology, 19(23), 4298-4304.

Shukeir, N., Arakelian, A., Kadhim, S., Garde, S., & Rabbani, S. A. (2003). Prostate secretory protein PSP-94 decreases tumor growth and hypercalcemia of malignancy in a syngenic in vivo model of prostate cancer. Cancer Research, 63(9), 2072-2078.

Shukeir, N., Arakelian, A., Chen, G., Garde, S., Ruiz, M., Panchal, C., & Rabbani, S. A. (2004). A synthetic 15-mer peptide (PCK3145) derived from prostate secretory protein can reduce tumor growth, experimental skeletal metastases, and malignancy-associated hypercalcemia. Cancer Research, 64(15), 5370-5377.

Siegel, R., Ma, J. M., Zou, Z. H., & Jemal, A. (2014).Cancer Statistics. CA: A Cancer Journal for Clinicians, 64(1), 9-29.

Sood, A. K. & Buller, R. E. (1996). Genomic instability in ovarian cancer: a reassessment using an arbitrarily primed polymerase chain reaction. Oncogene, 13(11), 2499-2504.

Stewart, D. J. (2007). Mechanisms of resistance to cisplatin and carboplatin. Critical Reviews in Oncology/Hematology, 63(1), 12-31.

Stoehlmacher, J., Park, D. J., Zhang, W., Yang, D., Groshen, S., Zahedy, S., & Lenz, H. J. (2004). A multivariate analysis of genomic polymorphisms: prediction of clinical outcome to 5-FU/oxaliplatin combination chemotherapy in refractory colorectal cancer. British Journal of Cancer, 91(2), 344-354.

Taverna, P., Hansson, J., Scanlon, K. J., & Hill, B. T. (1994). Gene expression in X-irradiated human tumour cell lines expressing cisplatin resistance and altered DNA repair capacity. Carcinogenesis, 15(9), 2053-2056.

Viswanathan, S. R., Daley, G. Q., & Gregory, R. I. (2008). Selective blockade of microRNA processing by Lin28. Science, 320(5872), 97-100.

Viswanathan, S. R., Powers, J. T., Einhorn, W., Hoshida, Y., Ng, T. L., Toffanin, S., … Daley, G. Q. (2009). Lin28 promotes transformation and is associated with advanced human malignancies. Nature Genetics, 41(7), 843-848.

Vogelstein, B., Lane, D., & Levine, A. (2000). Surfing the p53 network. Nature, 408(6810), 307-310.

Wakasugi, M. & Sancar, A. (1999). Order of assembly of human DNA repair excision nuclease. Journal of Biological Chemistry, 274(26), 18759-18768.

Weiber, H., Andersson, C., Murne, A., Rannevik, G., Lindstrom, C., Lilja, H., & Fernlund, P. (1990). Beta microseminoprotein is not a prostate-specific protein. Its identification in mucous glands and secretions. American Journal of Pathology, 137(3), 593-603.

Welsh, C., Day, R., McGurk, C., Masters, J. R., Wood, R. D., & Köberle, B. (2004). Reduced levels of XPA, ERCC1 and XPF DNA repair proteins in testis tumor cell lines. International Journal of Cancer, 110(3), 352-361.

Whitaker, H. C., Warren, A. Y., Eeles, R., Kote-Jarai, Z., & Neal, D. E. (2010). The potential value of microseminoprotein-beta as a prostate cancer biomarker and therapeutic target. Prostate, 70(3), 333-340.

Wood, R. D. (1997). Nucleotide excision repair in mammalian cells. Journal of Biological Chemistry, 272(38), 23465-23468.

Wright, J. A., Keegan, K. S., Herendeen, D. R., Bentley, N. J., Carr, A. M., Hoekstra, M. F., & Concannon, P. (1998) Protein kinase mutants of human ATR increase sensitivity to UV and ionizing radiation and abrogate cell cycle checkpoint control. Proceedings of the National Academy of Science of the United States of America, 95(13), 7445-7450.

Yan, B. X., Ma, J. X., Zhang, J., Guo, Y., Riedel, H., Mueller, M. D., Remick, S. C., & Yu, J. J. (2014). PSP94 contributes chemoresistance and its peptide derivative PCK3145 represses tumor growth in ovarian cancer. Oncogene, 33(45), 5288-5294.

Yan, Q. W., Reed, E., Zhong, X. S., Thornton, K., Guo, Y., & Yu, J. J. (2006). MZF1 possesses a repressively regulatory function in ERCC1 expression. Biochemical Pharmacology, 71(6), 761-771.

Yang, X. Q., Jin, X. L., Song, Q. H., Tang K. L., Yang Z. Y., Zhang, X. F., & Tang, Y. Q. (2010). Structural studies of dicycloplatin, an antitumor supramolecule. Science China Chemistry, 53(6), 1346-1351.

Yeung, J., Esposito, M. T., Gandillet, A., Zeisig, B. B., Griessinger, E., Bonnet, D., & So, C. W. (2010). beta-Catenin mediates the establishment and drug resistance of MLL leukemic stem cells. Cancer Cell, 18(6), 606-618.

Yu, J. J., Yang, X. Q., Song, Q. H., Mueller, M. D., & Remick, S. C. (2014). Dicycloplatin, a novel platinum analog in chemotherapy: Synthesis of Chinese preclinical and clinical profile and emerging mechanistic studies. Anticancer Research, 34(1), 455-464.

Yu, J. J. (2009). Unlocking the Molecular Mechanisms of DNA Repair and Platinum Drug Resistance in Cancer Chemotherapy. Current Drug Therapy, 4(1), 19-28.

Yu, J. J., Mu, C. J., Lee, K. B., Okamoto, A., Reed, E. L., Bostick-Bruton, F., ... Reed, E. (1997). A nucleotide polymorphism in ERCC1 in human ovarian cancer cell lines and tumor tissues. Mutation Research Genomics, 382(1-2), 13-20.

Yu, J. J., Dabholkar, M., Bennett, W. P., Welsh, J. A., Mu, C. J., Bostick-Bruton, F., & Reed, E. (1996). Platinum-sensitive and platinum-resistant ovarian cancer tissues show differences in the relationships between mRNA levels of p53, ERCC1 and XPA. International Journal of Oncology, 8(2), 313-317.

Yu, Q., Rose, J. H., Zhang, H., & Pommier, Y. (2001). Antisense inhibition of Chk2/hCds1 expression attenuates DNA damage-induced S and G2 checkpoints and enhances apoptotic activity in HEK-293 cells. FEBS Letters, 505(1), 7-12.

Zhang, Y., Cho, Y. Y., Petersen, B. L., Bode, A. M., Zhu, F., & Dong, Z. (2003). Ataxia telangiectasia mutated proteins, MAPKs and RSK2 are involved in the phosphorylation of STAT3. Journal of Biological Chemistry, 278(15), 12650-12659.

Zhen, W., Link, C. J., O'Connor, P. M., Reed, E., Parker, R. J., & Bohr, V. A. (1992). Increased gene-specific repair of cisplatin interstrand cross-links in cisplatin-resistant human ovarian cancer cell lines. Molecular and Cellular Biology, 12(9), 3689-3698.

X-ray Digital Tomosynthesis Imaging for Pulmonary Nodule Detection

Tsutomu Gomi[*]

1 Introduction

Lung cancer is currently the primary cause of cancer death, and its incidence continues to increase worldwide. Because of its high sensitivity, normal-dose helical computed tomography (CT) is currently considered the gold standard for lung cancer detection. Previous studies have shown that low-dose helical CT can detect early-stage lung cancer, thereby decreasing morbidity (Yankelevitz et al., 2000). CT is advantageous because it is not susceptible to the problem of reduced accuracy due to overlapping anatomy. However, CT has disadvantages, such as higher radiation doses and costs than chest radiography. The advantages of chest radiography include short examination time, low cost, and easy access; however, low sensitivity and specificity are its main disadvantages. In chest radiography, a three-dimensional view of the chest is projected onto a two-dimensional image; therefore, for many analyses, the detection of pathological findings is limited by overlapping anatomy rather than quantum noise. Chest radiography has relatively low sensitivity for the detection of pulmonary nodules. This poor sensitivity precludes its use as a screening method despite its low cost, low dose, and the widespread availability of radiographic devices.

Digital tomosynthesis (DT) imaging provides greater contrast than radiography for images of similarly sized nodules. Three recent studies found that the detectability of pulmonary nodules was considerably higher with chest DT than with chest radiography; and in one report, sensitivity was found to be increased, particularly for nodules smaller than 9 mm (Vikgren et al., 2008). Another study reported that DT is an advantageous technique for detecting pulmonary nodules (Zachrisson et al., 2009). DT was also shown to have considerably improved sensitivity for the detection of known small lung nodules in three size groups [< 5, 5 – 10, and > 10 mm] compared with chest radiography (Dobbins et al., 2008). According to these reports, DT is better than radiography for the detection of lung nodules.

DT is a limited angle method of image reconstruction. Furthermore, DT provides the benefits of digital imaging (Godwin, 1983; Littleton, 1983; Siegelman et al., 1980, 1986; Fraser et al., 1986; McLendon et al., 1985) and tomographic benefits of CT at decreased radiation doses and costs. In a recent review, chest DT was described on the basis of advantages and limitations, potential applications, and suggested indications, with supporting evidence from the medical literature (Johnsson et al., 2014; Chou et al., 2014). However, as the projection images in DT are acquired over a limited angle, the depth resolution in the reconstructed section images is limited, and complete removal of superimposed tissue cannot be obtained (Johnsson et al., 2014). There are other difficulties associated with the limited depth resolution of chest DT

[*] School of Allied Health Sciences, Kitasato University, Japan

(Johnsson *et al.*, 2014). Nodule lesion detection tends to be difficult because of the effects of quantum noise in chest imaging (Ullman *et al.*, 2010; Svalkvist *et al.*, 2010; Bath *et al.*, 2005). Against this background, we discuss the novel chest DT imaging technique [dual-energy subtraction (DES)-DT technique and new wavelet denoising processing] for the improvement of lesion detection accuracy.

2   Evaluation of Detected Pulmonary Nodules

2.2   Comparison between Tomosynthesis and Radiography

DES imaging has been proposed and investigated by many researchers to reduce the impact of anatomical "noise" during disease diagnosis by chest radiography. DES involves utilization of X-ray beams of different energies to form two radiographic projections of the patient. By exploiting the difference between energy dependence and bone and soft tissue attenuation, bone contrast can be reduced, thereby producing a soft-tissue only image in which the contrast can be reduced to produce a bone image (Brody *et al.*, 1981). Recent computed radiographic systems have been hampered by poor subtraction effectiveness, workflow inconveniences, and the detective quantum efficiency limitations of the technology. However, DES radiography (DES-R) is useful for detecting calcifications (Littleton, 1983; Zerhouni *et al.*, 1988; Hickey *et al.*, 1987; Ishigaki *et al.*, 1986, 1988; Nishitani *et al.*, 1986). Projected images acquired by DES techniques exhibit the disadvantage of overlapping anatomical features (e.g., lesions superimposed over the ribs or spine). Gomi *et al.* conducted a phantom study to compare the effectiveness of chest DES-DT imaging with that of DES-R for detecting simulated pulmonary nodules and found that DES-DT imaging exhibited greater sensitivity than DES-R (Gomi *et al.*, 2011).

In this chapter, we compared initial evaluations of chest DES-DT and DES-R for the detection of pulmonary nodules (Gomi *et al.*, 2013).

2.2.1   Conditions for Data Acquisition

The DES-DT system (SonialVision Safire II; Shimadzu Co., Kyoto, Japan) consists of a 432 × 432-mm amorphous selenium digital flat-panel detector with a detector element size of 150 × 150 μm. The motion of the collimator was synchronized with the tube motion constant measuring the misalignment of low- and high-kVp images. In DES-DT imaging, pulsed X-ray exposures were used with rapid switching between low (60 kVp) and high energies (120 kVp). Linear tomographic movement of the system, a scan time of 6.4 s, and a swing angle of 40° were used to perform tomography. Thirty-seven low- and high-voltage projection images were sampled during a single tomographic pass. A matrix size of 1280 × 1280 by 12 bits (0.27 mm/pixel) was used to sample the images, which were used to reconstruct low- and high-voltage tomograms of any desired layer height. Bone or soft-tissue tomograms were produced by weighted subtraction of each absorption coefficient (Gomi *et al.*, 2011). Each projection image was acquired at 280 mA and a 100-ms exposure time for low-voltage X-rays and at 368 mA and a ≤ 20-ms exposure time for high-voltage X-rays. The reconstructed images were obtained with a 5-mm slice thickness at 1-mm reconstruction intervals. Filtered back projection was used to reconstruct the DES-DT images (Gomi *et al.*, 2008). The effective dose was approximately 1.22 mSv.

The DES-R system (CXDI-50c; Canon Inc., Tokyo, Japan) consisted of a 352 × 427.52-mm amorphous silicon digital flat-panel detector with a detector element size of 160 × 160 μm. The DES-R images were processed from low- and high-voltage projection images by two double-exposure acquisitions. A matrix size of 2200 × 2672 by 12 bits (0.16 mm/pixel) was used to sample the images, which were used to reconstruct low- and high-voltage tomograms at any desired layer height. Bone or soft-tissue images were produced by weighted subtraction for each absorption coefficient (Gomi *et al.*, 2011). Each projection image was acquired at 400 mA and a 461-ms exposure time for low-voltage X-rays and at 250 mA and a ≤ 16-ms exposure time for high-voltage X-rays. The effective dose was approximately 0.39 mSv.

2.2.2   Reference Method

Our institutional review board approved this study, and written informed consent was obtained from all patients. From October 2011 to September 2012, 46 consecutive patients with pulmonary nodules who were referred for chest CT were prospectively included in this study. Normal volunteers without pulmonary nodules were also examined (32 men; mean age, 40.21 ± 2.39; median age, 39 years; age range, 24 – 57 years; 4 women; mean age, 29.00 ± 1.76; median age, 29 years; age range, 23 – 35 years). Of the 46 patients who were deemed initially eligible for the study, 10 were excluded because they had subdiagnostic DES-DT images caused by suspected respiration or inability to maintain the upright position. Thirty-six patients (age, 67.52 ± 1.45 years) who met the inclusion criteria, including 19 men (mean age, 69.31 ± 2.03; median age, 72 years; age range, 44 – 82 years) and 17 women (mean age, 65.52 ± 2.05; median age, 65 years; age range, 48 – 72 years), were studied (Table 1).

Diagnosis	n	Mean size (mm) SE
adenocarcinoma	22	14.4 ± 1.7
squamous cell carcinoma	2	23.3 ± 11.8
non-small cell carcinoma	1	10.3*
small cell carcinoma	4	16.4 ± 2.2
tuberculosis	2	10.5 ± 1.7
bronchioalveolar carcinoma	1	15.8*
mycobacterium avium complex	1	43.6*
metastasis from liver angiosarcoma	1	17.2*
inflammatory reactive change	1	7.9*
metastatic carcinoma from breast cancer	1	27.8*

SE, standard error
* No average

Table 1: Pattern of lesions.

For this study, DES-DT and DES-R examinations were performed for all patients. Multidetector CT (64-slice SOMATOM Definition scanner; Siemens Medical Systems, Forchheim, Germany) served as the reference method for nodule detection. CT scanning was performed on a multidetector CT scanner that used 120 kVp, 110 mA, 0.6 mm × 64 collimation, and a 0.5-s gantry rotation time at a beam pitch of 0.8. The axial images were obtained with a 5-mm slice thickness at 5-mm reconstruction intervals, and the coronal and sagittal images were obtained with a 2-mm slice thickness at 2-mm reconstruction intervals. The reference data were collected by two experienced thoracic radiologists after completion of the detection study. Differences in the assessments were resolved by discussion until consensus was reached. Two of the radiologists participated in the reference study (observers 1 and 5). Axial, coronal, and sagittal reformations were used in all cases to identify the nodules. The largest diameter in the transverse plane was assessed. Identical magnification was used for the measurements. The nodules were grouped for size in accordance with the guidelines for the management of small pulmonary nodules created by the Fleischner Society (MachMahon *et al.*, 2005) (≤ 4 mm, > 4 – 6 mm, > 6 – 8 mm, and > 8 mm). According to nodule localization on the multidetector CT images, the nodules were marked on the DES-DT images and radiographs to obtain the true locations.

2.2.3   Detection Study

To evaluate the images for the presence of pulmonary nodules, receiver operating characteristic (ROC) paradigm was used by two radiologists and three doctors of pulmonary medicine who had 28 (observer 1), 26 (observer 2), 14 (observer 3), 13 (observer 5), and 10 (observer 4) years of experience in chest radiography, respectively. We examined 36 samples with and 36 samples without pulmonary nodules by both DES-DT imaging and DES-R. Each case occurred only once in each group. The radiologists and doctors of pulmonary medicine were presented with both the DES-R and DES-DT images at different times. Each observer was instructed to detect pulmonary nodules on the DES-DT and DES-R images and use a continuous scale from 1 to 50 to assess the presence of a nodule. For both situations (with and without pulmonary nodules), a score of 50 represented the highest degree of confidence (probably a nodule) and a score of 0 represented the lowest degree of confidence (probably not a nodule). ROC analysis software, DBM MRMC version 2.2, was used (Derbaum, 2009). The accuracy of detection of pulmonary nodules was described by the area under the ROC curves (Hanley *et al.*, 1982, 1983).

2.2.4   Statistical Analysis

ROC analysis was used to assess the true-positive fraction versus the false-positive fraction. The average area under the curve (AUC) and standard deviation were obtained by individually fitting the ROC curves into the confidence ratings of each observer and averaging the estimated areas across observers. The AUC values were used to test the significance of the differences in detection accuracy between the two methods using the paired F-test. The multireader multicase ROC method, in which a mixed effects model is used to analyze pseudovalues based on jackknifing, was used to determine the significance of the differences observed between modalities.

2.2.5   Results

A high-contrast detectability case with clear contrast detectability by DES-DT imaging was produced for identical planes (Figure 1). Greater image contrast for similarly sized nodules was obtained by DES-DT than by DES-R. When the nodules were no longer superimposed over the normal structures, their characteristics and distribution could be observed much more clearly.

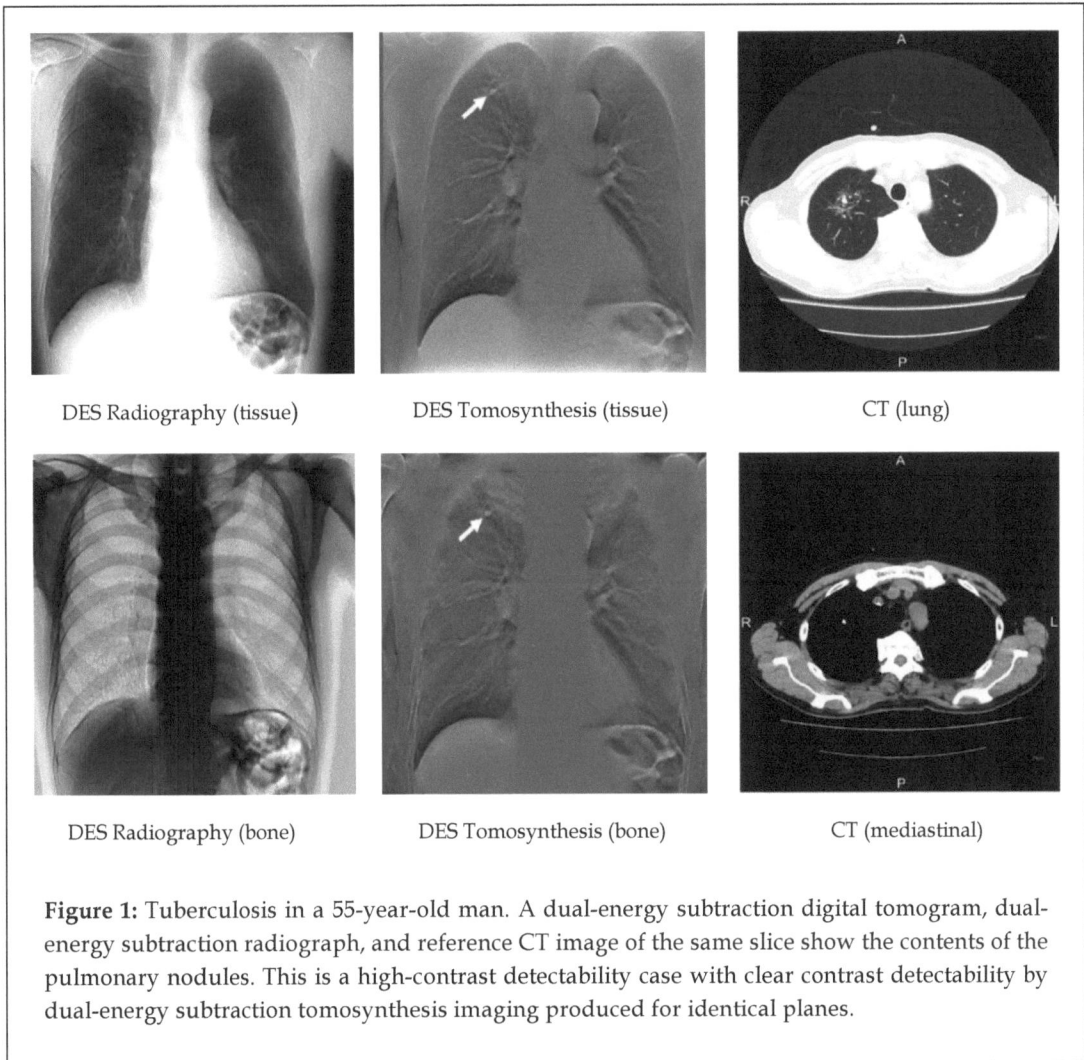

| DES Radiography (tissue) | DES Tomosynthesis (tissue) | CT (lung) |
| DES Radiography (bone) | DES Tomosynthesis (bone) | CT (mediastinal) |

Figure 1: Tuberculosis in a 55-year-old man. A dual-energy subtraction digital tomogram, dual-energy subtraction radiograph, and reference CT image of the same slice show the contents of the pulmonary nodules. This is a high-contrast detectability case with clear contrast detectability by dual-energy subtraction tomosynthesis imaging produced for identical planes.

The results of ROC performance analysis (Figure 2) showed that the detection accuracy was significantly better for DES-DT imaging than for DES-R [$P < 0.0001$; 95% confidence interval: DES-DT, 0.94 (95% confidential interval: CI; 0.83 – 0.99); DES-R, 0.76 (CI; 0.68 – 0.85)]. The ROC analysis showed a tendency toward easy detection of larger pulmonary nodules by DES-DT.

The sensitivity, specificity, and overall diagnostic accuracy of the two techniques differed between observers. Agreement among all observers improved from moderate with DES-R to very good with DES-DT (sensitivity: DES-DT, 87.7 ± 2.9%; DES-R, 53.8 ± 3.5%; specificity: DES-DT, 78.3 ± 5.6%; DES-R, 78.4 ± 3.4%; accuracy: DES-DT, 83.1 ± 3.8%, DES-R, 66.1 ± 2.0%).

With the multidetector CT reference, 36 nodules were found (≤ 4 mm, n = 0; > 4 – 6 mm, n = 2; > 6 – 8 mm, n = 2; and > 8 mm, n = 32). Of these nodules, 79.58% could be seen on the DES-DT images and 57.5% could be seen on the DES-R images when determining the true locations (Figure 3).

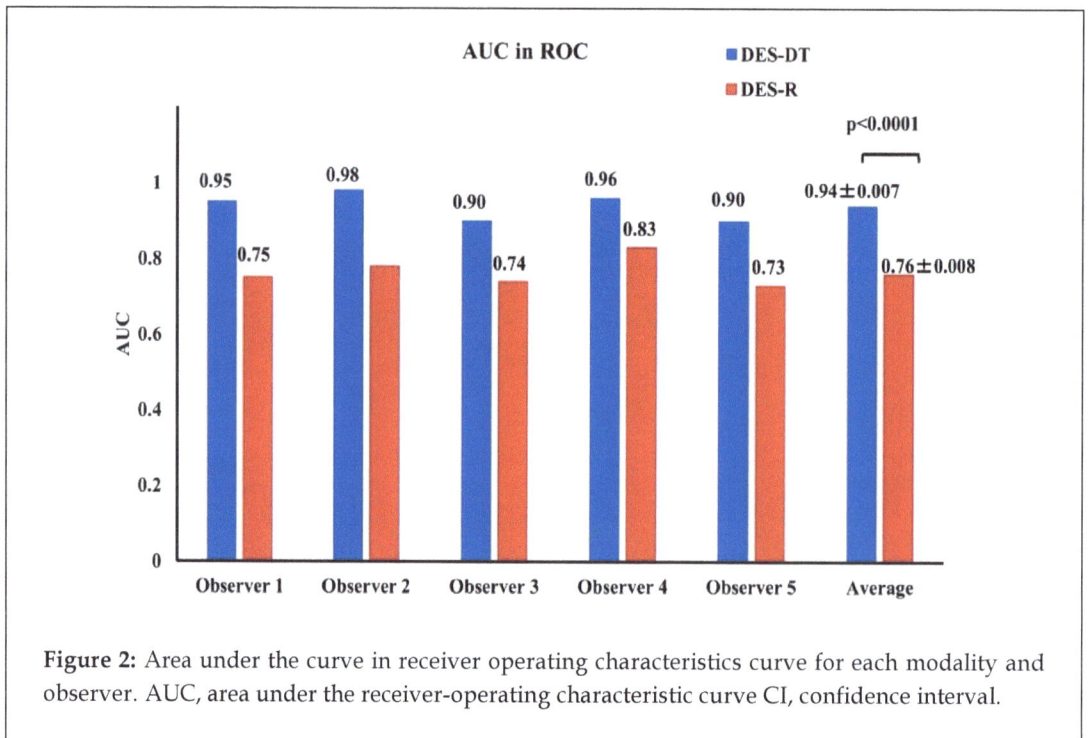

Figure 2: Area under the curve in receiver operating characteristics curve for each modality and observer. AUC, area under the receiver-operating characteristic curve CI, confidence interval.

2.3   New Image Processing for the Improvement of Image Quality

DT reconstruction also suffers from quantum noise or inconsistent reconstructed images that suffer from a low signal-to-noise ratio because of the superposition of several low-exposure projection images. Several methods have been proposed to suppress this irrelevant plane in formation and enhance the DT image quality, including sampling geometry optimization (Ghosh *et al.*, 1985), pre-filtering projections (Matsuo *et al.*, 1993; Knutsson *et al.*, 1980; Petersson *et al.*, 1980), and post-processing of reconstructed images (Sone *et al.*, 1995; Chakraborty *et al.*, 1984; Ruttiman *et al.*, 1984; Kolitsi *et al.*, 1993; Sone *et al.*, 1993). Post-processing can be further classified into two basic approaches: denoising through predictable noise reconstruction followed by subtraction from the tomographic images (Chakraborty *et al.*, 1984; Ruttiman *et al.*, 1984; Kolitsi *et al.*, 1993; Sone *et al.*, 1993) and post-reconstruction filtering techniques that specifically address artifact streaking that introduces tomosynthetic noise into DT images (Sone *et al.*, 1995). Obviously, no single method can be generally and effectively applied to all DT imaging cases. Reconstruction using inverse filtering yields images with few superimposed details but a low spatial resolution along the rotational axis (Matsuo *et al.*, 1993; Knutsson *et al.*, 1980; Petersson *et al.*, 1980). Noise reconstruction methods can be used to remove the noise attributed to all classes of structures. However, blurred out-of-plane structures must be removed from several planes (Chakraborty *et al.*, 1984; Ruttiman *et al.*, 1984; Kolitsi *et al.*, 1993; Sone *et al.*, 1993), and noise subtraction is associated with poor contrast in the resulting images because of the concurrent loss of details relevant to planes. In addition, post-reconstruction filtering techniques are only efficient for specific types of images (Sone *et al.*, 1995).

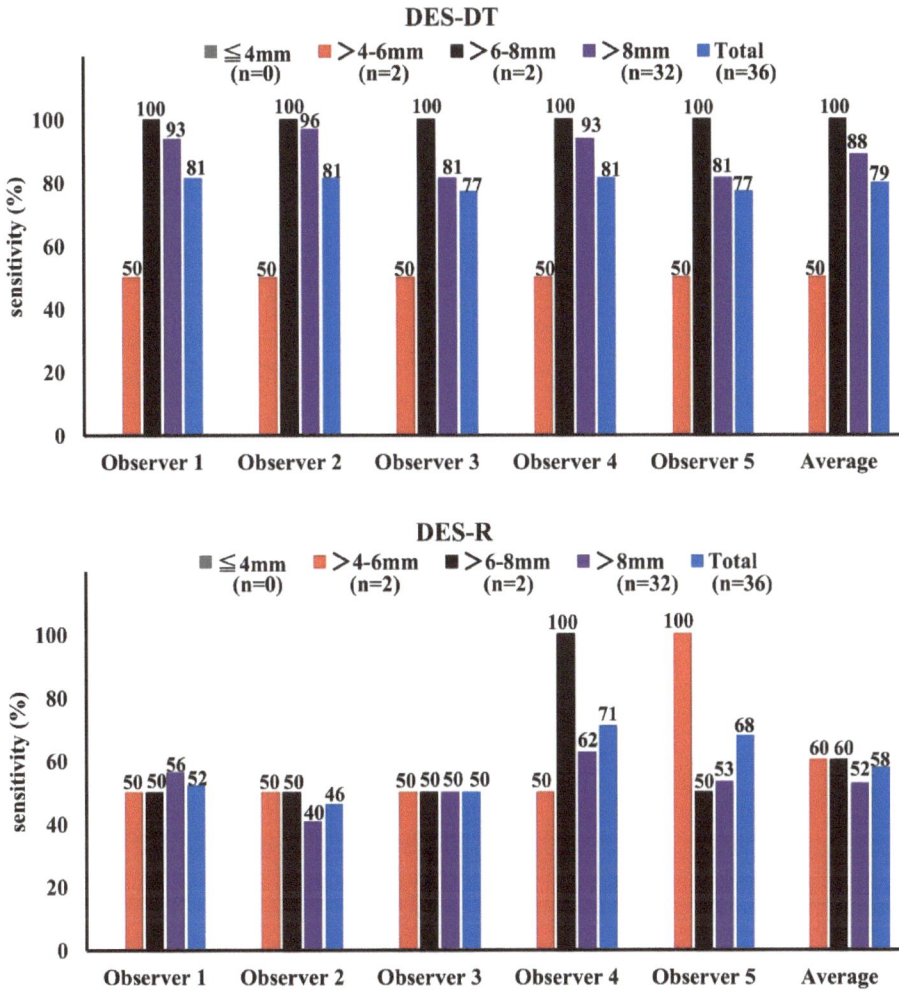

Figure 3: Subgroup analysis of the sensitivity (%) by the size of the nodules.

Wavelets have been widely used to analyze the characteristics of signals for irregular structures such as those included in biomedical images. Therefore, it is entirely reasonable to analyze such signals using wavelets (Michael *et al.*, 1996). Donoho *et al.* developed a theoretical framework of discrete wavelet transforms to estimate signals degraded by additive noise in their wavelet shrinkage method (Donoho *et al.*, 1994). This method has been used for denoising because of its simplicity and effectiveness. A previous study investigated the use of this method for two-dimensional tomography reconstruction (Kolaczyk, 1996) and other modalities (Nitzken *et al.*, 2012, 2013). However, appropriate threshold estimation is often difficult and *a priori* knowledge of the noise intensity is necessary to determine the optimal threshold. Furthermore, the signal edge information might be removed during this denoising process. Badea *et al.* developed a wavelet that could be applied to the reconstructed plane for DT (Badea *et al.*, 1998). This technique can discriminate and subsequently remove unrelated structures from the reconstructed plane. In Badea's wavelet approach, thresholding is based on location, and the local maxima that account for the blurred edges are discarded inside the noise map created at each wavelet scale. However, the effect of this technique on large structures is limited to further blurring with incomplete residual noise removal.

To resolve incomplete residual noise removal, we suggest a balance sparsity-norm (Antoniadis *et al.*, 1999; Hall *et al.*, 1997; Donoho *et al.*, 1996) wavelet denoising processing method. This method produces a calculated norm of the spectrum, which balances thresholding with loss in image quality. The novel aspect of our technique is that it is a hybrid method that exploits both the predictability of quantum noise generation and the signal locality of the wavelet domain. Therefore, we anticipate that both conserved spatial resolution and effective quantum noise reduction will be achieved with the balance sparsity-norm technique. Against this background, we developed a wavelet-based method using a balance sparsity-norm algorithm to generate reconstructed images that would conserve spatial resolution and effectively decrease the quantum noise (Figure 4).

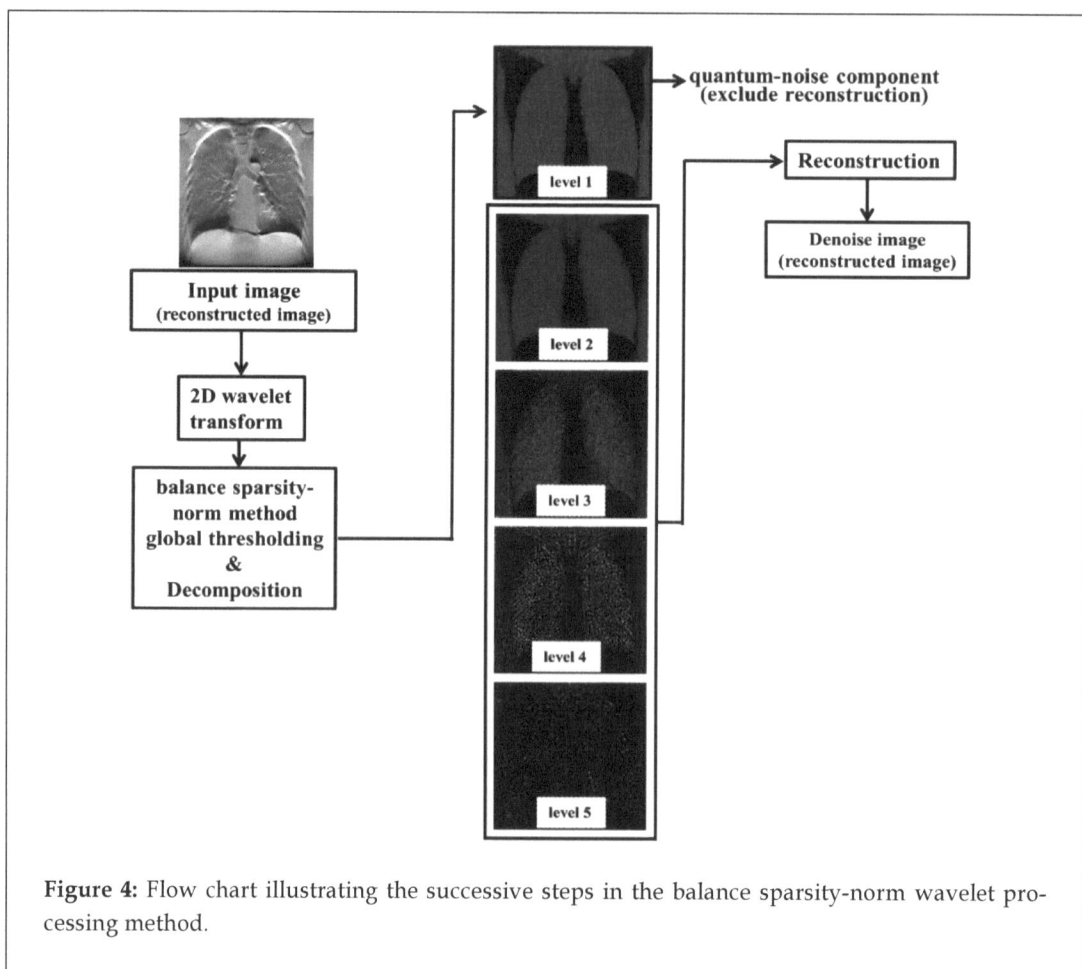

Figure 4: Flow chart illustrating the successive steps in the balance sparsity-norm wavelet processing method.

The developed DT technique has been used to conduct diagnostic studies in hospitals, where it enables the visualization of fine body structures with a shorter scan time than traditional methods. Despite these merits, all DT systems present the problem of exposing patients to radiation. Therefore, it becomes necessary to remove the noise for improving the DT image quality.

This chapter discusses a novel balance sparsity-norm wavelet denoising algorithm for chest DT to selectively remove quantum noise structures and possibly improve the image quality and compares this method with the existing Badea algorithm. The method was implemented on a DT system and experimentally evaluated using chest measurements of contrast resolution in a clinical case (71-year-old woman with brochioalveolar carcinoma). We evaluated the possibility that this balance sparsity-norm wavelet denoising algorithm would enhance the clinical applications of chest DT in medical imaging fields,

2.3.1 Conditions for Data Acquisition

The DT system (SonialVision Safire II; Shimadzu Co.) comprised an X-ray tube with a 0.4-mm focal spot and a 362.88 × 362.88-mm digital flat-panel detector composed of amorphous selenium. Each projection image was acquired at 120 kVp, 200 mA, and with a 5-ms exposure time for X-rays. The size of each detector element was 150 × 150 μm. Tomography was performed using a linear tomographic movement, a total acquisition time of 6.4 s, and an acquisition angle of 40°. Projection images were sampled during a single tomographic pass (74 projections) using a matrix size of 1440 × 1440 by 12 bits per image and were used to reconstruct tomograms of a desired layer height. Reconstructed images (0.252 mm/pixel) were obtained with a 5-mm slice thickness at 5-mm reconstruction intervals. The DT images were reconstructed using filtered back projection with the conventional Shepp–Logan filter kernel (Gomi *et al.*, 2008).

2.3.2 Contrast-to-noise Ratio

Our analysis considered the contrast-to-noise ratio (CNR) of the pulmonary nodules. CNR is defined in equation (1).

$$CNR = \frac{N_1 - N_0}{\sigma_0} \tag{1}$$

where N_1 is the mean pixel value in the region of pulmonary nodules, N_0 is the mean pixel value in the background area, and σ_0 is the standard deviation of pixel values in the background area. Throughout these results, σ_0 includes structure noise that can obscure the object besides photon statistics and electronic noise.

2.3.3 Results

Intensity profiles along the sweep (vertical) and horizontal directions with wavelet denoising processing were investigated (Figure 5). Wavelet denoising processing effectively decreased the quantum noise in the reconstructed images obtained with balance sparsity-norm wavelet denoising processing. Furthermore, with balance sparsity-norm wavelet denoising processing, contrast detectability (CNR) was highly relative to that of the existing Badea algorithm. In the reconstructed images obtained using wavelet denoising processing techniques, the quantum noise structure exhibited reduced and the noise structure was slightly smoothed (Figure 6 and 7). In the reconstructed images obtained using the existing Badea algorithm, the noise structure was reduced and smoothed, and the normal structure was not preserved (Figure 6).

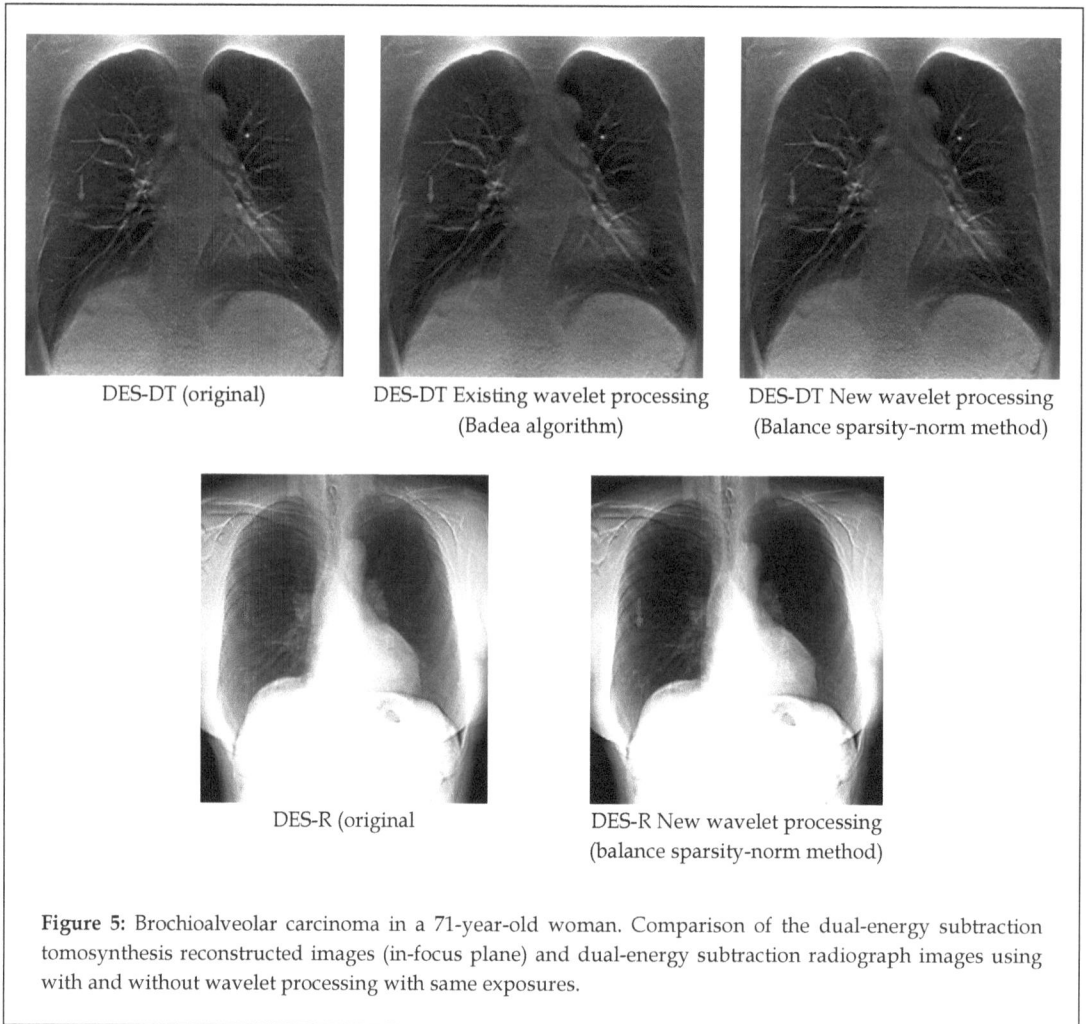

| DES-DT (original) | DES-DT Existing wavelet processing (Badea algorithm) | DES-DT New wavelet processing (Balance sparsity-norm method) |

DES-R (original

DES-R New wavelet processing (balance sparsity-norm method)

Figure 5: Brochioalveolar carcinoma in a 71-year-old woman. Comparison of the dual-energy subtraction tomosynthesis reconstructed images (in-focus plane) and dual-energy subtraction radiograph images using with and without wavelet processing with same exposures.

3   Discussion

3.1   DES-DT Imaging

The initial data from our clinical study suggested that DES-DT imaging exhibited substantially enhanced sensitivity for the detection of pulmonary nodules. Despite its potential, DES-DT is a new technique; therefore, there is no history of evidence to support its integration into clinical practice as a method for chest radiography. Because there is no radiographic characteristic that is specific for characterizing masses, it is important to specifically detect pulmonary lesions. DES-DT imaging can be used to assess the presence, distribution, and characteristics of lung nodules to an extent that is not possible with currently available projection-type DES techniques.

In this study, DES-DT was able to decisively confirm pulmonary lesions and differentiate between true pulmonary opacities and pulmonary pseudolesions. The method provided a clear improvement in diagnostic accuracy, confidence, and inter-reader agreement relative to those obtained by DES-R, with only a modest increase in the radiation dose and interpretation time. DES-R showed low sensitivity for most of these pulmonary lesions and gave false nega-

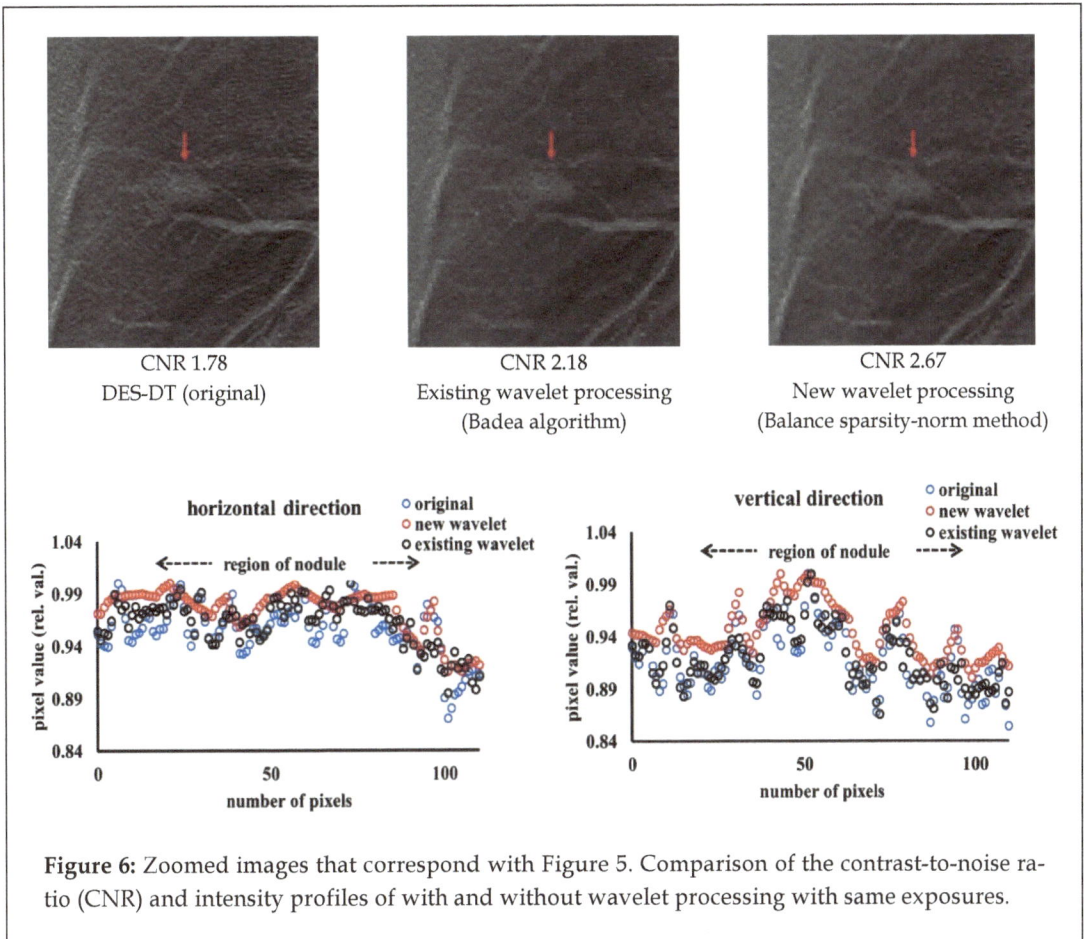

Figure 6: Zoomed images that correspond with Figure 5. Comparison of the contrast-to-noise ratio (CNR) and intensity profiles of with and without wavelet processing with same exposures.

tive findings as confirmed by the CT reference method analyses. This has a strong clinical impact because, in general, approximately only 53% of pulmonary nodules are detected by DES-R. In our study, we found greater sensitivity because we were able to detect 87% of CT-confirmed pulmonary lesions on average by DES-DT. These results indicated that DES-DT could be used as a problem-solving technique for the confirmation of suspected pulmonary lesions identified at preliminary assessments made by DES-R.

Many nodules identified by chest radiography or CT require follow-up to determine if they are malignant (MachMahon et al., 2005). Most of such follow-ups are currently performed using CT. Considering our results and those of a previous phantom study in which the detection of artificial pulmonary nodules (5 and 8 mm in diameter) on DT images was similar to that on CT images (Gomi et al., 2012), DES-DT may be used in the future for the follow-up of pulmonary nodules identified on chest radiography or CT.

Another feature of the DES technique is that the most reliable signs for discriminating between benign and malignant masses are the growth rate and presence or absence of calcifications within the mass. Because calcifications are commonly observed in benign masses and no other radiographic characteristic is specific for characterizing masses, it is important to detect and characterize calcification within lesions (Littleton, 1983). To further demonstrate the DES technique, we believe that the method should be tested by clinically examining.

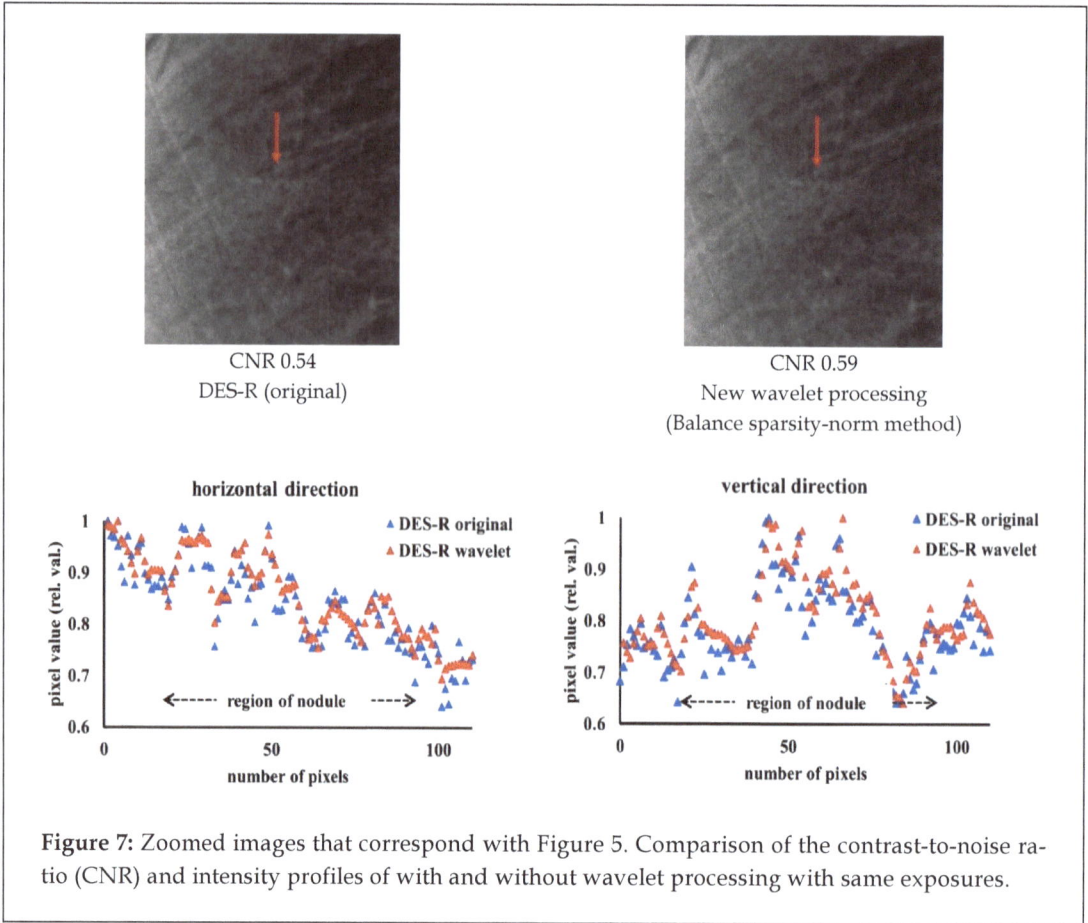

Figure 7: Zoomed images that correspond with Figure 5. Comparison of the contrast-to-noise ratio (CNR) and intensity profiles of with and without wavelet processing with same exposures.

3.2   New Image Processing for the Improvement of Image Quality

Our experimental results clearly demonstrate the ability of balance sparsity-norm wavelet denoising processing to remove quantum noise from chest DT images. In this study, the in-focus plane intensities of the normal structures remained unchanged, whereas the superimposed quantum noise was removed and replaced with the average background intensity level.

However, the influence of the Badea algorithm on low-dose exposure patterns was limited to incomplete residual quantum noise removal. The selective behavior of this technique was expected because the last wavelet decomposition approximation actually contained the background alone; therefore, the undesirable superimposed structures were effectively removed by eliminating the local maxima that accounted for the quantum noise (Badea *et al.*, 1998). However, large structures constituted low-frequency elements and could be filtered because they were present in the coarse wavelet transformation approximations.

Balance sparsity-norm wavelet denoising processing could successfully eliminate in-focus plane denoising. However, on a heterogeneous background, it could not achieve good CNR values for pulmonary nodules with high inherent CNR.

Noise removal during wavelet denoising processing is attained by subtracting the noise mask from the DT reconstruction plane. This noise mask is the sum of the restored set of all blurred replicas in the DT plane, weighted accordingly. Therefore, this sum contains the image that has been added as quantum noise to the plane of interest. However, it also contains a directionally blurred version of the tomogram of interest. The effect of this blurred post-noise mask subtraction version is similar to that of unsharpened filters such that the edges of the reconstructed structures in the plane of interest are enhanced in the direction of the line intersecting the tomogram with the trajectory plane.

4   Conclusion

We concluded that DES-DT is superior to DES-R for the detection of pulmonary nodules. The imaging quality of DES-DT should improve the detection of pulmonary nodules when applied in clinical practice.

Balance sparsity-norm wavelet denoising processing involved a wavelet technique specifically for chest DT images and has been demonstrated to effectively remove quantum mottle noise from chest DT images of structures with features of high-frequency components. Furthermore, this approach suggests that the image quality could be improved.

References

Antoniadis A, Gregoire G, Nason G. (1999). Density and harzard rate estimation for right-censored data using wavelet methods. Journal of the Royal Statistical Society: Series B 61, 63-84.

Badea C, Kolitsi Z, Pallikarakis N. (1998). A wavelet method for removal of out-of-plane structures in digital tomosynthesis. Computerized Medical Imaging and Graphics 22, 309-315.

Bath M, Hakansson A, Tingberg A, Månsson LG. (2005). Method of simulating dose reduction for digital radiographic systems. Radiation Protection Dosimetry 114, 253-259.

Brody WR, Butt G, Hall A, Macovski A. (1981). A method for selective tissue and bone visualization using dual-energy scanned projection radiography. Medical Physics 8, 353-357.

Chakraborty DP, Yester MV, Barnes GT, Lakshminarayanan AV. (1984). Self-masking subtraction tomosynthesis. Radiology 150, 225-229.

Chou SH, Kicska GA, Pipavath SN, Reddy GP. (2014). Digital tomosynthesis of the chest: current and emerging applications. Radiographics 34, 359-372.

Derbaum K. DBM MRMC software 2.2. URL: http://perception.radiology.uiowa.edu (published June 24, 2008; accessed January 7, 2009).

Dobbins JT, Mcadams HP, Song JW, Li CM, Godfrey DJ, Delong DM, Paik SH, Martinez-Jimenez S. (2008). Digital tomosynthesis of the chest for lung nodule detection: interim sensitivity results from an ongoing NIH-sponsored trial. Medical Physics 35, 2554-2557.

Donoho DL, Johnstone IM, Kerkyacharian G, Picard D. (1996). Density estimation by wavelet thresholding. The Annals of Statistics 24, 508-539.

Donoho DL, Johnstone JM. (1994). Ideal spatial adaptation by wavelet shrinkage. Biometrika 81, 425-455.

Fraser RG, Hickey NM, Niklason LT, Sabbagh EA, Luna RF, Alexander CB, Robinson CA, Katzenstein AL, Barnes GT. (1986). Calcification in pulmonary nodules. detection with dual-energy digital radiography. Radiology 160, 595-601.

Ghosh Roy DN, Kruger RA, Yih B, Del Rio P. (1985). Selective plane removal in limited angle tomographic imaging. Medical Physics 12, 65-70.

Godwin JD. (1983). The solitary pulmonary nodule. Radiologic Clinics of North America 21, 709-21.

Gomi T, Hirano H. (2008). Clinical potential of digital linear tomosynthesis imaging of total joint arthroplasty. Journal of Digital Imaging 21, 312-322.

Gomi T, Nakajima M, Fujiwara H, Takeda T, Saito K, Umeda T, Sakaguchi K. (2012). Comparison between chest digital tomo-synthesis and CT to detect artificial pulmonary nodules for screening: a phantom study. The British Journal of Radiology 85, e622-e629.

Gomi T, Nakajima M, Fujiwara H, Umeda T. (2011). Comparison of chest dual-energy subtraction digital tomosynthesis imaging and dual-energy subtraction radiography to detect simulated pulmonary nodules with and without calcifications. Academic Radiology 18, 191-196.

Gomi T, Nozaki M, Takeda T, Umeda T, Takahashi K, Nakajima M. (2013). Comparison of chest dual-energy subtraction digital tomosynthesis and dual-energy subtraction radiography for detection of pulmonary nodules: initial evaluations in human clinical cases. Academic Radiology 20, 1357-1363.

Hall P, Penev S, Kerkyacharian G, Picard D. (1997). Numerical performance of block thresholded wavelet estimators. Statistics and Computing 7, 115-124.

Hanley JA, McNeil BJ. (1982). The meaning and use of the area under receiver operating characteristic (ROC) curves. Radiology 143, 29-36.

Hanley JA, McNeil BJ. (1983). A method of comparing the areas under receiver operating characteristic curves derived from the same cases. Radiology 148, 839-843.

Hickey NM, Niklason LT, Sabbagh E, Fraser RG, Barnes GT. (1987). Dual-energy digital radiographic quantification of calcium in simulated pulmonary nodules. American Journal of Roentgenology 148, 19-24.

Ishigaki T, Sakuma S, Horikawa Y, Ikeda M, Yamaguchi H. (1986). One-shot dual-energy subtraction imaging. Radiology 161, 271-3.

Ishigaki T, Sakuma S, Ikeda M. (1988). One-shot dual-energy subtraction chest imaging with computed radiography. Radiology 168, 67-72.

Johnsson AA, Vikgren J, Bath M. (2014). Chest tomosynthesis: technical and clinical perspectives. Seminars in Respiratory and Critical Care Medicine 35, 17-26.

Knutsson HE, Edholm P, Granlund HG, Petersson CU. (1980). Ectomography – a new radiographic reconstruction method I Theory and error estimates. IEEE Transaction on Biomedical Engineering 27, 640-648.

Kolaczyk ED. (1996). A Wavelet shrinkage approach to tomographic image reconstruction. Journal of the American Statistical Association 91, 1079-1090.

Kolitsi Z, Panayiotakis G, Pallikarakis N. (1993). A method for selective removal of out-of-plane structures in digital tomosynthesis. Medical Physics 20, 47-50.

Littleton JT. (1983). Pluridirectional tomography in diagnosis and management of early bronchogenic carcinoma. In: sectional imaging methods. A comparison, edited by Little JT & Durizch ML. University Park Press, 155.

MachMahon H, Austin JH, Gamsu G, Herold CJ, Jett JR, Naidich DP, Patz EF Jr, Swensen SJ. (2005). Guidelines for management of small pulmonary nodules detected on CT scans: a statement from the Fleischer Society. Radiology 237, 395-400.

Matsuo H, Iwata A, Horiba I, Suzumura N. (1993). Three-dimensional image reconstruction by digital tomosynthesis using inverse filtering. IEEE Transaction on Medical Imaging 12, 307-313.

McLendon RE, Roggli VL, Foster WL Jr, Becsey D. (1985). Carcinoma of the lung with osseous stromal metaplasia. Arcjhives of Pathology & Laboratory Medicine 109, 1051-3.

Michael U, Akram A. (1996). A review of wavelets in biomedical application. Proceedings of the IEEE 84, 626-638.

Nishitani H, Umezu Y, Ogawa K, Yuzuriha H, Tanaka H, Matsuura K. (1986). Dual-energy projection radiography using condenser X-ray generator and digital radiography apparatus. Radiology 161, 533-5.

Nitkzen M, Beache G, Elnakib A, Khalifa F, Gimel'farb G, El-Baz A. (2012). Improving Full-Cardiac Cycle Strain Estimation from Tagged CMR by Accurate Modeling of 3D Image Appearance Characteristics. Proc IEEE International Symposium on Biomedical Imaging (ISBI'12) Barcelona Spain May 2-5, 462-465.

Nitzken M, Bajaj N, Aslan S, Gimel'farb G, El-Baz A, Ovechkin A. (2013). Local Wavelet-Based Filtering of Electromyographic Signals to Eliminate the Electrocardiographic-Induced Artifacts in Patients with Spinal Cord Injury. Journal of Biomedical Science and Engineering 6, 1-13.

Peloschek P, Sailer J, Weber M, Herold CJ, Prokop M, Schaefer-Prokop C. (2007). *Pulmonary nodules: sensitivity of maximum intensity projection versus that of volume rendering of 3D multidetector CT data. Radiology 2007, 243:561-569.*

Petersson CU, Edholm P, Granlund HG, Knutsson HE. (1980). *Ectomography – a new radiographic reconstruction method II computer-simulated experiments. IEEE Transaction on Biomedical Engineering 27, 649-655.*

Ruttiman UE, Groenhuis RA, Webber RL. (1984). *Restoration of digital multi-plane tomosynthesis by a constrained iteration method. IEEE Transaction on Medical Imaging 3, 141-148.*

Siegelman SS, Khouri NF, Leo FP, Fichman EK, Braverman RM. Zerhouni EA. (1986). *Solitary pulmonary nodules: CT assessment. Radiology 160, 307-312.*

Siegelman SS, Zerhouni EA, Loe FP, Khouri NF, Stitik FP. (1980). *CT of the solitary pulmonary nodule. American Journal of Roentgenology 135, 1-13.*

Sone S, Kasuga T, Sakai F, Hirano H, Kubo K, Morimoto M, Takemura K, Hosoba M. (1993). *Chest imaging with dual-energy subtraction digital tomosynthesis. Acta Radiologica 34, 346-350.*

Sone S, Kasuga T, Sakai F, Kawai T, Oguchi K, Hirano H, Li F, Kubo K, Honda T, Haniuda M. (1995). *Image processing in the digital tomosynthesis for pulmonary imaging. European Radiology, 5, 96-101.*

Svalkvist A, Bath M. (2010). *Simulation of dose reduction in tomosynthesis. Medical Physics 37, 258-269.*

Ullman G, Dance DR, Sandborg M, Carlsson GA, Svalkvist A, Båth M. (2010). *A monte carlo-based model for simulation of digital chest tomosynthesis. Radiation Protection Dosimetry 139, 159-163.*

Valencia R, Denecke T, Lehmkuhl L, Fischbach F, Felix R, Knollmann F. (2006). *Value of axial and coronal maximum intensity projection (MIP) images in the detection of pulmonary nodules by multislice spiral CT: comparison with axial 1-mm and 5-mm slices. European Radiology 16, 325-332.*

Vikgren J, Zachrisson S, Svalkvist A, Johnsson AA, Boijsen M, Flink A, Kheddache S, Båth M. (2008). *Comparison of chest tomosynthesis and chest radiography for detection of pulmonary nodules: human observer study of clinical cases. Radiology 217, 251-256.*

Yankelevitz DF, Reeves AP, Kostis WJ, Zhao B, Henschke CI. (2000). *Small pulmonary nodules: volumetrically determined growth rates based on CT evaluation. Radiology 217, 251-56.*

Zachrisson S, Vikgren J, Svalkvist A, Johnsson AA, Boijsen M, Flinck A, Månsson LG, Kheddache S, Båth M. (2009). *Effect of clinical experience of chest tomosynthesis on detection of pulmonary nodules. Acta Radiologica 50, 884-891.*

Zerhouni EA, Caskey C, Khouri NF. (1988). *The pulmonary nodules. Seminars in Ultrasound, CT, and MRI 9, 67-78.*

Carcinoma of the Gallbladder: Current State and Future Directions in Diagnosis and Treatment

Thy Bao Ngoc Tran[*], Sonia John[†], Huong Giang Tran[‡], Shubham Pant[†] and Lewis Hassell[*]

1 Introduction

Gallbladder cancer (GBC) was first reported in 1777 (Lazcano-Ponce *et al.*, 2001). Today it is most often found in two situations which are late stage with constitutional symptoms and positive imaging findings, and early stage, incidentally diagnosed after cholecystectomy for other disease. The incidence of GBC has declined over the last few decades and the survival time is also better than in the past. With the improvement of treatment and imaging techniques, the future promises more late stage cases will survive longer and more early stage cases will be discovered. We are optimistic this will lead to increased survival times on the whole and eliminate the current fear of GBC as a highly mortal cancer (Gourgiotis *et al.*, 2008).

2 Epidemiology

Gallbladder cancer is uncommon in the US with an incidence of about 1.2/100,000, according to the Surveillance, Epidemiology, and End Results Program (SEER). The incidence of GBC during the last three decades has declined, primarily due to declining incidence among the elderly aged 65+ (Figure 1); while it has remained unchanged in the younger aged groups. GBC is rarely seen before age 35 and as seen in Figure 3, increases dramatically with age especially after the age of 60. Women are nearly 1.5 times more likely to get GBC than men.

The SEER database just has cancer data from 1975 to the most recent year of 2010. However Siegel et al made an effort to project estimated new cases for most of the cancers which will be diagnosed in 2014. From their efforts, GBC and extrahepatic bile duct cancers in 2014 are the seventh most common cancers in the gastrointestinal tract with a projected 10,650 new cases, higher than cancers in the small intestine and in the anus, anal canal and anorectum, but dwarfed by projected colon cancer cases which are approximately 9.5 times greater than GBC and extrahepatic bile duct cancers, (Figure 2) (Siegel *et al.*, 2014).

In the US, Hispanic and American Indian/Alaska Native have greater incidence rates than other ethnic groups. Some of the reasons potentially behind this variance in ethnic incidence will be discussed below.

Fifty percent of GBC patients had a survival time of only one year after diagnosis. The survival time after 3 years plateaus at less than 20% (Figure 6).

[*] Department of Pathology, University of Oklahoma Health Sciences Center, Oklahoma City, Oklahoma, USA

[†] Department of Medicine, Hematology/Oncology, University of Oklahoma Health Sciences Center/Oklahoma City, Oklahoma, USA

[‡] Department of Pathology, University of Medicine and Pharmacy, Ho Chi Minh City, Vietnam

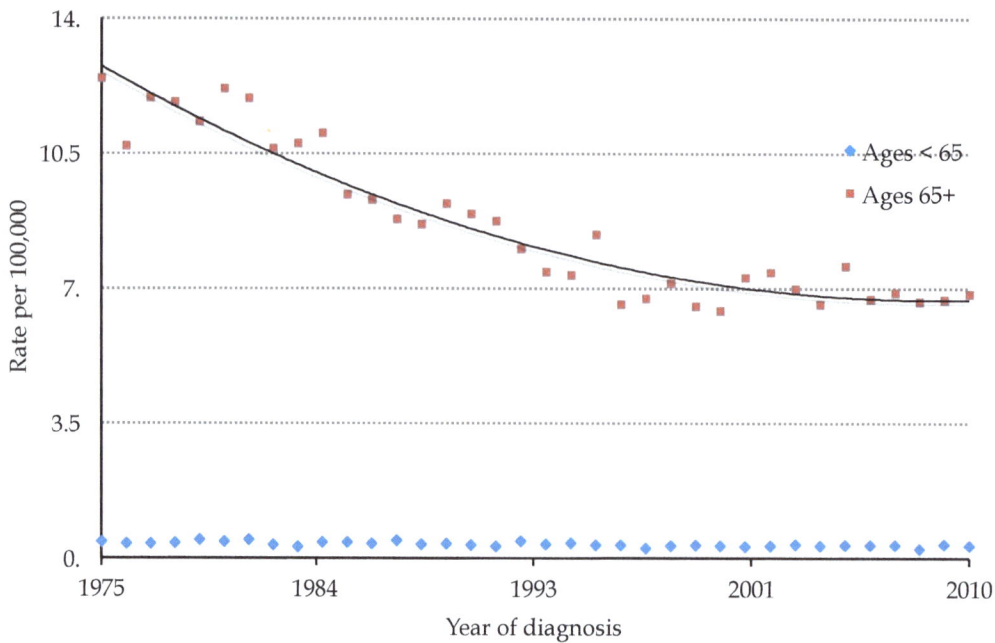

Figure 1: Age-Adjusted SEER Incidence Rates Gallbladder All Races, Both Sexes, 1975-2010 (SEER 9).

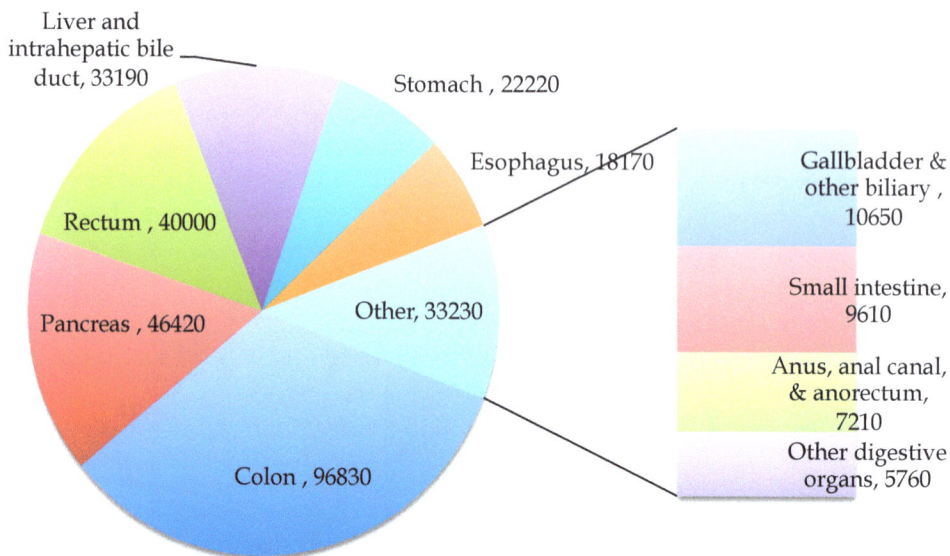

Figure 2: Estimated New Cancer Cases In Digestive System, United States, 2014.

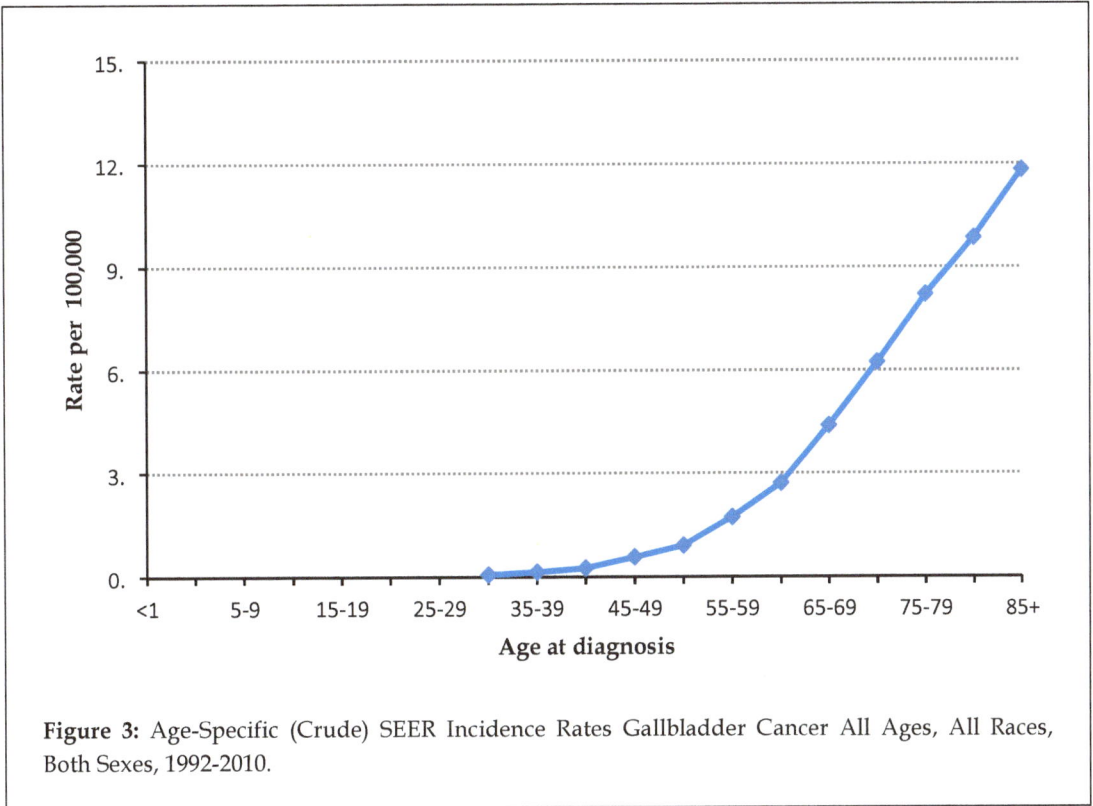

Figure 3: Age-Specific (Crude) SEER Incidence Rates Gallbladder Cancer All Ages, All Races, Both Sexes, 1992-2010.

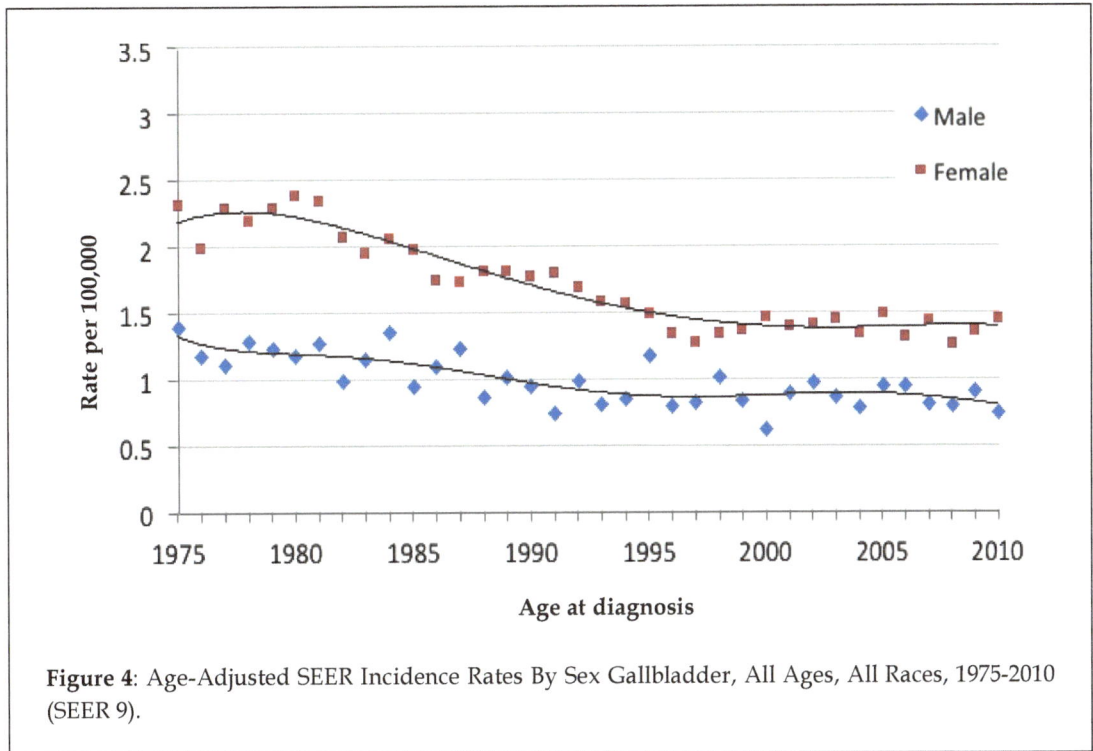

Figure 4: Age-Adjusted SEER Incidence Rates By Sex Gallbladder, All Ages, All Races, 1975-2010 (SEER 9).

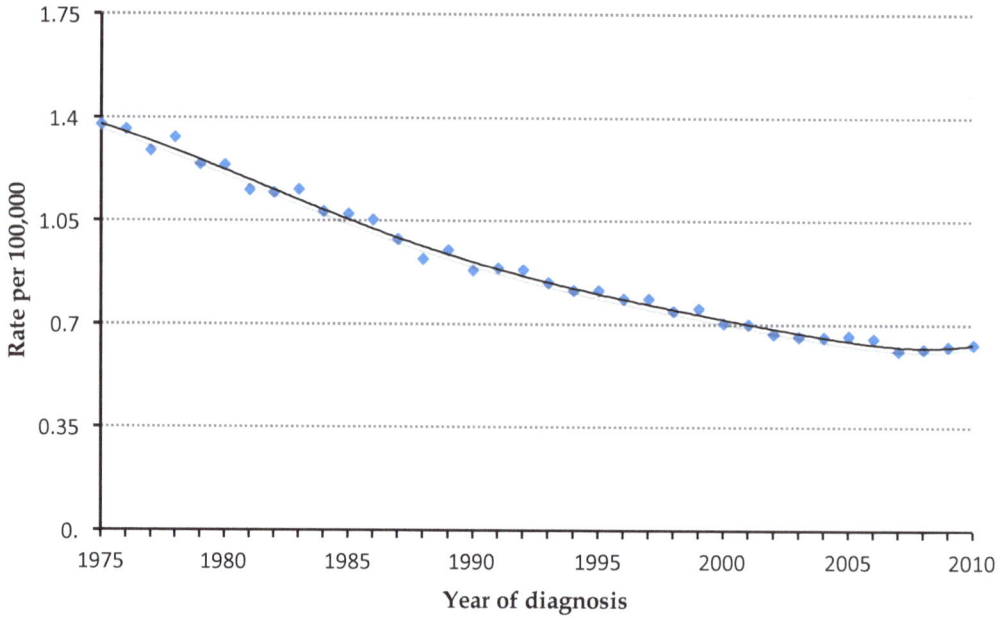

Figure 5: Age-Adjusted U.S. Mortality Rates for GBC, All Ages, All Races, Both Sexes, 1975-2010.

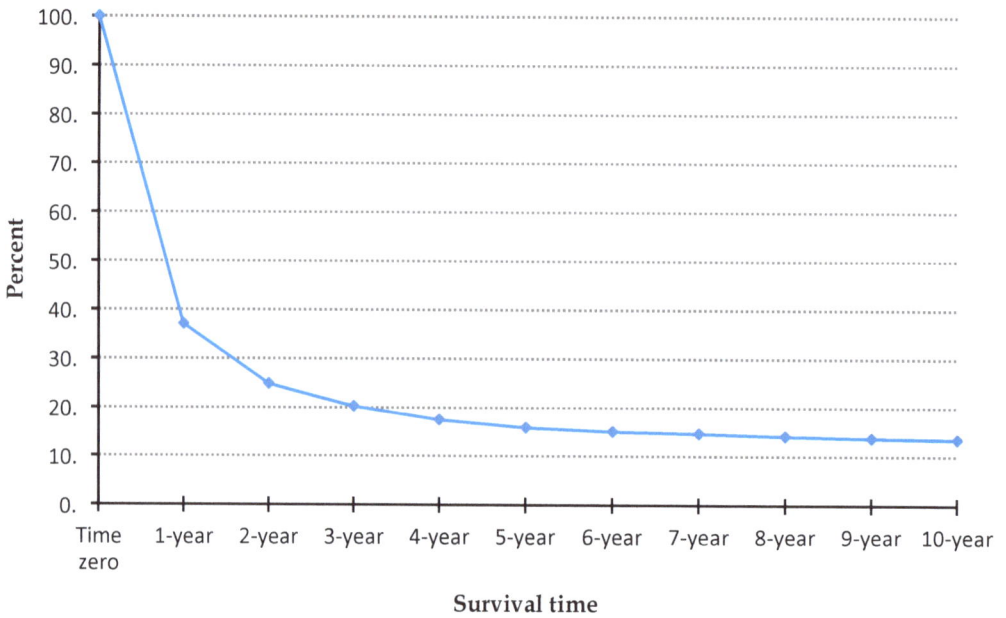

Figure 6: Relative Survival of Gallbladder Cancer By Survival Time – All Ages, All Races, Both Sexes, 1992-2009.

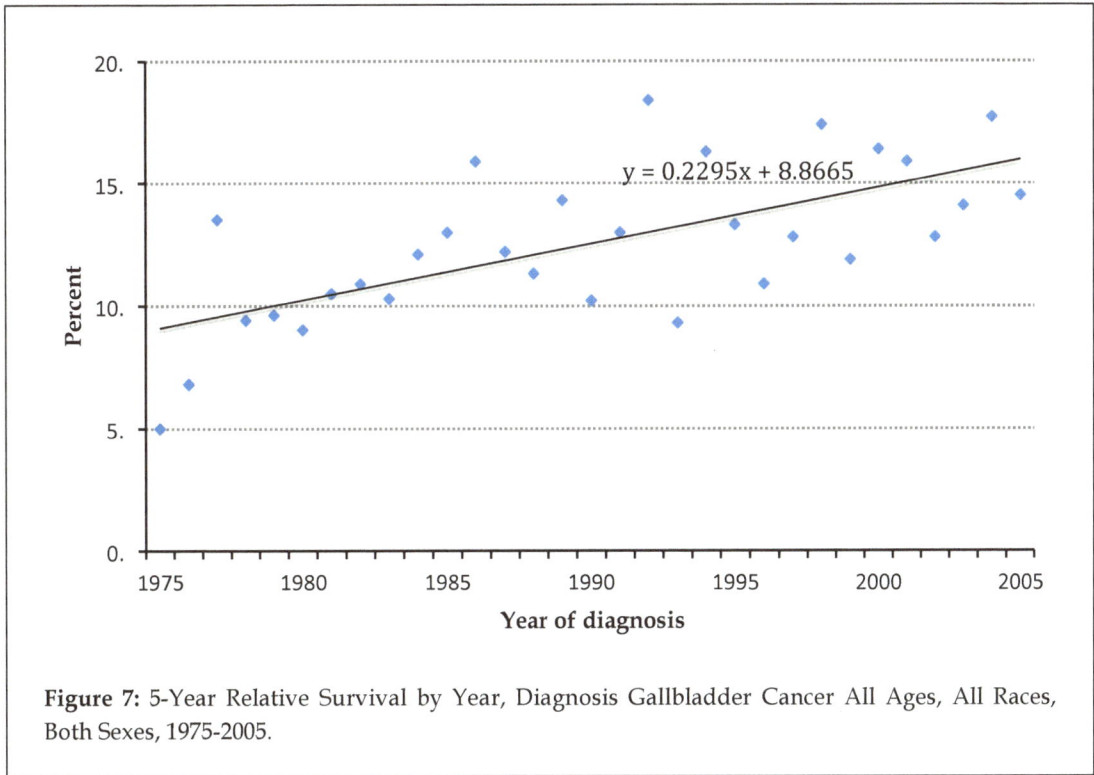

$y = 0.2295x + 8.8665$

Figure 7: 5-Year Relative Survival by Year, Diagnosis Gallbladder Cancer All Ages, All Races, Both Sexes, 1975-2005.

The 5-year relative survival for gallbladder cancer in the US has increased about 5% every 15 years, from 5% in 1975 to 10.2% in 1990, and 14.5% in 2005 (Figure 7).

The age standardized mortality rate of gallbladder cancer across the world also appears to be declining (Hariharan *et al.*, 2008). In the US during a period from 1975 to 2010, there was also a dramatic decline by fifty percent in the mortality rate of GBC from approximately 1.4/100,000 to 0.6/100,000 (Figure 5).

There is, however, a wide variation in the rate of gallbladder cancer globally. This could be due to environmental exposure which is different in parts of the world, and the genetics aspect of different ethnicities such as the Native American variance above (Hundal & Shaffer, 2014). Despite this regional and ethnic variation, GBC generally has similar female to male ratio from 1.5 to 2.5 (Figure 4). Noted exceptions to this are Denmark, Spain, Pakistan, and Colombia where the ratio exceeds 5. Gallbladder cancer incidence is highest in areas of Asia (India, Pakistan, Korea, Japan), followed by Eastern Europe (Slovakia, Poland, Czech Republic, Yugoslavia), South America (Ecuador, Uruguay), Southern and Central Europe, Northern Europe (except Sweden), and Northern America and Australia (Randi *et al.*, 2006).

3 Etiology

3.1 Gallstones

Cholelithiasis is the strongest risk factor for GBC, according to a meta-analysis of studies with relative risk of 4.9% [95% confidence interval (CI): 3.3-7.4] (Randi *et al.*, 2006). This risk factor is supported by many other studies (Hamdani *et al.*, 2012; Scott *et al.*, 1999; Zatonski *et al.*, 1997).

Gallstones greater than 3 cm increased the risk of GBC 9-10 times compared with the size less than 1 cm (Diehl, 1983; Lowenfels *et al.*, 1989).

Frequency of surgical intervention for gallstone disease may account for some of the decline in incidence of GBC, particularly with the advent of improved diagnostic techniques such as nuclear medicine functional scans and ultrasound. Advanced laparoscopic techniques have furthered this. The decrease in incidence of GBC started decades prior to the application of laparoscopic cholecystectomy (Hundal & Shaffer, 2014).

3.2   Polypoid Lesions

Gallbladder polyps are usually found incidentally since they are asymptomatic. Most of them are cholesterol polyps and benign, but the adenoma-carcinoma sequence may occur in some cases. When the diagnosis of polyp is made pre-operatively features predicting malignancy include age >50 years, sessile polyps, size >10 mm and rapid growth on serial ultrasonography (Andrén-Sandberg *et al.*, 2012; Myers *et al.*, 2002).

3.3   Porcelain Gallbladder

Porcelain gallbladder is a term describing diffuse fibrous thickening and calcification of GB wall. It is uncommon with an incidence of no greater than 0.2% (Hayes & Muldoon, 2014; Kim *et al.*, 2008; Towfigh *et al.*, 2001). One study found that there were 2 types of GB calcification: selective mucosal calcification and diffuse intramural calcification, the latter being understood as porcelain GB. Only selective calcification had a significant association with GBC [Odd ratio (OR) =13.89, p<0.01] (Stephen & Berger, 2001). This is supported by other studies finding that no cases of true diffuse porcelain GB had GBC and none of the GBC cases had the features of porcelain GB (Kim *et al.*, 2008; Towfigh *et al.*, 2001).

3.4   Anomalous Junction of the Pancreaticobiliary Duct (AJPBD)

Anomalous junction of the pancreaticobiliary duct is a congenital malformation in which the pancreatic duct and the distal common bile duct unite outside or before they reach the duodenal wall. This anomaly is seen more commonly in Asian than Western patients (Nuzzo *et al.*, 2004). An experimental model showed that the reflux and stasis of pancreatic juice in the bile duct stimulated inflammation and induced chronic cholecystitis with intestinal metaplasia (Nagata *et al.*, 1985). GBC associated with AJPBD were not associated with gallstones (Kang *et al.*, 2007; Nagata *et al.*, 1985). Most of the pathological findings were adenocarcinoma, both poorly-differentiated and well-differentiated. The well-differentiated tumors appeared with intestinal types such as papillary, tubular, and mucinous carcinoma (Nagata *et al.*, 1985; Tanaka *et al.*, 1998). These histological subtypes have been seen with less invasion and longer survival time than other subtypes of adenocarcinoma of GBC, possibly due to earlier symptomatic presentation (Henson *et al.*, 1992; Hundal & Shaffer, 2014; Nuzzo *et al.*, 2004). This association further supports a role for chronic irritation in carcinogenesis in GBC.

3.5   Obesity

Larsson and Wolk identified obesity as a risk factor in GBC. They based this on their meta-analysis of GBC cases from the MEDLINE and EMBASE databases from 1966 to 2007. They found from eight cohort studies and three case control studies with 3288 cases that the over-weight and obese have higher risks of developing GBC with 1.15 (95% CI, 1.01-1.30) and 1.66 (95% CI, 1.47-1.88), respectively. Women had a significantly increased risk (relative risk, 1.88; 95% CI, 1.6-2.13) than did men (relative risk, 1.35, 95% CI, 1.09-1.68). In addition, their data showed that a body mass index (BMI) equal or greater than 25 kg/m² accounts for 30% of female GBC patients but only 12% of males (Larsson & Wolk, 2007).

In their prospective cohort studies from Norway, Australia, and Sweden with data collected from 1972 to 2006, Borena et al performed a multivariable adjusted analysis of z-score and found that higher BMI and blood glucose increased the risk of developing GBC, with the relative risk per unit increment of z-score for BMI of 1.35 (95% CI, 1.11-1.57) and for blood glucose 1.76 (95% CI, 1.10-2.85) (Borena *et al.*, 2014).

3.6   Genetics

According to Fernandez et al from their study conducted in Milan, the relative risk of developing GBC in patients with a first degree relative who had a history of GBC was 13.9 (95% CI, 1.2-163.9) (Fernandez *et al.*, 1994). The total number of GBC cases in this study was only 58 which explains why the confidence interval is widened. Another study from Sweden also showed an increased risk of familial GBC with the standardized incidence ratio of 5.21 (95% CI, 2.07-10.08) (Hemminki & Li, 2003). Counterbalancing these very high relative risks Goldgar et al found from multigenerational linked genealogical records that familial risk from first degree relatives of GBC in Utah was only 2.1 (95% CI, 0.2-6.1) (Goldgar *et al.*, 1994).

Cholesterol excreted from the liver is regulated by adenosine triphosphate-binding cassette transporter ABCG8. Many data support the hypothesis that the polymorphism D19H of ABCG8 might affect ABCG5/G8 transporter function. 19H carriers had lower serum cholesterol suggesting that D19H increases ABCG5/G8 mediated removal of cholesterol into bile and intestine. The increased secretion of cholesterol from the liver stimulates the saturation of cholesterol in bile and formation of cholesterol gallstones. This is substantiated by studies showing that gallstones are strongly associated with the D19H variant of the ABCG8 gene and cholesterol cholelithiasis is due to hypersecretion of cholesterol from the liver (Grunhage *et al.*, 2007; Buch *et al.*, 2007; Srivastava *et al.*, 2009). Thus gallstone susceptibility, in turn, plays a role in GBC.

3.7   Toxins

Tobacco use is found to be one of the risk factors of GBC in a few studies – Jain et al [OR: 4.1 (1.8-9.7); p<0.001)], Yagyu et al [Hazard ratio (HR): 2.00 (0.91-4.42) for women, and HR: 2.27 (1.05-4.90 for men], Dutta et al [OR: 11 (2-71)] (Jain *et al.*, 2013; Yagyu *et al.*, 2008; Dutta *et al.*, 2000). There are also some reports showing no significant increase in risk with smoking (Scott *et al.*, 1999; Zatonski *et al.*, 1997).

Drinking more than 72g per day of alcohol has a hazard ratio of 3.60 (1.29-9.85) for men, while there was no association between alcohol intake and GBC in women according to Yagyu et al (2008). Some occupations with reported high alcohol intake such as cooks, stewards and journalists had a 2-3 fold increase in standardized incidence ratio of GBC according to Ji et al (2005). However, there are other studies that have not found evidence of that association (Scott *et al.*, 1999; Zatonski *et al.*, 1997).

3.8   Micro-Organisms

There are many studies showing that a chronic typhoid carrier state can be an important risk factor for GBC (Dutta *et al.*, 2000; Shukla *et al.*, 2000; Tewari *et al.*, 2010). Nagaraja and Eslick found from their meta-analysis that there was a strong association between chronic *S.typhi* carrier state and GBC in Southeast Asia (OR: 4.13, 95% CI: 2.87-5.94, P <0.01), and more prominent between GBC and controls without gallstones (OR: 5.86, 95% CI: 3.84-8.95, P <0.01) versus   GBC and controls with gallstones (OR: 2.71, 95% CI: 1.92–3.83, P <0.01) (Nagaraja & Eslick, 2014).

Individuals, regardless of gallstones status, with positive typhoid culture have 8.47 times higher risk of developing GBC than ones with negative culture (Shukla *et al.*, 2000).

Helicobacter species colonize the gastrointestinal tract of both human and animals. Gastric and enterohepatic *Helicobacter* spp are the two classes of this organism species; while *H. pylori* is included in the former, *H. bilis* belongs to the latter (Fox & Lee, 1997).

The first report of an association between *Helicobacter* sp in the gallbladder and gallstone disease came in 1998 from Fox et al (Fox *et al.*, 1998). The following year Rudi et al reported that there was no evidence of *Helicobacter* sp in the bile of German patients with biliary disease (Rudi *et al.*, 1999), and Bohr et al found only one case with PCR positive *Helicobacter* spp in over 99 cases including GSD, GBC and control group (Bohr *et al.*, 2007). In 2001, Méndez-Sánchez et al showed in their study that there was no association of *Helicobacter* in Mexican patients, but did not exclude the possibility that an uncommon *Helicobacter* sp could be causative (Méndez-Sánchez *et al.*, 2001). From these studies it was concluded that the presence of *Helicobacter* sp in the biliary tract mostly depends on ethnicity and geography (Murata *et al.*, 2004).

This potential association between *Helicobacter* spp and biliary tract malignances was made clearer when Zhou et al reported from their meta-analysis of ten studies published from 2002 to 2011 about infection of *Helicobacter* spp and biliary tract cancer that *H. pylori, H. bilis, H. hepaticus* and *H. ganmani* were significantly more highly represented in the biliary tract malignancy group than in the benign disease and normal groups with P=0.0001 (Zhou *et al.*, 2013).

There have been a few studies restricted to *H. pylori* and biliary diseases. Bulajic et al published two studies about the association between *H. pylori* and benign and malignant biliary diseases. In the first study they found that the prevalence of *H. pylori* in benign biliary diseases was not significantly different compared to that of *H. pylori* in the control group (Bulajic *et al.*, 2002). The second study, published the same year, showed that patients with gallstones were 3.5 times more likely to have *H. pylori* than a control group with p value >0.05 (95% CI, 0.8-15.8; P=0.100), and *H. pylori* was 9.9 times more frequent in biliary tract malignancies than in the control group (95% CI, 1.4-70.5; P=0.022) (Bulajic *et al.*, 2002; Cariati *et al.*, 2003).

In GBC patients, 32.5% of patients with gallstones had *H. pylori* versus 35.7% of those patients without gallstones. This suggests there might not be an association between gallstone formation and *H. pylori* per se. Mishra et al also found *H. pylori* present 33% of the time in GBC and 28% in GSD (control group) with P>0.05, suggesting that *H. pylori* has high prevalence in endemic regions without a resultant significant difference in GBC and GSD patients (Mishra *et al.*, 2011). For example, in Africa there is a high rate of *H. pylori* infection, but a low rate of GBC and other biliary tract cancers (Bulajic *et al.*, 2002).

Using PCR only to detect the presence of *Helicobacter* spp in the bile of patients with gallstone disease, Jahani Sherafat et al found that *H. pylori* was only discovered in the absence

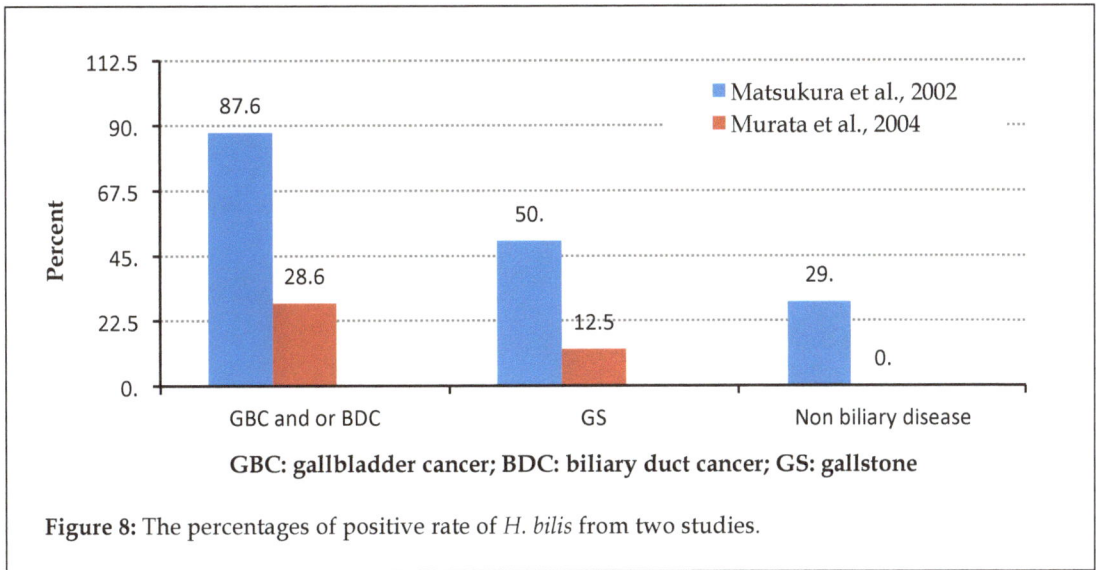

GBC: gallbladder cancer; BDC: biliary duct cancer; GS: gallstone

Figure 8: The percentages of positive rate of *H. bilis* from two studies.

of non-*H. pylori* species. They found no association between *H. pylori* and biliary tract diseases though the positive rate was 3.92% (Jahani *et al.*, 2012).

With IHC and PCR, Yakoob et al found that there was a significantly higher incidence of *H. pylori* in benign and malignant gallbladder diseases than the control group, and no positive results for *H. bilis* and *H. hepaticus* (Yakoob *et al.*, 2011).

In conclusion, evidence of an association between *H. pylori* and GBC is not clearly defined.

With other *helicobacter* species however, the story appears to be developing differently. Hamada et al found that there was a significantly higher rate (P=0.029) of *H. hepaticus* in cholelithiasis and cholecystitis compared to patients with gallbladder polyps and nonbiliary diseases (Hamada *et al.*, 2009); while it was not found in bile samples from many studies (Kobayashi *et al.*, 2005; Jahani *et al.*, 2012; Yakoob *et al.*, 2011). At the present, few studies show any consistent association between *H. hepaticus* and biliary diseases.

Very careful studies on the association between *Helicobacter bilis* and biliary tract cancer were conducted by using PCR with a primer specific for 16S rRNA of *H. bilis*. These found that *H. bilis* presented at a high incidence in biliary tract and gallbladder cancer patients compared to patients with gallstone or non-biliary disease. As seen in Figure 8 the positive rates from Murata's study were all lower than those from Matsukura's, a fact explained by Murata's et al use of DNA extracted from archival specimens rather than collected fresh and stored immediately as in the latter's study. In addition, Matsukura et al controlled for confounding factors due to use of no antibiotics in the week before collecting bile samples. Their data suggests that *H. bilis* could play a role in the pathogenesis of biliary malignancies (Matsukura *et al.*, 2002; Murata *et al.*, 2004).

In 2010, Takayama et al made an effort to discover the effect of *H. bilis* infection on a human bile duct cancer cell line. They found that *H. bilis* infection in a human bile duct cancer cell line activates NF-κB, one of the transcription factors which in turn stimulate the production of vascular endothelial growth factor (VEGF) leading to angiogenesis, further supporting the hypothesis of *H. bilis'* role in bile duct cancer (Takayama *et al.*, 2010).

Tumor type		
Epithelial tumors	Carcinoma in situ	
	Adenocarcinoma	
	Papillary adenocarcinoma	
	Adenocarcinoma, intestinal type	
	Mucinous adenocarcinoma	
	Clear cell adenocarcinoma	
	Signet ring cell carcinoma	
	Adenosquamous carcinoma	
	Squamous cell carcinoma	
	Small cell carcinoma (oat cell carcinoma)	
	Undifferentiated carcinoma	
Nonepithelial tumors	Sarcoma	
Endocrine tumors	Carcinoid tumor	
	Mixed carcinoid-adenocarcinoma	
	Paraganglioma	
Miscellaneous tumors	Carcinosarcoma	
	Malignant melanoma	
	Malignant lymphomas	
Unclassified tumors		
Secondary tumors		

Table 1: WHO classification of gallbladder cancer (Albores-Saavedra *et al.*, 1992).

4   Pathology

Current histological classification of GBC is given in Table 1 below. Adenocarcinoma is the most common histological type of GBC (Hamdani *et al.*, 2012; Henson *et al.*, 1992; Yamaguchi & Enjoji, 1988), which together with intestinal and mucinous variants accounts for over 85% of the malignancies in this organ. Neuroendocrine tumors of the gallbladder have not been extensively studied, though presumably their behavior, particularly for the well-differentiated forms, would be as difficult to predict in the GB as they are in other intestinal sites. Metastatic tumors involving the gallbladder are not infrequent, and may occasionally present as the initial presentation, particularly low grade tumors such as well-differentiated lymphoma. Papillary adenocarcinoma has the best prognosis among all histological types of GBC (Henson *et al.*, 1992). Small cell carcinoma and undifferentiated carcinoma have the worst prognosis (Compton *et al.*, 2012).

5   Clinical Diagnosis

Patients with GBC usually are asymptomatic; most cases are found incidentally. When symptomatic, clinical findings include weight loss, right upper quadrant abdominal pain, nausea, vomiting, anorexia, and jaundice (Hamdani *et al.*, 2012; Mitchell *et al.*, 2014). Laboratory findings often include low hemoglobin, high liver enzyme levels and bilirubin. GBC are diagnosed by imaging and endoscopically directed fine needle biopsy (Hamdani *et al.*, 2012). Incidental cases (50-72% of cases) are diagnosed after cholecystectomy for acute cholecystitis or gallstone diseases or rarely from occult metastatic disease (Compton *et al.*, 2012; Kalita *et al.*, 2013). Preoperative diagnosis is challenging for radiologists and even more so for clinicians. One study reported that of 63 unsuspected GBC cases diagnosed with acute cholecystitis before imaging had only 16 cases switched to GBC after imaging studies (Lam *et al.*, 2005). So while the role of radiology in diagnosis of GBC is imperative, there are many imaging pitfalls reported after retrospective studies of this cancer. In one study with 18 cases of GBC in which 6 cases were incorrectly preoperatively diagnosed, 4 of these 6 cases showed focal wall thickening with jaundice as a symptom, 1 patient with polypoid mass clinically presented as acute cholecystitis, and the remainder with diffuse circumferential wall thickening (Mitchell *et al.*, 2014). Another study showed GBC only correctly diagnosed preoperatively in 20%, mistaken for benign diseases in 50%, and with biliary tract tumors in another 30% (Giang *et al.*, 2012). A study in Italy found that during a period of 8 years, there were 5 patients correctly preoperatively diagnosed with GBC and 6 cases were incidentally recognized following resection (Panebianco *et al.*, 2012). To increase the sensitivity of imaging diagnosis of GBC, it needs to be recalled that GBC can have a variety of radiological appearances, which when combined with clinical findings will help radiologists not exclude GBC prematurely (Mitchell *et al.*, 2014). One of the reported pitfalls is that well-differentiated adenocarcinoma with cystic component within the tumor on MRI may mimic benign adenomyomatosis. The imaging cystic pattern in adenomyomatosis has a linear, flat, round, and regular surface characteristic (Yoshimitsu *et al.*, 2005). Differentiation of areas of wall thickening in order to diagnose GBC or benign lesions is another key in avoiding misdiagnosis. A new technique using contrast-enhanced harmonic endoscopic ultrasonography (CH-EUS) to differentiate wall thickening is superior, and significantly increased the accuracy and the agreement among different observers compared with the conventional harmonic EUS (Imazu *et al.*, 2014). In addition, improved diagnosis with histological evidence via EUS-guided FNA is found to be more sensitive (100%), specific (100%) and accurate (100%) with fewer adverse events than cytological study of bile juice obtained from endoscopic transpapillary gallbladder drainage (Ogura *et al.*, 2014). Among imaging techniques, high resolution ultrasound and magnetic resonance imaging (MRI) with MR cholangiopancreatography (MRCP) were similar in their sensitivity and accuracy, while contrast-enhanced computed tomography (CT) had lower sensitivity (Bang *et al.*, 2014). Positron emission tomography (PET) with fluorine-18-labeled fluoro-deoxyglucose (FDG) was not superior to other imaging techniques with a sensitivity and specificity of 75% and 87.5%, respectively (Koh *et al.*, 2003).

6 Pathological Diagnosis

Macroscopically, finding a GB mass is more common overall than wall thickening, though the latter may be more frequent in occult and potentially overlooked cases. The masses are located mostly in the body and the fundus (Hamdani *et al.*, 2012). A pathologic sampling scheme that includes three random sections representing a full longitudinal sample is more sensitive in finding metaplasia, hyperplasia, and dysplasia than one random section from the fundus or in any other GB site. With only one random section, the likelihood of discovering subtle lesions was less than one third (Duarte *et al.*, 1993). A recent study has shown that careful macroscopic examination with no identifiable lesions had a high negative predictive value in excluding GB dysplasia and GBC (Hayes & Muldoon, 2014).

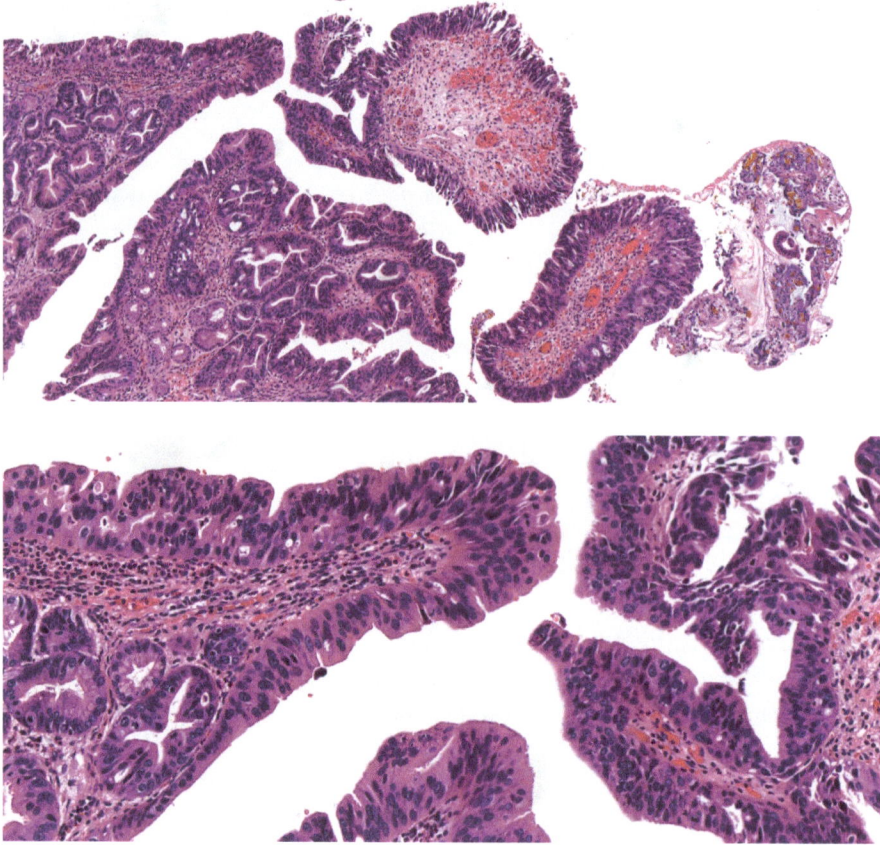

Figure 9: Low and high magnification images of surface dysplasia and carcinoma in situ of gallbladder. Invasive adenocarcinoma is often found in association with these kinds of surface changes.

Several studies suggest a pathogenetic pathway of GBC progressing from intestinal metaplasia to dysplasia, then to carcinoma. A significant association between intestinal metaplasia and dysplasia has been found. Hyperplasia and dysplasia are both seen more frequently in association with GBC both within the neoplasm and in adjacent mucosa (Duarte *et al.*, 1993). (Figure 9)

While making a correct preoperative GBC diagnosis is more challenging than postoperative diagnosis, there are still many pitfalls microscopically in terms of underdiagnosis, overdiagnosis and misinterpretation. For example, Rokitansky-Aschoff sinuses (RAS) often demonstrate deep penetration of the GB wall which may be diagnosed as tumor invasion, or if distended by mucin may be confused with extracellular mucin in mucinous carcinoma. Acute cholecystitis with parietal necrosis can induce epithelial atypia suggestive of an aggressive neoplastic process (Albores-Saavedra *et al.*, 2009). (Figure 10).

Underdiagnosis occurs when a well-differentiated invasive carcinoma is confused with benign disease such as adenomyomatosis, or in a high grade tumor when extensive tumor necrosis with minimal residual viable tumor may mimic acute gangrenous cholecystitis. Thus

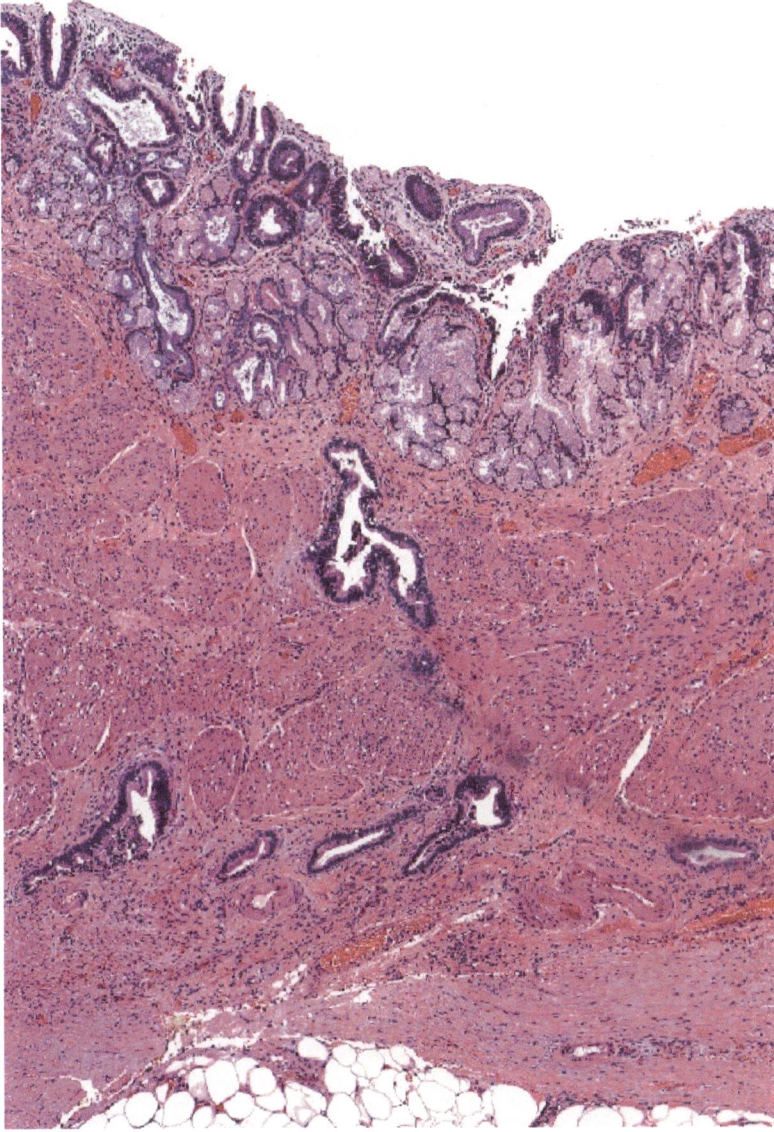

Figure 10: Surface Dysplasia involving Rokitansky-Aschoff sinuses, extending fully through gallbladder wall. Note the small benign residual gland of the RAS on the lower right.

thorough histologic sampling including areas without necrosis is critical in cases with extensive necrosis to reveal diagnostic viable tumor (Figure 11). When patients present with other malignancies making the diagnosis of primary GBC less likely, the possibility of a second neoplasm of the GB should not be overlooked if focal high grade glandular dysplasia or intramucosal adenocarcinoma within the gallbladder are present. GBC may also present as seemingly primary tumors metastatic to the other abdominal sites (omentum, ovary, pancreas, etc.) (Giang *et al.*, 2012).

GBC has many modes of spread including direct spread or extension, intra-lumenal, lymphatic, vascular, neural and intraperitoneal (Fahim *et al.*, 1962). There are three levels of lymph nodes which drain the GB: 1- the lymph nodes along the biliary duct system which is the initial site of spread, 2- the lymph nodes surrounding the pancreas and the duodenum,

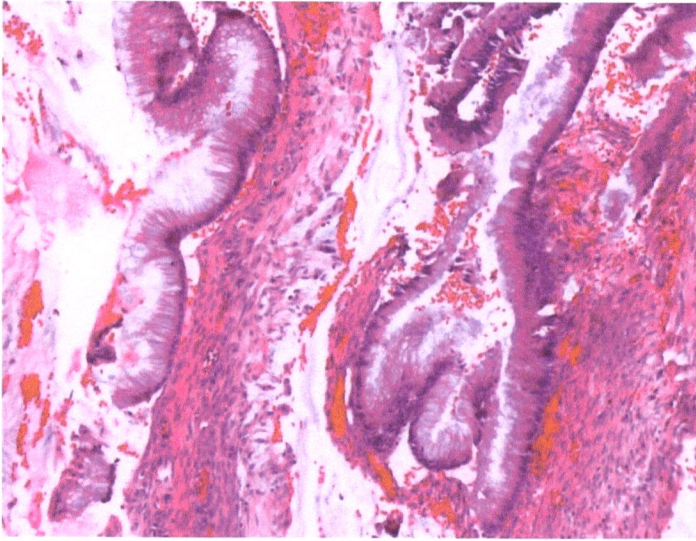

Figure 11: Primary mucinous carcinoma of the gallbladder may distend the gallbladder with mucin and leave only a few areas of identifiable tumor cells.

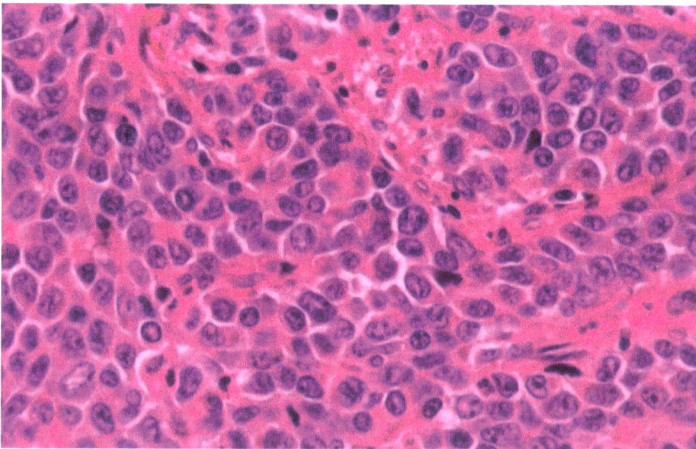

Figure 12: High grade neuroendocrine carcinoma of the gallbladder that was associated with extensive mural necrosis, almost totally masking the presence of neoplasia.

those posterior to the portal vein, and around the common hepatic artery, and 3- the lymph nodes of the para-aortic, superior mesenteric, and celiac vessels which, according to the American Joint Committee on Cancer (AJCC) 7th edition (2009), are considered as distant metastatic disease (Misra *et al.*, 2003). The frequency of lymph nodes spread is strongly correlated with the depth of invasion. Lymph node spread is considered as a prognostic factor in GBC (Tsukada *et al.*, 1997).

7   Staging

The AJCC 7th edition was released in 2009 with changes in stage grouping and reclassification of regional lymph nodes compared with the 6th edition, though the primary tumor definitions remained the same. The stage groupings in the 5th and 7th edition are similar, but differ in

TNM definition. In the 7th edition, metastasis to regional lymph nodes plays a big role in treatment and prognosis. N1 is limited to hepatic hilar nodes not excluding nodes adjacent to portal vein, and N2 has nodes in other regions such as periaortic, pericaval, superior mesenteric artery, and/or celiac artery which are considered distant metastatic disease and classified as stage IVB (Compton *et al.*, 2012).

Primary Tumor (T)	
TX	Primary tumor cannot be assessed
T0	No evidence of primary tumor
Tis	Carcinoma in situ
T1	Tumor invades lamina propria or muscular layer
T1a	Tumor invades lamina propria
T1b	Tumor invades muscular layer
T2	Tumor invades perimuscular connective tissue; no extension beyond serosa or into liver
T3	Tumor perforates the serosa (visceral peritoneum) and/or directly invades the liver and/or one other adjacent organ or structure, such as the stomach, duodenum, colon, pancreas, omentum, or extrahepatic bile ducts
T4	Tumor invades main portal vein or hepatic artery or invades two or more extrahepatic organs or structures
Regional Lymph Nodes (N)	
NX	Regional lymph nodes cannot be assessed
N0	No regional lymph node metastasis
N1	Metastases to nodes along the cystic duct, common bile duct, hepatic artery, and/or portal vein

Continued on next page...

... Continued from previous page

N2	Metastases to periaortic, pericaval, superior mesenteric artery, and/or celiac artery lymph nodes
Distant Metastasis (M)	
M0	No distant metastasis
M1	Distant metastasis

Anatomic Stage/Prognostic Groups			
Stage 0	Tis	N0	M0
Stage I	T1	N0	M0
Stage II	T2	N0	M0
Stage IIIA	T3	N0	M0
Stage IIIB	T1-3	N1	M0
Stage IVA	T4	N0-1	M0
Stage IVB	Any T	N2	M0
	Any T	Any N	M1

Table 2: GBC staging in the AJCC 7th edition (2009).

8   Molecular Pathology of GBC

Abundant research has sought to unravel the molecular tumorigenesis of GBC to identify potential targets for treatment and prevention. We will summarize the key learnings to date in this evolving field.

The Cadherins include a group of homologous transmembrane proteins mediating intercellular interaction of variable cell types (Hoschuetzky *et al.*, 1994). E (epithelial)-cadherin is a Ca^{2+} ion-dependent glycoprotein belonging to the cadherin family, critical in epithelial cells adherence, suppressing invasion. Its gene (CDH1) is located on chromosome 16q22.1 (Berx *et al.*, 1995). This protein is absent in GBC and present in chronic cholecystitis (Priya *et al.*, 2010).

Catenins are cytoplasmic anchorage proteins, playing a key role in cadherin function by mediating connection of cadherins to the actin filament network. α-catenin does not bind directly to the cytoplasmic domain of cadherins, but mediates the cadherin-catenin complex connecting with actin filament. But β-catenin, a component of desmosomal plaques and adherens junctions, binds directly to the cytoplasmic domain of E-cadherin (Hoschuetzky *et al.*, 1994). Both reduced E-cadherin and β-catenin expression can be seen with tumor progression and with decreased apoptosis (Hirata *et al.*, 2007). Other studies have found that β-catenin is expressed on the cell membrane in most benign gallbladder tissues, while it appears in the cytoplasm and/or nuclei in cancerous tissues (Ghosh *et al.*, 2013; Kimura *et al.*, 2003; Moon *et al.*, 2005). This suggests that alteration of β-catenin quantitatively or in its expression patterns such as shifting from membranous staining to cytoplasmic and/or nuclear staining could be a factor in GBC carcinogenesis.

Normal microvessels in tissue are composed of endothelial cells and pericytes. Pericytes help mature microvessels to be stable. Their absence is found in the leaky microvessels in tumor tissues. The intercellular complexes adhering endothelium and pericytes contain N (neural)-cadherin. The pericytes in tumor microvessels are poorly attached to the endothelium which suggests dysfunction of N-cadherin (Blaschuk & Devemy, 2009). P (placental)-cadherin is an intercellular adhesion molecule associated with undifferentiated cells in both normal adult epithelia and carcinoma (Albergaria *et al.*, 2011). N-cadherin absence and P-cadherin presence are found to be independent factors predicting poor prognosis in adenocarcinoma, squamous cell/adenosquamous carcinoma type of GBC. They are strongly associated with tumor size, lymph metastasis and invasion (Yi *et al.*, 2014).

P53 overexpression is found in GBC and not seen in chronic cholecystitis (Ghosh *et al.*, 2013; Priya *et al.*, 2010). Mutation in the p53 gene produces in abnormal p53 protein which appears to be antigenic, resulting in detectable circulating antibodies against p53. One study from India showed that one third of GBC patients significantly positive with p53 antibodies compared with the cholelithiasis (Nigan *et al.*, 2010). Loss of the p53 tumor suppressor functionality (due either to a defective protein, or loss of function following Ab-Ag interaction) may also contribute to GBC carcinogenesis.

The tumor suppressor gene Ras association domain family 1A (RASSF1A) is hypermethylated in GB adenocarcinomas. RASSF1A has a Ras association domain; however, loss of RASSF1A expression by methylation in cancerous tissues does not require Ras activation. Hypermethylation of RASSF1A gene could be helpful for early detection as serum methylation analysis is sensitive. It also presents a potential treatment target using demethylation agents (Kee *et al.*, 2007). There have been many studies conducted in several countries with variable findings with most of them showing low frequency of Kras expression in GBC, showing the controversy about the role of Kras in GBC pathway. (Kee *et al.*, 2007; Pai *et al.*, 2011).

COX-2, an isoform of cyclooxygenase enzymes, is induced by mitogens, cytokines, and growth factors. Its function is to produce prostaglandin-related inflammation and cell growth. COX-2 mRNA expression is highly increased in colorectal carcinoma tissues, and also overexpressed in 80% of invasive GBC suggesting a potential role of COX-2 in tumorigenesis and tumor progression (Asano *et al.*, 2002; Moon *et al.*, 2005). mRNA levels of COX-2 and concentration of prostaglandin E2 (PGE2), which is a product related to that enzyme, are significantly higher in pT3 and pT4 compared with those in pT1 and pT2 (Asano *et al.*, 2002). COX-2 may be an important factor, when interacting with c-Met, beta-catenin and C-erbB2 proteins, in promoting tumor invasion. COX-2 together with c-Met, beta-catenin were found to be present in cancerous cells at the invasive tumor front but not in the central parts of the tumor, significantly associated with the depth of invasion (Moon *et al.*, 2005).

The S100 protein (SP) family comprises more than 20 members involved in many cellular functions, especially in regulating cell growth, cell cycle, differentiation, transcription and secretion. Overexpression of SPs have been found in many types of tumors. Haptoglobin is an acute-phase protein produced in the liver to respond to inflammation, infection, injuries and also malignancies (Tan *et al.*, 2011). Elevated concentration of haptoglobin and its altered glycoforms is reported to be associated with hepatocellular carcinoma (Ang *et al.*, 2006). Haptoglobin-hemoglobin complex has a cytotoxic effect on liver cancer cells and prevented proliferation of cancerous cell via the apoptotic pathway (Kim *et al.*, 1995). One study showed that increased S100A10 and haptoglobin are found in GBC tissues compared with benign GB tissues, and associated with advanced stage and poor prognosis (Tan *et al.*, 2011).

Connective tissue growth factor (CTGF) is a key element in wound repair processing, promoting myofibroblast differentiation and angiogenesis which are similar to the desmoplastic stromal response in cancer. There is no general consensus about the role of CTGF in tumor behavior since it is associated with both suppression and progression of many types of tumors (Jacobson & Cunningham, 2012). A study in GBC showed CTGF was increased most in advanced stage, followed by early stage, then dysplasia and least in chronic cholecystitis. Ironically, high expression of CTGF was significantly associated with increased 5-year survival time compared with the low or absent expression. The authors suggested that desmoplastic action is usually seen in advanced GBC, and increased expression of CTGF in GBC cells may act as paracrine to the stromal composition that possibly reduces the tumor growth. The suggested these changes are related to the expression of some important cancer progression/suppression-related molecules or pathways, such as TGF-b, HIF-1a, b-catenin/Tcf/MMP-7, and PI3K/AKT and offer further support for the role of inflammatory responses in GBC pathogenesis (Garcia *et al.*, 2013).

9   Predisposition from Genetic Factors

Xeroderma pigmentosum complementation group C (XPC) is one of the nucleotide excision repair (NER) genes. Its protein recognizes and binds to damaged DNA and initiates the NER pathway. It is thought to play a role in suppression of tumorigenesis (Jiao *et al.*, 2011). Jiao et al showed that the allele T of XPC Ala499Val polymorphism was associated with GBC in the Chinese population (Jiao *et al.*, 2011).

Abnormal apoptosis can also lead to development of cancer. Single nucleotide polymorphisms (SNP) of death receptor DR4 haplotypes play an important role in GBC susceptibility without the influence of their ligands such as FASL (Rai *et al.*, 2014).

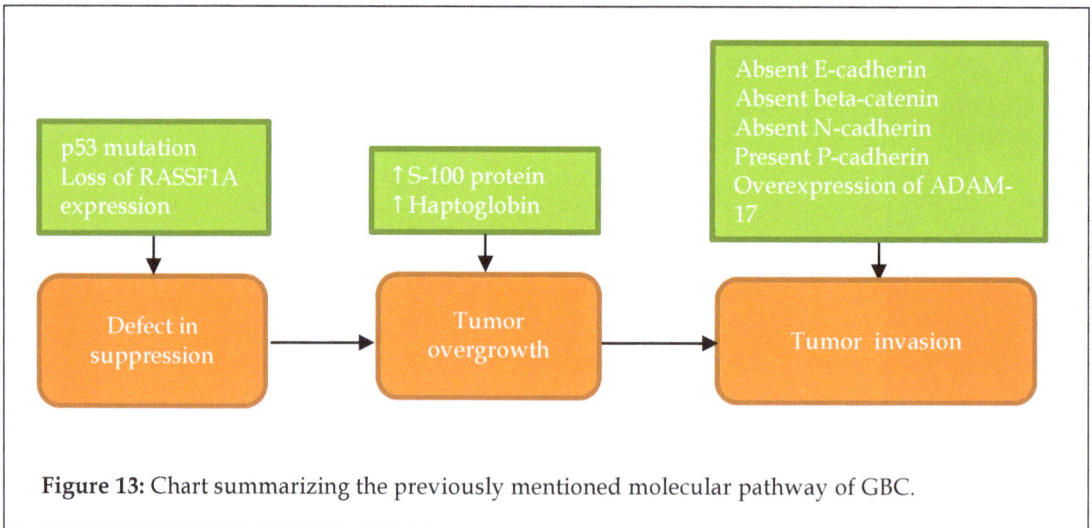

Figure 13: Chart summarizing the previously mentioned molecular pathway of GBC.

ADR is an adrenergic receptor found to be related to hypomotility disorder of GSD, which, in turn, is one of the main risk factors of GBC. ADRβ3 T190C polymorphism is significantly related to GBC and GSD susceptibility with the possible mechanism of both gallstone dependent and independent pathways (Rai *et al.*, 2014a).

CYP17 is an enzyme in sex hormone biosynthesis, and GBC has known female predilection. Rai et al found that CYP17 rs743572 is associated with GBC susceptibility in smokers only (Rai *et al.*, 2014b). Also another polymorphism of CYP1A1-MspI [CT] was shown to increase risk of GBC in those tobacco users and in women (Sharma *et al.*, 2014). CYP1A1 polymorphisms increase the risk of GBC as it possibly impairs xenobiotic metabolism via pathway unrelated to gallstones (Sharma *et al.*, 2014).

10   Prognostic Markers

The markers discussed below are recently studied and mostly for assessing prognosis of GBC rather than exploring pathogenesis. Undoubtedly further investigations may however provide links in that story as well.

Transmembrane protease, serine 4 (TMPRSS4), a member of the transmembrane serine proteases is upregulated in many cancers. It is found to be significantly increased in GBC with a positive correlation with tumor stage, histologic grade, lymph node metastasis and lymphatic invasion. It is also an independent prognostic factor for GBC (Wu *et al.*, 2014).

Reduced E-cadherin expression has a significant correlation with poor prognosis in GBC (Hirata *et al.*, 2007). PML and p53 are also possible independent prognostic factors when both of them are normal; the 5 year survival is longer (60 months vs 11 months) when they are normal (Chang *et al.*, 2007). Another study showed the opposite with p53 expression not correlating with survival period. But they did find mucin correlated with survival time and suggested that mucin could be a more important prognostic marker than p53 (Takagawa *et al.*, 2005).

Mucins are glycoproteins with a mucin core protein and O-linked carbohydrates. MUC1 is thought to be an anti-adhesion molecule promoting metastasis and is expressed in many types of human tumors. Many studies have shown MUC1 expressed in GBC has an association with lymph node metastasis, lymphatic invasion and poor outcome (Ghosh *et al.*, 2005; Kashiwagi *et al.*, 2001; S. M. Kim *et al.*, 2012; Xiong *et al.*, 2012), while MUC5AC and MUC4 are inconsistent prognostic factors in GBC (S. M. Kim *et al.*, 2012; Lee *et al.*, 2012; Sasaki *et al.*, 1999; Xiong *et al.*, 2012).

The ADAMs are a multi-functional gene family of membrane proteins, regulating the extracellular matrix remodeling and cell migration. Among them, ADAM-17, known as tumor necrosis factor-alpha converting enzyme, stimulates the release of many growth factors, namely EGFR ligands, transforming growth factor (TGF-alpha), amphiregulin, heparin-binding epidermal growth factor (HB-EGFR) which are related to tumor behavior (Brou *et al.*, 2000). Significantly increased expression of ADAM-17 is found in tumor tissues with high histological grade and pT stage. Also, over expression of ADAM-17 is associated with short survival compared with low expression. It is found to be an independent prognostic factor in GBC (Wu, *et al.*, 2011).

The high mobility group A2 (HMGA2) protein is a nonhistone chromosomal protein highly expresssed during embryogenesis, and minimally expressed or undetectable in normal adult tissues. Overexpression of HMGA2 has been found in some benign tumors such as lipoma, leiomyoma and pituitary adenoma in transgenic mice as well as in several cancers such as lung, breast, pancreatic, thyroid, and ovarian cancers.(Motoyama *et al.*, 2008). One study shows the HMGA2 expression rate is higher in poorly differentiated GBC than in the well differentiated and associated with a shorter survival period than cases with negative HMGA2 expression.(Zou *et al.*, 2012). Another study shows HMGA2 is a direct target of miR-26a which is a single-stranded, non-coding RNA molecule. It has a negative correlation with HMGA2 in GBC and can be considered as a therapeutic target for GBC patients (Zhou *et al.*, 2014).

Tetraspanins are a family of transmembrane proteins crossing the membrane four times and interacting with many types of molecules especially integrins producing multiple functions related to cancer behavior such as spread, migration and cell adhesion. Two tetraspanins, CD82 and CD9, play roles in tumor suppression, while the other two CD151 and tetraspanin 8 are involved in promoting tumor progression (Zoller, 2009). Recently there are several studies showing the role of CD9 and CD151 in GBC. Low or absent expression of CD9 was found in poorly differentiated GBC associated with short survival period (Zou *et al.*, 2012). Matsumoto *et al.* found that there was a significant difference between 5 year survival of CD151 positive and negative (P< 0.006) and by using multivariate analysis the authors showed CD151 was an independent prognostic factor with hazard ratio of 2.97 (P< 0.02) (Matsumoto *et al.*, 2014).

CD146 is a member of immunoglobulin (Ig) gene superfamily recognized as a cell adhesion molecule (CAM) and has several names such as MUC18, A32 antigen, MCAM, Mel-CAM (melanoma cell adhesion molecule due to first being seen in melanoma cell), and S-Endo-1. CD146 is overexpressed in melanoma, while it is absent in carcinoma in situ and invasive carcinoma in breast cancer. Its role in cancer behavior is variable in different types of cancers. (Shih, 1999). There have been four CAM families identified including integrins, cadherins, selectins and Ig gene superfamily. Among of them, CD146 has a weaker adhesion activity than the other two families or other CAMs such as ICAMs, VCAM-1, and PECAM-1. Recently CD146 has been found to have more functions beyond cell adhesion which involve development, immune response, signal transduction, mesenchymal stem cell differentiation, cell migration, and angiogenesis (Z. Wang & Yan, 2013). Wang *et al.* found in their study that positive expression of CD146 is higher in poorly differentiated GBC than in well differentiated GBC, and overexpression of CD146 along with high average microvessel and lymph vessel counts are correlated with poor overall survival. Moreover, CD146 was an independent prognostic factor in GBC from their study (W. Wang *et al.*, 2012).

Polycomb group (PcG) genes are transcriptional repressors modifying chromatin state during embryogenesis by contributing to maintenance of appropriate spatial and temporal expression of homeotic genes. Those PcG genes transcribe two polycomb repressive complexes PRC1-containing more than 10 subunits including oncoprotein BMI-1 (B cell-specific Moloney murine leukemia virus integration site 1) and HPC protein family and PRC2-containing EZH2 (enhancer of Zeste homolog 2), EED (embryonic ectoderm development), SUZ12 (suppressor of zeste 12 protein homolog) and RbAp48. PRC1, PRC2 and their related product trimethylated histone involve more than 1000 silenced genes which determine cell differentiation during embryogenesis (Bracken *et al.*, 2006). PRC2 is one of the histone methyltransferases functioning in transcriptional silencing of differentiation genes. Among the PRC2 components, EZH2 is a catalytic subunit mainly contributing to the enzyme active site when assembling with at last two other noncatalytic subunits-EED and SUZ12. EZH2 is the first subunit documented as overexpression in prostate and breast cancers compared with the other subunits, leading to hypersilencing of genes that promote differentiation (Simon & Lange, 2008). Based on the positive correlation between overexpression of EZH2 and histologic grade of many cancers, Liu and Yang searched for and found that EZH2 is overexpressed in poorly differentiated GBC with lymph node metastasis and invasion, and there was a correlation between EZH2 overexpression and shorter survival periods. It is also found that EZH2 is an independent prognostic predictor (Liu & Yang, 2011). Inhibition of PRC2 by targeting EZH2, which plays a main part in the enzyme active site or its interaction with other subunits, is a promising treatment approach. There was a study using EZH2 methyltransferase inhibitor combined with histone deacetylase (HDAC) such as suberoylanilide hydroxamic acid (SAHA), one of the most clinically advanced anticancer agent, on GBC cultured cells with a significant decrease in cancer cells (Yamaguchi *et al.*, 2010).

Phosphatase and tensin homolog (PTEN) first discovered in 1997 has been recognized as a tumor suppressor. Its main function is dephosphorylating phosphatidylinositol-3,4,5-trisphosphate leading to activating the phosphoinositide 3-kinase (PI3K)–AKT–mammalian target of rapamycin (mTOR) pathway, which will stimulate cell growth and survival. PTEN was found to be related with PTEN hamartoma tumor syndromes including Cowden syndrome, Bannayan–Riley–Ruvalcaba syndrome, Proteus syndrome, Proteus-like syndrome and autism disorder with macrocephaly. PTEN is one of the most common suppressor genes mutated or suppressed in various cancers such as breast, lung, prostate, colon, endometrial and glioblastoma (Leslie & Downes, 2004; Song *et al.*, 2012). Due to its central role in cancer processes, PTEN has been extensively studied and the increasing knowledge about PTEN promises a hopeful targeted therapeutic treatment. One study shows loss of PTEN is related to high grade, metastatic GBC and short survival period. The authors also found that PTEN was a prognostic predictor for GBC (Liu & Yang, 2011).

Epithelial cell adhesion molecule (EPCAM or MK-1) is a transmembrane protein found in epithelial cells responsible for the function of adhering cell to cell. Two studies show overexpression of EPCAM is related to increased overall survival and is a prognostic predictor (Ikeda *et al.*, 2009; L. Yang *et al.*, 2011).

Excision repair cross-complementation group 1 (ERCC1) is a nucleotide excision repair enzyme which is widely studied in cancer science due to its relationship to survival and chemotherapy treatment. ERCC1 has been studied deeply in lung cancers but with inconsistent findings about the relation between ERCC1 and overall survival in a meta-analysis study (Smirnov *et al.*, 2015). However, a study in Chile, where GBC in women has high incidence rate, reveals that patients with ERCC1 expression have survival period of 6 times longer than do patients without ERCC1 expression (P=0.005) (Roa *et al.*, 2011).

Raf kinase inhibitor protein (RKIP) is an inhibitor of Raf-MEK (Mitogen-activated protein kinase)-ERK (extracellular signal-regulated kinase), binding and inhibiting the kinase activity of Raf-1. Its expression is low in metastatic cancer, and meets the criteria of metastasis suppressor gene. Loss of RKIP has been shown to be related to resistance to chemotherapy and radiotherapy.(Escara-Wilke *et al.*, 2012). A GBC study shows that reduced or loss expression of RKIP was significantly higher in GBC versus non GBC (P< 0.001), lymph node metastasis versus non lymph node metastasis (P= 0.009) and in lower overall survival versus in longer survival period (P=0.011). Also RKIP was found to be a prognostic marker for GBC. (H. S. Kim *et al.*, 2010).

Hypoxia-inducible factor-1 (HIF-1) is a transcription factor mediating cell response to hypoxia. It has subunits alpha and beta, with the former playing a main role in this response. Hypoxia-inducible factor-1 alpha (HIF-1α) is degraded when interacting with von Hippel-Lindau (VHL), a tumor suppressor, under normoxic conditions. During hypoxia, the alpha subunit becomes stable and translocates to the nucleus to dimerize with beta subunit. The heterodimer then binds to the hypoxia response element in the promoters of targeted genes which promote cell proliferation, angiogenesis and metabolic responses to adapt with hypoxic conditions. (Kitajima & Miyazaki, 2013). Studies show that overexpression of HIF-1α and reduced expression of VHL in GBC correlate with tumor stage, lymph node metastasis, lymphatic invasion and lower overall survival period (Batmunkh *et al.*, 2010; Z. Yang *et al.*, 2011). A study suggests a panel using the profile of pVHL−/IMP3+/maspin+/S100P+ by immunohistochemistry staining helps to distinguish between GBC-adenocarcinoma type and benign conditions (Shi *et al.*, 2013). Recently there are two studies using hispidulin and cordycepin as HIF-1α targeted therapeutic agents with positive results which give hope for future GBC treatment. (Gao *et al.*, 2014; Wu *et al.*, 2014).

These prognostic markers in GBC are summarized in Table 3 and 4

Poor Prognostic Markers (Overexpression)	
ADAM-17	Membrane protein
CD146	Member of Immunoglobulin gene superfamily (other names Mel-CAM or MCAM)
CD151	Tetraspanin protein
EZH2	Enhancer of Zeste homolog 2
HIF-1α	Hypoxia-inducible factor 1 alpha
HMGA2	High mobility group protein A2
MUC1	Mucin 1
TMPRSS4	Transmembrane protease, serine 4

Table 3: Poor prognostic markers (overexpression)

Better Prognostic Markers (Overexpression)	
CD9	Mobility related protein 1/tetraspanin protein
E-cadherin	Transmembrane protein
ERCC1	Excision repair cross-complementing group 1
EPCAM	Epithelial cell adhesion molecule (MK-1)
PTEN	Phosphatase and tensin homologue
RKIP	Raf-1 kinase inhibitory protein
pVHL	Von Hippel-Lindau protein

Table 4: Better prognostic markers (overexpression)

From a pragmatic standpoint however, the use of these newer markers has not yet penetrated routine clinical practice. Certain patients presenting for treatment at our facility may be tested for one or more of these but this is usually always in the context of a clinical trial or other study, and while a few of the markers (MUC-1, E-cadherin) might be on the routine test menu by IHC or other means, the remainder are not widely available for use.

11   Treatment

Treatment of GBC is varied and can involve surgical resection, radiation and/or chemotherapy dependent on the stage of disease at presentation.

11.1   Surgical management:

Surgical resection is the only curative treatment in GBC. Patients with stage I and II have potentially resectable disease while stage III or IVA can also occasionally be resected. Stage IVB patients have unresectable disease and are candidates for medical management. Ideally, surgery should be performed at high volume centers with availability of multidisciplinary care. Surgical options include cholecystectomy or extended cholecystectomy (resection of surrounding hepatic tissue segment IVB and V) and are dependent on the Tumor (T) stage of the patient. Cholecystectomy is the treatment of choice in patients with T1 disease with extended cholecystectomy an option in patients with T1b disease. This can be curative for a majority of the patients. Radical cholecystectomy (resection of the gallbladder, gallbladder fossa and lymph node dissection) was found to improve overall survival in patients with T2N0, T2N1, and T3N0 disease, but not in those patients presenting with T3N1 and T4 disease. (Foster *et al.,* 2006). A retrospective analysis of the SEER registry showed that evaluation of lymph node (LN) status in patients with T1b, T2 and T3 disease at surgery was associated with improvement in survival. (Jensen *et al.,* 2009). Major liver and common bile duct resection is associated with significant morbidity with no impact on survival and is recommended only in cases that warrant extensive resection to obtain clear surgical margins. (D'Angelica *et al.,*2009).

11.2   Adjuvant treatment

Patients with resected disease are at a risk of recurrence, especially those with positive surgical margins or node positive disease. They can present with locoregional recurrence involving the resection margin, porta hepatis or retroperitoneal lymph nodes or distant metastasis to the peritoneum, liver and lungs. In a study 66 % of patients with resected GBC recurred, with a median time to recurrence of 11.5 months (Jarnagin *et al.*,2003). Thus, adjuvant therapy may have a role in decreasing the risk of recurrence. However, on account of the low incidence and prevalence of GBC, randomized studies are limited and majority of the evidence is based on retrospective analysis that can suffer from bias. Jarnagin et al, in a retrospective analysis of patients demonstrated a worse prognosis for patients with GBC vs. hilar cholangiocarcinoma (85 % vs. 41 %). This study concluded that the use the locoregional therapy like radiation was probably more beneficial in patients with hilar cholangiocarcinoma as they had higher locoregional recurrence rate compared to GBC (Jarnagin *et al.*, 2003). In contrast, a retrospective analysis of the SEER database in patients with locally advanced gall bladder cancer or gall bladder cancer with tumor spread to the regional lymph nodes demonstrated an improvement in overall survival in patients who received adjuvant radiation (14 months vs. 8 months, $p \leq 0.001$) (Mojica *et al.*, 2007). The benefit of concurrent chemoradiation with 5-Fluoropyrimidine (5FU) after adequate surgical resection has been evaluated in numerous trials that have demonstrated a possible improvement in survival in patients with locally advanced GBC, though the number of patients enrolled in these trails was small (Czito *et al.*, 2005, Kresl *et al.*, 2002). In addition, a large meta-analysis of adjuvant therapy in the treatment of biliary cancer demonstrated a nonsignificant improvement in overall survival with any adjuvant therapy vs. surgery alone (P = .06). There was no difference between gallbladder and bile duct tumors, with a statistically significant improvement in patients who received chemotherapy or chemo-radiation vs. radiation treatment alone (OR, 0.39, 0.61, and 0.98, respectively; P = .02). Patients with lymph node positive and R1 disease seemed to derive the maximum benefit (OR, 0.49; P = .004 and OR, 0.36; P = .002, respectively) (Horgan *et al.*,2012).

Adjuvant chemotherapy with gemcitabine or a 5FU backbone has also been evaluated in several trials. A phase III trial randomized patients with gall bladder cancer to adjuvant treatment with 5FU and Mitomycin C or observation after surgery. There was a significant improvement in the 5 year survival rate (26 % vs. 14.4%, p = 0.0367) and the 5-year disease-free survival (DFS) (20.3% vs. 11.6%, p = 0.0210) in patients who received adjuvant therapy vs. observation respectively. Significant improvements were also seen in body weight compared with the control. (Takada *et al.*, 2002). Based on the available data, adjuvant external beam radiation and/or chemotherapy is recommended in patients with stage II and III GBC according to the National Comprehensive Cancer Network (NCCN) guidelines (Category 2A recommendation) (NCCN, 2014).

11.3   Unresectable/Metastatic GBC:

Chemotherapy is the mainstay for patients with metastatic or unresectable disease. The prognosis of such patients is poor and is reported to be less than 1 year across most trials. Chemotherapy has the potential to improve the survival and quality of life in patients with advanced cancer. Gimelus, et al randomized patients with pancreaticobiliary tumors to 5FU/Leucovorin, Etoposide and best supportive care vs. best supportive care. Chemotherapy led to significant improvements in overall survival (6 vs. 2.5 months) and quality-adjusted survival (Glimelius *et al.*,1996). Based on such studies, it is appropriate to offer chemotherapy to patients with good performance status. The most common chemotherapeutic agents used include 5FU and Gemcitabine. A combination of 5FU and cisplatin in 25 patients with biliary tract tumors resulted in a partial response in 24 % of patients. (Ducreux *et al.*,1998). Fifty four patients with advanced biliary tract tumors were randomized in a phase II trial to 5FU, cisplatin and epirubicin or 5FU, etoposide and leucovorin. The patient reported symptom relief and survival was similar in both arms, but patients in the ECF arm reported less toxicities (Rao *et al.*, 2005). Gemcitabine, an analog of deoxycytidine is active in biliary tumors, both as a single agent or in combination with other agents. (Gallardo *et al.*, 2001). A phase III study randomized 410 patients with locally advanced or metastatic cholangiocarcinoma, gallbladder cancer, or ampullary cancer to Cisplatin and Gemcitabine vs. Gemcitabine as single agent therapy. Patients in the combination arm had a statistically significant benefit in the median overall survival (11.7 months vs. 8.1 months), median progression-free survival (8.0 months vs. 5.0 months) and the rate of tumor control (81.4% vs. 71.8%, P=0.049). The patients in the combination group experienced more neutropenia, but the incidence of neutropenia associated infections was similar in both groups (Valle *et al.*, 2010). Based on this data, chemotherapy with Gemcitabine and Cisplatin is the standard of care in front line therapy of patients with advanced biliary cancer. Gemcitabine has also been combined with other chemotherapeutic agents like carboplatin and oxaliplatin with encouraging results.

Cholangiocarcinoma is associated with multiple genetic changes including the RAS-RAF-MEK or the PI3K-AKT-mTOR pathways amongst others. Hence, targeted agents have been used as single agents or combined with chemotherapy in an effort to improve outcomes. Erlotinib, an EGFR inhibitor, was studied as a single agent in patients with advanced biliary tract tumors who had received one prior systemic or locoregional therapy. Patients had a response rate of 8%, with 43 % achieving stable disease (Philip *et al.*, 2006). Phase II trials of Bevacizumab (a VEGF inhibitor) in combination with gemcitabine and oxaliplatin demonstrated a partial response of 40% with a median overall survival (OS) of 12.7 months. (Zhu et al, 2010). The BINGO trial randomized 150 patients to chemotherapy (gemcitabine+oxliplatin) plus cetuximab vs. chemotherapy alone. Median progression-free survival was 6·1 months vs. 5·5 months and the median overall survival was 11·0 months (9·1-13·7) vs. 12·4 months (8·6-16·0) in the chemotherapy plus cetuximab group vs. the chemotherapy alone group (Malka *et al.*, 2009). More data is required to determine the impact of targeted agents on this disease.

12   Conclusions

Because of its worldwide distribution and propensity to present at an advanced stage, or be missed by current diagnostic methods at an early stage, control or prevention of GBC is a challenge. Surgical interventions to remove the GB in cases with problematic stones or other risk factors appears to have had some impact in reducing overall incidence, but there are still cases that present treatment issues. Broader understanding of the molecular pathogenesis and the beginnings of screening programs using circulating biomarkers appear to offer the best hope of further impacting the burden of this malignancy for society.

References

Albergaria, A., Ribeiro, A.-S., Vieira, A.-F., Sousa, B., Nobre, A.-R., Seruca, R., Schmitt, F., et al (2011). P-cadherin role in normal breast development and cancer. Int J Dev Biol, 55(7-9), 811-822.

Albores-Saavedra, J., Galliani, C., Chable-Montero, F., Batich, K., Henson, D.E. (2009). Mucin-containing Rokitansky-Aschoff sinuses with extracellular mucin deposits simulating mucinous carcinoma of the gallbladder. The American Journal of Surgical Pathology, 33(11), 1633-1638.

Albores-Saavedra, J., Henson, D.E., Sobin, L.H. (1992). The WHO histological classification of tumors of the gallbladder and extrahepatic bile ducts. Cancer, 70(2), 410-414.

Andrén-Sandberg, A. et al (2012). Diagnosis and management of gallbladder polyps. N Am J Med Sci, 4(5), 203-211.

Ang, I.L., Poon, T.C., Lai, P.B., Chan, A.T., Ngai, S.-M., Hui, A.Y., Johnson, P.J., et al (2006). Study of serum haptoglobin and its glycoforms in the diagnosis of hepatocellular carcinoma: a glycoproteomic approach. Journal of Proteome Research, 5(10), 2691-2700.

Asano, T., Shoda, J., Ueda, T., Kawamoto, T., Todoroki, T., Shimonishi, M., Tanabe, T., et al (2002). Expressions of cyclooxygenase-2 and prostaglandin E-receptors in carcinoma of the gallbladder: crucial role of arachidonate metabolism in tumor growth and progression. Clinical Cancer Research, 8(4), 1157-1167.

Bang, S.H., Lee, J.Y., Woo, H., Joo I., Lee, E.S., Han, J.K., Choi, B.I. (2014). Differentiating between adenomyomatosis and gallbladder cancer: revisiting a comparative study of high-resolution ultrasound, multidetector CT, and MR imaging. Korean Journal of Radiology, 15(2), 226-234.

Batmunkh, E., Shimada, M., Morine, Y., Imura, S., Kanemura, H., Arakawa, Y., Nishi, M. (2010). Expression of hypoxia-inducible factor-1 alpha (HIF-1alpha) in patients with the gallbladder carcinoma. Int J Clin Oncol, 15(1), 59-64. doi: 10.1007/s10147-009-0011-7

Berx, G., Staes, K., van Hengel, J., Molemans, F., Bussemakers, M.J., van Bokhoven, A., Van Roy, F. (1995). Cloning and characterization of the human invasion suppressor gene E-cadherin (CDH1). Genomics, 26(2), 281-289.

Blaschuk, O.W. & Devemy, E. (2009). Cadherins as novel targets for anti-cancer therapy. European Journal of Pharmacology, 625(1), 195-198.

Bohr, U.R.M., Kuester, D., Meyer, F., Wex, T., Stillert, M., Csepregi, A., Lippert, H., et al (2007). Low prevalence of Helicobacteraceae in gall-stone disease and gall-bladder carcinoma in the German population. Clinical Microbiology and Infection: The Official Publication of the European Society of Clinical Microbiology and Infectious Diseases, 13(5), 525-531. Doi:10.1111/j.1469-0691.2007.01690.x

Borena, W., Edlinger, M., Bjøge, T., Häggström, C., Lindkvist, B., Nagel, G., Engeland, A., et al (2014). A prospective study on metabolic risk factors and gallbladder cancer in the metabolic syndrome and cancer (me-can) collaborative study. PloS one, 9(2), e89368. doi:10.1371/journal.pone.0089368.

Bracken, A. P., Dietrich, N., Pasini, D., Hansen, K. H., Helin, K., et al (2006). Genome-wide mapping of Polycomb target genes unravels their roles in cell fate transitions. Genes & Development, 20(9), 1123-1136. doi: Doi 10.1101/Gad.381706

Brou, C., Logeat, F., Gupta, N., Bessia, C., LeBail, O., Doedens, J.R., Cumano, A., et al (2000). A novel proteolytic cleavage involved in notch signaling: the role of the disintegrin-metalloprotease TACE. Molecular Cell, 5(2), 207-216.

Buch, S., Schafmayer, C., Völzke, H., Becker, C., Franke, A., von Eller-Eberstein, H., Kluck, C., et al (2007). A genome-wide association scan identifies the hepatic cholesterol transporter ABCG8 as a susceptibility factor for human gallstone disease. Nature Genetics, 39(8), 995-999.

Bulajic, M., Maisonneuve, P., Schneider-Brachert, W., Müller, P., Reischl, U., Stimec, B., Lehn, N., et al (2002). Helicobacter pylori and the risk of benign and malignant biliary tract disease. Cancer, 95(9), 1946-1953.

Bulajic, M., Stimec, B., Milicevic, M., Loehr, M., Mueller, P., Boricic, I., Kovacevic, N., et al (2002). Modalities of testing Helicobacter pylori in patients with nonmalignant bile duct diseases. World Journal of Gastroenterology: WJG, 8(2), 301-304.

Cariati, A., Puglisi, R., Zaffarano, R., Accarpio, F.T., Cetta, F. (2003). Helicobacter pylori and the risk of benign and malignant biliary tract disease. Cancer, 98(3), 656-657.

Chang, H.J., Yoo, B.C., Kim, S.W., Lee, B.L., Kim, W.H. (2007). Significance of PML and p53 protein as molecular prognostic markers of gallbladder carcinomas. Pathology & Oncology Research, 13(4), 326-335.

Compton, C.C., Byrd, D.R., Garcia-Aguilar, J., Kurtzman, S.H., Olawaiye, A., Washington, M.K. (2012). Gallbladder. AJCC Cancer Staging Atlas (pp. 259-268).

Czito, B.G., Hurwitz, H.I., Clough, R.W., Tyler, D.S., Morse, M.A., Clary, B.M., Pappas, T.N., Fernando, N.H., Willett, C.G. (2005). Adjuvant external-beam radiotherapy with concurrent chemotherapy after resection of primary gallbladder carcinoma: a 23-year experience. Int J Radiat Oncol Biol Phys, 62, 1030.

D'Angelica, M., Dala, K., DeMatteo, R., (2009). Analysis of the extent of resection for adenocarcinoma of the gall bladder. Ann Surg Onco, 16, 806-816.

Diehl, A.K. (1983). Gallstone size and the risk of gallbladder cancer. JAMA, 250(17), 2323-2326.

Doval, D.C., Sekhon, J.S.Gupta, S.K., Fuloria, J., Shukla, V.K., Gupta, S., Awasthy, B.S. (2004). *A phase II study of gemcitabine and cisplatin in chemotherapy-naive, unresectable gall bladder cancer. Br J Cancer, 90(8), 1516-1520.*

Duarte, I., Llanos, O., Domke, H., Harz, C., Valdivieso, V. (1993). *Metaplasia and precursor lesions of gallbladder carcinoma. Frequency, distribution, and probability of detection in routine histologic samples. Cancer, 72(6), 1878-1884.*

Ducreux, M., Rougier, P., Fandi, A., et al. (1998). *Effective treatment of advanced biliary tract carcinoma using 5-fluorouracil continuous infusion with cisplatin. Ann Oncol, 9, 653.*

Dutta, U., Garg, P.K., Kumar, R., Tandon, R.K. (2000). *Typhoid carriers among patients with gallstones are at increased risk for carcinoma of the gallbladder. The American Journal of Gastroenterology, 95(3), 784-787.*

Ellis, P.A., Norman, A., Hill, A., O'Brien, M.E., Nicolson, M., Hickish, T., Cunningham, D. (1995). *Epirubicin, cisplatin and infusional 5-fluorouracil (5-FU) (ECF) in hepatobiliary tumours. Eur J Cancer, 31A(10), 1594.*

Escara-Wilke, J., Yeung, K., Keller, E. T., et al (2012). *Raf kinase inhibitor protein (RKIP) in cancer. Cancer Metastasis Rev, 31(3-4), 615-620. doi: 10.1007/s10555-012-9365-9*

Fahim, R.B., McDonald, J.R., Richards, J.C., Ferris, D.O. (1962). *Carcinoma of the gallbladder: a study of its modes of spread. Annals of Surgery, 156(1), 114.*

Fernandez, E., La Vecchia, C., D'Avanzo, B., Negri, E., Franceschi, S. (1994). *Family history and the risk of liver, gallbladder, and pancreatic cancer. Cancer Epidemiology Biomarkers & Prevention, 3(3), 209-212.*

Foster, J.M., Hoshi, H., Gibbs, J.F., Iyer, R., Javle, M., Chu, Q., Kuvshinoff, B (2006). *Gallbladder cancer: Defining the indications for primary radical resection and radical re-resection. Ann Surg Oncol, 2007 Feb, 14(2), 833-840.*

Fox, J.G. & Lee, A. (1997). *The role of Helicobacter species in newly recognized gastrointestinal tract diseases of animals. Laboratory Animal Science, 47(3), 222-255.*

Fox, J.G., Dewhirst, F.E., Shen, Z., Feng, Y., Taylor, N.S., Paster, B.J., Ericson, R.L., et al (1998). *Hepatic Helicobacter species identified in bile and gallbladder tissue from Chileans with chronic cholecystitis. Gastroenterology, 114(4), 755-763.*

Gallardo, J., Rubio, B., Fodor, M., Orlandi, L., Yanez, M., Gamargo, C., Ahumada, M. (2001). *A phase II study of gemcitabine in gallbladder carcinoma. Annuls of Oncology, 12, 1403-1406.*

Gao, H., Xie, J., Peng, J., Han, Y., Jian, Q., Han, M., Wang, C., et al (2014). *Hispidulin inhibits proliferation and enhances chemosensitivity of gallbladder Cancer cells by targeting HIF-1alpha. Exp Cell Res. doi: 10.1016/j.yexcr.2014.11.021*

Garcia, P., Leal, P., Alvarez, H., Brebi, P., Ili, C., Tapia, O., Roa, J.C. (2013). *Connective tissue growth factor immunohistochemical expression is associated with gallbladder cancer progression. Archives of Pathology & Laboratory Medicine, 137(2), 245-250.*

Ghosh, M., Kamma, H., Kawamoto, T., Koike, N., Miwa, M., Kapoor, V. K., Todoroki, T. (2005). *MUC 1 core protein as a marker of gallbladder malignancy. Eur J Surg Oncol, 31(8), 891-896. doi: 10.1016/j.ejso.2005.03.008*

Ghosh, M., Sakhuja, P., Singh, S., Agarwal, A.K. (2013). *p53 and beta-catenin expression in gallbladder tissues and correlation with tumor progression in gallbladder cancer. Saudi Journal of Gastroenterology: Official Journal of the Saudi Gastroenterology Association, 19(1), 34.*

Giang, T.H., Ngoc, T.T., Hassell, L.A. (2012). *Carcinoma involving the gallbladder: a retrospective review of 23 cases – pitfalls n diagnosis of gallbladder carcinoma. Diagnostic Pathology, 7, 10. doi:10.1186/1746-1596-7-10.*

Glimelius, B., Hoffman, K., Sjödén, P.O., Jacobsson, G., Sellström, H., Enander, L.K., Linné, T., Svensson, C. (1996). *Chemotherapy improves survival and quality of life in advanced pancreatic and biliary cancer. Ann Oncol, 7(6), 593-600.*

Goldgar, D.E., Easton, D.F., Cannon-Albright, L.A., Skolnick, M.H. (1994). *Systematic population-based assessment of cancer risk in first-degree relatives of cancer probands. Journal of the National Cancer Institute, 86(21), 1600-1608.*

Gourgiotis, S., Kocher, H.M., Solaini, L., Yarollahi, A., Tsiambas, E., Salemis, N.S. (2008). *Gallbladder cancer. The American Journal of Surgery, 196(2), 252-264.*

Grünhage, F., Acalovschi, M., Tirziu, S., Walier, M., Wienker, T.F., Ciocan, A., Mosteanu, O., et al (2007). *Increased gallstone risk in humans conferred by common variant of hepatic ATP-binding cassette transporter for cholesterol. Hepatology, 46(3), 793-801.*

Hamada, T., Yokota, K., Ayada, K., Hirai, K., Kamada, T., Haruma, K., Chayama, K., et al (2009). *Detection of Helicobacter hepaticus in human bile samples of patients with biliary disease. Helicobacter, 14(6), 545-551.*

Hamdani, N.H., Qadri, S.K., Aggarwalla, R., Bhartia, V.K., Chaudhuri, S., Debakshi, S., Baig, S.J., et al (2012). Clinicopathological study of gall bladder carcinoma with special reference to gallstones: our 8-year experience from eastern India. Asian Pac J Cancer Prev, 13, 5613-5617.

Hariharan, D., Saied, A., Kocher, H.M. (2008). Analysis of mortality rates for gallbladder cancer across the world. HPB: The Official Journal of the International Hepato Pancreato Biliary Association, 10(5), 327-331. doi:10.1080/13651820802007464.

Hayes, B.D. & Muldoon, C. (2014). Seek and ye shall find: the importance of careful macroscopic examination and thorough sampling in 2522 cholecystectomy specimens. Annals of Diagnostic Pathology. 18(3), 181-186.

Hemminki, K. & Li, X. (2003). Familial liver and gall bladder cancer: a nationwide epidemiological study from Sweden. Gut, 52(4), 592-596.

Henson, D.E., Albores-Saavedra, J., code, D. (1992). Carcinoma of the gallbladder. Histologic types, stage of disease, grade, and survival rates. Cancer, 70(6), 1493-1497.

Hirata, K., Ajiki, T., Okazaki, T., Horiuchi, H., Fujita, T., Kuroda, Y. (2006). Frequent occurrence of abnormal E-cadherin/beta-catenin protein expression in advanced gallbladder cancers and its association with decreased apoptosis. Oncology, 71(1-2), 102-110.

Horgan, A.M., Amir, E., Walter, T., Knox, J.J. (2012). Adjuvant therapy in the treatment of biliary tract cancer: a systematic review and meta-analysis. J Clin Oncol, 30(16), 1934-1940.

Hoschuetzky, H., Aberle, H., Kemler, R. (1994). Beta-catenin mediates the interaction of the cadherin-catenin complex with epidermal growth factor receptor. The Journal of Cell Biology, 127(5), 1375-1380.

Hundal, R. & Shaffer, E.A. (2014). Gallbladder cancer: epidemiology and outcome. Clinical Epidemiology, 6, 99.

Ikeda, T., Nakayama, Y., Hamada, Y., Takeshita, M., Iwasaki, H., Maeshiro, K., Ikeda, S. (2009). FU-MK-1 expression in human gallbladder carcinoma: an antigenic prediction marker for a better postsurgical prognosis. Am J Clin Pathol, 132(1), 111-117. doi: 10.1309/AJCP5HPHG6NGBWZO

Imazu, H., Mori, N., Kanazawa, K., Chiba, M., Toyoizumi, H., Torisu, Y., Koyama, S., et al (2014). Contrast-enhanced harmonic endoscopic ultrasonography in the differential diagnosis of gallbladder wall thickening. Digestive diseases and Sciences, doi:10.1007/x10620-014-3115-5.

Jacobson, A. & Cunningham, J.L. (2012). Connective tissue growth factor in tumor pathogenesis. Fibrogenesis & Tissue Repair, 5(Suppl 1), S8.

Jahani Sherafat, S., Ajeddin, E., Reza Seyyed Majidi, M., Vaziri, F., Alebouyeh, M., Mohammad Alizadeh, A.H., Nazemalhosseini Mojarad, E., et al (2012). Lack of association between Helicobacter pylori infection and biliary tract diseases. Polish Journal of Microbiology / Polskie Towarzystwo Mikrobiologów = the Polish Society of Microbiologists, 61(4), 319-322.

Jain, K., Sreenivas, V., Velpandian, T., Kapil, U., Garg, P.K. (2013). Risk factors for gallbladder cancer: A case-control study. International Journal of Cancer, 132(7), 1660-1666.

Jarnagin, W., Ruo, L., Little, S., Klimstra, D., D'Angelica, M., DeMatteo, R., Wagman, R., Blumgart, L., Fong Y.I. (2003). Patterns of initial disease recurrence after resection of gallbladder carcinoma and hilar cholangiocarcinoma: implications for adjuvant therapeutic strategies. Cancer, 98, 1689.

Jensen, E., Abraham, A., Jarosek, S., Habermann, E., Al-Refaie, W., Vickers, S., Virnig, B., Tuttle, T. (2009). Lymph node evaluation is associated with improved survival after surgery for early stage gallbladder cancer. Surgery, 146(4), 706-711.

Ji, J., Couto, E., Hemminki, K. (2005). Incidence differences for gallbladder cancer between occupational groups suggest an etiological role for alcohol. International Journal of Cancer. Journal International du Cancer, 116(3), 492-493. doi:10.1002/ijc.21055.

Jiao, X., Ren. J., Chen, H., Ma, J., Rao, S., Huang, K., Wu, S., et al (2011). Ala499Val (C> T) and Lys939Gln (A> C) polymorphisms of the XPC gene: their correlation with the risk of primary gallbladder adenocarcinoma – a case-control study in China. Carcinogenesis, 32(4), 496-501.

Kalita, D., Pant, L., Singh, S., Jain, G., Kudesia, M., Gupta, K., Kaur, C. (2013). Impact of routine histopathological examination of gall bladder specimens on early detection of malignancy – A study of 4,115 cholecystectomy specimens. Asian Pacific Journal of Cancer Prevention, 14(5), 3315-3318.

Kang, C.M., Kim, K.S., Choi, J.S., Lee, W.J., Kim, B.R. (2007). Gallbladder carcinoma associated with anomalous pancreaticobiliary duct junction. Canadian Journal of Gastroenterology, 21(6), 383.

Kashiwagi, H., Kijima, H., Dowaki, S., Ohtani, Y., Tobita, K., Yamazaki, H., Makuuchi, H. (2001). MUC1 and MUC2 expres-

sion in human gallbladder carcinoma: a clinicopathological study and relationship with prognosis. Oncol Rep, 8(3), 485-489.

Kee, S. K., Lee, J. Y., Kim, M. J., Lee, S. M., Jung, Y. W., Kim, Y. J., Kim, D. S. (2007). Hypermethylation of the Ras association domain family 1A (RASSF1A) gene in gallbladder cancer. Mol Cells, 24(3), 364-371.

Kim, H. S., Kim, G. Y., Lim, S. J., Park, Y. K., & Kim, Y. W. (2010). Reduced expression of Raf-1 kinase inhibitory protein is a significant prognostic marker in patients with gallbladder carcinoma. Hum Pathol, 41(11), 1609-1616. doi: 10.1016/j.humpath.2010.04.012

Kim, I., Lee, J., Kim, H., Kwon, O., Shim, B. (1995). A novel function of haptoglobin: haptoglobin-haemoglobin complex induces apoptosis of hepatocarcinomatous Hep 3B cells. Scandinavian Journal of Clinical and Laboratory Investigation, 55(6), 529-535.

Kim, J.H., Kim, W.H., Yoo, B.M., Kim, M. (2008). Should we perform surgical management in all patients with suspected porcelain gallbladder? Hepato-Gastroenterology, 56(93), 943-945.

Kim, K., Chie, E.K., Jang, J.Y., Kim, S.W., Han, S.W., Oh, D.Y., Im, S.A., Kim, T.Y., Bang, Y.J., Ha, S.W. (2012). Postoperative chemoradiotherapy for gallbladder cancer. Strahlenther Onkol, 188(5), 388-392.

Kim, S. M., Oh, S. J., & Hur, B. (2012). Expression of MUC1 and MUC4 in gallbladder adenocarcinoma. Korean J Pathol, 46(5), 429-435. doi: 10.4132/KoreanJPathol.2012.46.5.429

Kimura, Y., Furuhata, T., Mukaiya, M., Kihara, C., Kawakami, M., Akita, K., Yanai, Y., et al (2003). Frequent beta-catenin alteration in gallbladder carcinomas. Journal of Experimental and clinical Cancer Research, 22(2), 321-328.

Kitajima, Y., & Miyazaki, K. (2013). The Critical Impact of HIF-1a on Gastric Cancer Biology. Cancers (Basel), 5(1), 15-26. doi: 10.3390/cancers5010015

Kobayashi, T., Harada, K., Miwa, K., Nakanuma, Y. (2005). Helicobacter genus DNA fragments are commonly detectable in bile from patients with extrahepatic biliary diseases and associated with their pathogenesis. Digestive Diseases and Sciences, 50(5), 862-867.

Koh, T., Taniguchi, H., Yamaguchi, A., Kunishima, S., Yamagishi, H. (2003). Differential diagnosis of gallbladder cancer using positron emission tomography with fluorine-18-labeled fluoro-deoxyglucose (FDG-PET). Journal of Surgical Oncology, 84(2), 74-81.

Kresl, J.J., Schild, S.E., Henning, G.T., Gunderson, L.L., Donohue, J., Pitot, H., Haddock, M.G., Nagorney, D. (2002). Adjuvant external beam radiation therapy with concurrent chemotherapy in the management of gallbladder carcinoma. Int J Radiat Oncol Biol Phys, 52(1), 167-175.

Lam, C., Yuen, A., Wai, A., Leung, R., Lee, A., Ng, K., Fan, S. (2005). Gallbladder cancer presenting with acute cholecystitis: a population-based study. Surgical Endoscopy and Other Interventional Techniques, 19(5), 697-701.

Larsson, S. & Wolk, A. (2007). Obesity and the risk of gallbladder cancer: a meta-analysis. British Journal of Cancer, 96(9), 1457-1461.

Lazcano-Ponce, E.C., Miquel, J., Muñoz, N., Herrero, R., Ferrecio, C., Wistuba, I.I., de Ruiz, P.A., et al (2001). Epidemiology and molecular pathology of gallbladder cancer. CA: A Cancer Journal for Clinicians, 51(6), 349-364.

Lee, H. K., Cho, M. S., & Kim, T. H. (2012). Prognostic significance of muc4 expression in gallbladder carcinoma. World J Surg Oncol, 10, 224. doi: 10.1186/1477-7819-10-224

Leslie, N. R., & Downes, C. P. (2004). PTEN function: how normal cells control it and tumour cells lose it. Biochemical Journal, 382, 1-11.

Liu, D. C., & Yang, Z. L. (2011). Overexpression of EZH2 and loss of expression of PTEN is associated with invasion, metastasis, and poor progression of gallbladder adenocarcinoma. Pathol Res Pract, 207(8), 472-478. doi: 10.1016/j.prp.2011.05.010

Lowenfels, A., Walker, A., Althous, D., Townsend, G., Domellöf, L. (1989). Gallstone growth, size, and risk of gallbladder cancer: an interracial study. International Journal of Epidemiology, 18(1), 50-54.

Malik, I.A., Aziz, Z., Zaidi, S.H., Sethuraman, G. (2003). Gemcitabine and Cisplatin is a highly effective combination chemotherapy in patients with advanced cancer of the gallbladder. Am J Clin Oncol, 26(2), 174-177.

Malka, D., Trarbach, T., Fartoux, L., Mendiboure, J., de la Fouchardière, C., Viret, F., Assenat, E., Boucher, E., Rosmorduc, O., Greten, T. (2009). A multicenter, randomized phase II trial of gemcitabine and oxaliplatin (GEMOX) alone or in combination with biweekly cetuximab in the first-line treatment of advanced biliary cancer: Interim analysis of the BINGO trial. J Clin Oncol, 27(15 suppl), 4520.

Matsukura, N., Yokomuro, S., Yamada, S., Tajiri, T., Sundo, T., Hadama, T., Kamiya, S., et al (2002). *Association between Helicobacter bilis in bile and biliary tract malignancies: H. bilis in bile from Japanese and Tai patients with benign and malignant diseases in the biliary tract.* Cancer Science, 93(7), 842-847.

Matsumoto, N., Morine, Y., Utsunomiya, T., Imura, S., Ikemoto, T., Arakawa, Y., Shimada, M. (2014). *Role of CD151 expression in gallbladder carcinoma.* Surgery, 156(5), 1212-1217. doi: 10.1016/j.surg.2014.04.053

Méndez-Sánchez, N., Pichardo, R., González, J., Sánchez, H., Moreno, M., Barquera, F., Estevez, H.O., et al (2001). *Lack of association between Helicobacter sp colonization and gallstone disease.* Journal of Clinical Gastroenterology, 32(2), 138-141.

Mishra, R.R., Tewari, M., Shukla, H.S. (2011). *Helicobacter pylori and pathogenesis of gallbladder cancer.* Journal of Gastroenterology and Hepatology, 26(2), 260-266.

Misra, S., Chaturvedi, A., Misra, N.C., Sharma, I.D. (2003). *Carcinoma of the gallbladder.* The Lancet Oncology, 4(3), 167-176.

Mitchell, C.H., Johnson, P.T., Fishman, E.K., Hruban, R.H., Raman, S.P. (2014). *Features suggestive of gallbladder malignancy: Analysis of T1, T2, and T3 tumors on cross-sectional imaging.* Journal of Computer Assisted Tomography, 38(2), 235-241

Mojica, P., Smith, D., Ellenhorn, J. (2007). *Adjuvant radiation therapy is associated with improved survival for gallbladder carcinoma with regional metastatic disease.* J Surg Onco, 96, 8.

Moon, W.S., Park, H.S., Lee, H., Pai, R., Tarnawski, A.S., Kim, K.R., Jang, K.Y. (2005). *Co-expression of Cox-2, C-Met and β-catenin in cells forming invasive front of gallbladder cancer.* Cancer Research and Treatment, 37(3), 171-176.

Motoyama, K., Inoue, H., Nakamura, Y., Uetake, H., Sugihara, K., & Mori, M. (2008). *Clinical significance of high mobility group A2 in human gastric cancer and its relationship to let-7 microRNA family.* Clin Cancer Res, 14(8), 2334-2340. doi: 10.1158/1078-0432.ccr-07-4667

Murata, H., Tsuji, S., Tsujii, M., Fu, H., Tanimura, H., Tsujimoto, M., Matsuura, N., et al (2004). *Helicobacter bilis infection in biliary tract cancer.* Alimentary Pharmacology & Therapeutics, 20(s1), 90-94.

Myers, R.P., Shaffer, E.A., Beck, P.L. (2002). *Gallbladder polyps: epidemiology, natural history and management.* Canadian Journal of Gastroenterology = Journal Canadien de Gastroenterologie, 16(3), 187-194.

Nagaraja, V. & Eslick, G. (2014). *Systematic review with meta-analysis: the relationship between chronic Salmonella typhi carrier status and gall-bladder cancer.* Alimentary Pharmacology & Therapeutics, 39(8), 745-750.

Nagata, E., Sakai, K., Kinoshita, H., Kobayashi, Y. (1985). *The relation between carcinoma of the gallbladder and an anomalous connection between the choledochus and the pancreatic duct.* Annals of Surgery, 202(2), 182.

National Comprehensive Cancer Network. *Hepatobiliary Cancer.* (Version 2.2014) http://www.nccn.org/professionals/physician_gls/pdf/hepatobiliary.pdf (Accessed June 6, 2014)

Nigam, P., Misra, U., Negi, T., Mittal, B., Choudhuri,, G. (2010). *Alterations of p53 gene in gallbladder cancer patients of North India.* Tropical Gastroenterology, 31(2), 96-100.

Nuizzo, G., Clemente, G., Cadeddu, F., Ardito, F., Ricci, R., Vecchio, F.M. (2004). *Papillary carcinoma of the gallbladder and anomalous pancreatico-biliary junction. Report of three cases and review of the literature.* Hepato-Gastroenterology, 52(64), 1034-1038.

Ogura, T., Kurisu, Y., Masuda, D., Imoto, A., Onda, S., Kamiyama, R., Hayashi, M., et al (2014). *Can endoscopic ultrasound-guided fine needle aspiration offer clinical benefit for thick-walled gallbladders?* Digestive Diseases and Sciences, doi:10.1007/s10620-014-3100-z.

Pai, R. K., Mojtahed, K., & Pai, R. K. (2011). *Mutations in the RAS/RAF/MAP kinase pathway commonly occur in gallbladder adenomas but are uncommon in gallbladder adenocarcinomas.* Appl Immunohistochem Mol Morphol, 19(2), 133-140. doi: 10.1097/PAI.0b013e3181f09179

Panebionco, A., Volpi, A.., Lozito, C., Prestera, A., Ialongo, P., Palasciano, N. (2012). *Incidental gallbladder carcinoma: our experience.* Il Giornale di Chirurgia, 34(5-6), 167-169.

Philip, P.A., Mahoney, M.R., Allmer, C., Thomas, J., Pitot, H.C., Kim, G., Donehower, R.C., Fitch, T., Picus, J., Erlichman, C. (2006). *Phase II study of erlotinib in patients with advanced biliary cancer.* J Clin Oncol, 24(19), 3069-3074.

Priya, T.P., Kapoor, V., Krishnani, N., Agrawal, V., Agrawal, S. (2010). *Role of E-cadherin gene in gall bladder cancer and its precursor lesions.* Virchows Archiv, 456(5), 507-514.

Rai, R., Sharma, K.L., Misra, S., Kumar, A., Mittal, B. (2014). *CYP17 polymorphism (rs743572) is associated with increased risk of gallbladder cancer in tobacco users.* Tumor Biology, doi:10.1007/s13277-014-1876-2.

Rai, R., Sharma, K.L., Misra, S., Kumar, A., Mittal, B. (2014). Association of adrenergic receptor gene polymorphisms in gallbladder cancer susceptibility in a North Indian population. Journal of Cancer Research and Clinical Oncology, 140(5), 725-735.

Rai, R., Sharma, K.L., Sharma, S., Misra, S., Kumar, A., Mittal, B. (2014). Death receptor (DR4) haplotypes are associated with increased susceptibility of gallbladder carcinoma in North Indian population. PloS One, 9(2), e90264.

Randi, G., Franceschi, S., La Vecchia, C. (2006). Gallbladder cancer worldwide: geographical distribution and risk factors. International Journal of Cancer. Journal International du Cancer, 118(7), 1591-602. doi:10.1002/ijc.21683.

Rao, S., Cunningham, D., Hawkins, R.E., Hill, M.E., Smith, D., Daniel, F., Ross, P.J., Oates, J., Norman, A.R. (2005). Phase III study of 5FU, etoposide and leucovorin (FELV) compared to epirubicin, cisplatin and 5FU (ECF) in previously untreated patients with advanced biliary cancer. Br J Cancer, 92(9), 1650.

Roa, I., de Aretxabala, X., Lantadilla, S., & Munoz, S. (2011). ERCC1 (Excision repair cross-complementing 1) expression in pT2 gallbladder cancer is a prognostic factor. Histology and Histopathology, 26(1), 37-43.

Rudi, J., Rudy, A., Maiwald, M., Stremmel, W. (1999). Helicobacter sp. are not detectable in bile from German patients with biliary disease. Gastroenterology, 116(4), 1016-1017.

Sasaki, M., Yamato, T., Nakanuma, Y., Ho, S. B., Kim, Y. S., et al (1999). Expression of MUC2, MUC5AC and MUC6 apomucins in carcinoma, dysplasia and non-dysplastic epithelia of the gallbladder. Pathol Int, 49(1), 38-44.

Scott, T.E., Carroll, M., Cogliano, F.D., Smith, B.F., Lamorte, W.W. (1999). A case-control assessment of risk factors for gallbladder carcinoma. Digestive Diseases and Sciences, 44(8), 1619-1625.

Sharma, K.L., Agarwal, A., Misra, S., Kumar, A., Kumar, V., Mittal, B. (2014). Association of genetic variants of xenobiotic and estrogen metabolism pathway (CYP1A1 and CYP1B1) with gallbladder cancer susceptibility. Tumor Biology, doi:10.107/s13277-014-1708-4.

Shi, J., Liu, H., Wang, H. L., Prichard, J. W., Lin, F., et al (2013). Diagnostic utility of von Hippel-Lindau gene product, maspin, IMP3, and S100P in adenocarcinoma of the gallbladder. Hum Pathol, 44(4), 503-511. doi: 10.1016/j.humpath.2012.06.010

Shih, I. M. (1999). The role of CD146 (Mel-CAM) in biology and pathology. J Pathol, 189(1), 4-11. doi: 10.1002/(SICI)1096-9896(199909)189:1<4::AID-PATH332>3.0.CO;2-P

Shukla, V.K., Singh, H., Pandey, M., Upadhyay, S., Nath, G. (2000). Carcinoma of the gallbladder – is it a sequel of typhoid? Digestive Diseases and Sciences, 45(5), 900-903.

Siegel, R., Ma, J., Zou, Z., Jemal, A. (2014). Cancer statistics, 2014. CA: A Cancer Journal for Clinicians, 64(1), 9-29.

Simon, J. A., & Lange, C. A. (2008). Roles of the EZH2 histone methyltransferase in cancer epigenetics. Mutat Res, 647(1-2), 21-29. doi: 10.1016/j.mrfmmm.2008.07.010

Smirnov, S., Pashkevich, A., Liundysheva, V., Babenko, A., Smolyakova, R., et al (2015). Heterogeneity of excision repair cross-complementation group 1 gene expression in non-small-cell lung cancer patients. Mol Clin Oncol, 3(1), 227-331. doi: 10.3892/mco.2014.415

Song, M. S., Salmena, L., & Pandolfi, P. P. (2012). The functions and regulation of the PTEN tumour suppressor. Nature Reviews Molecular Cell Biology, 13(5), 283-296. doi: Doi 10.1038/Nrm3330

Srivastava, A., Tulsyan, S., Pandey, S.N., Choudhuri, G., Mittal, B. (2009). Single nucleotide polymorphism in the ABCG8 transporter gene is associated with gallbladder cancer susceptibility. Liver International, 29(6), 831-837.

Stephen, A.E. & Berger, D.L. (2001). Carcinoma in the porcelain gallbladder: a relationship revisited. Surgery, 129(6), 699-703.

Takada, T., Amano, H., Yasuda, H., Nimura, Y., Matsushiro, T., Kato, H., Nagakawa, T., Nakayama. (2002). Is postoperative adjuvant chemotherapy useful for gallbladder carcinoma? A phase III multicenter prospective randomized controlled trial in patients with resected pancreaticobiliary carcinoma. Cancer, 95(8), 1685-1695.

Takagawa, M., Muguruma, N., Oguri, K., Imoto, Y., Okamoto, K., Kunio, I, Ito, S. (2005). Prediction of prognosis in gallbladder carcinoma by mucin and p53 immunohistochemistry. Digestive Diseases and Sciences, 50(8), 1410-1413.

Takayama, S., Takahashi, H., Matsuo, Y., Okada, Y., Takeyama, H. (2010). Effect of Helicobacter bilis infection on human bile duct cancer cells. Digestive Diseases and Sciences, 55(7), 1905-1910.

Tan, Y., Ma, S.-Y., Wang, F.-Q., Meng, H.-P., Mei, C., Liu, A., Wu, H.-R. (2011). Proteomic-based analysis for identification of potential serum biomarkers in gallbladder cancer. Oncolog Reports, 26(4), 853-859.

Tanaka, K., Ikoma, A., Hamada, N., Nishida, S., Kadono, J., Taira, A. (1998). Biliary tract cancer accompanied by anomalous junction of pancreaticobiliary ductal system in adults. The American Journal of Surgery, 175(3), 218-220.

Tewari, M., Mishra, R.R., Shukla, H.S. (2010). *Salmonella typhi and gallbladder cancer: report from an endemic region.* Hepatobiliary Pancreat Dis Int, 9(5), 524-530.

Towfigh, S., McFadden, D.W., Cortina, G.R., Thompson Jr., J.E., Tompkins, R.K., Chandler, C., Hines, O.J. (2001). *Porcelain gallbladder is not associated with gallbladder carcinoma. The American Surgeon, 67(1), 7-10.*

Tsukada, K., Kurosaki, I., Uchida, K., Shirai, Y., Oohashi, Y., Yokoyama, N., Watanabe, H., et al (1997). *Lymph node spread from carcinoma of the gallbladder. Cancer, 80(4), 661-667.*

Valle, J., Wasan, H., Palmer, D.H., Cunningham, D., Anthoney, A., Maraveyas, A., Madhusudan, S., Iveson, T., Hughes, S., Pereira, S.P., Roughton, M., Bridgewater, J. (2010). *Cisplatin plus gemcitabine versus gemcitabine for biliary tract cancer. N Engl J Med, 362(14), 1273-1281.*

Wang, W., Yang, Z. L., Liu, J. Q., Jiang, S., & Miao, X. Y. (2012). *Identification of CD146 expression, angiogenesis, and lymphangiogenesis as progression, metastasis, and poor-prognosis related markers for gallbladder adenocarcinoma. Tumour Biol, 33(1), 173-182. doi: 10.1007/s13277-011-0260-8*

Wang, Z., & Yan, X. (2013). *CD146, a multi-functional molecule beyond adhesion. Cancer Lett, 330(2), 150-162. doi: 10.1016/j.canlet.2012.11.049*

Wu, K., Liao, M., Liu, B., Deng, Z. (2011). *ADAM-17 over-expression in gallbladder carcinoma correlates with poor prognosis of patients. Medical Oncology, 28(2), 475-480.*

Wu, W. D., Hu, Z. M., Shang, M. J., Zhao, D. J., Zhang, C. W., Hong, D. F., Huang, D. S., et al (2014). *Cordycepin downregulates multiple drug resistant (MDR)/HIF-1alpha through regulating AMPK/mTORC1 signaling in GBC-SD gallbladder cancer cells. Int J Mol Sci, 15(7), 12778-12790. doi: 10.3390/ijms150712778*

Wu, X.-Y., Zhang, L., Zhang, K.-M., Zhang, M.-H., Ruan, T.-Y., Liu, C.-Y., Xu, J.-Y. (2014). *Clinical implication of TMPRSS4 expression in human gallbladder cancer. Tumor Biology, doi:10.1007/s13277-014-1716-4.*

Xiong, L., Yang, Z., Yang, L., Liu, J., & Miao, X. (2012). *Expressive levels of MUC1 and MUC5AC and their clinicopathologic significances in the benign and malignant lesions of gallbladder. J Surg Oncol, 105(1), 97-103. doi: 10.1002/jso.22055*

Yagyu, K., Kikuchi, S., Obata, Y., Lin, Y., Ishibashi, T., Kurosawa, M., Inaba, Y., et al (2008). *Cigarette smoking, alcohol drinking and the risk of gallbladder cancer death: a prospective cohort study in Japan. International Journal of Cancer, 122(4), 924-929.*

Yakoob, J., Khan, M.R., Abbas, Z., Jafri, W., Azmi, R., Ahmad, Z., Naeem, S., et al (2011). *Helicobacter pylori: association with gall bladder disorders in Pakistan. British Journal of Biomedical Science, 68(2), 59-64.*

Yamaguchi, J., Sasaki, M., Sato, Y., Itatsu, K., Harada, K., Zen, Y., Nakanuma, Y. (2010). *Histone deacetylase inhibitor (SAHA) and repression of EZH2 synergistically inhibit proliferation of gallbladder carcinoma. Cancer Sci, 101(2), 355-362. doi: 10.1111/j.1349-7006.2009.01387.x*

Yamaguchi, K. & Enjoji, M. (1988). *Carcinoma of the gallbladder: a clinicopathology of 103 patients and a newly proposed staging. Cancer, 62(7), 1425-1432.*

Yang, L., Lan, S., Liu, J., & Yang, Z. (2011). *Expression of MK-1 and RegIV and its clinicopathological significances in the benign and malignant lesions of gallbladder. Diagn Pathol, 6, 100. doi: 10.1186/1746-1596-6-100*

Yang, Z., Yang, Z., Xiong, L., Huang, S., Liu, J., Yang, L., Miao, X., et al (2011). *Expression of VHL and HIF-1alpha and Their Clinicopathologic Significance in Benign and Malignant Lesions of the Gallbladder. Appl Immunohistochem Mol Morphol, 19(6), 534-539. doi: 10.1097/PAI.0b013e318212f001*

Yi, S., Yang, Z., Miao, X., Zou, Q., Li, J., Liang, L., Zeng, G., et al (2014). *N-cadherin and P-cadherin are biomarkers for invasion, metastasis, and poor prognosis of gallbladder carcinomas. Pathology-Research and Practice, 210(6), 363-368.*

Yoshimitsu, K., Irie, H., Aibe, H., Tajima, T., Nishie, A., Asayama, Y., Matake, K., et al (2005). *Well-differentiated adenocarcinoma of the gallbladder with intratumoral cystic components due to abundant mucin production: a mimicker of adenomyomatosis. European Radiology, 15(2), 229-233.*

Zatonski, W.A., Lowenfels, A.B., Boyle, P., Maisonneuve, P., Bueno de Mesquita, H.B., Ghadirian, P., Jain, M., et al (1997). *Epidemiologic aspects of gallbladder cancer: A case-control study of the SEARCH Program of the International Agency for Research on Cancer. Journal of the National Cancer Institute, 89(15), 1132-1138.*

Zhou, D., Wang, J., Weng, M., Zhang, Y., Wang, X., Gong, W., Quan, Z. (2013). *Infections of Helicobacter spp. In the biliary system are associated with biliary tract cancer: a meta-analysis. European Journal of Gastroenterology & Hepatology, 25(4), 447-454. doi:10.1097/MEG.0b013e32835c0362.*

Zhou, H., Guo, W., Zhao, Y., Wang, Y., Zha, R., Ding, J., Ma, B. (2014). *MicroRNA-26a acts as a tumor suppressor inhibiting gallblader cancer cell proliferation by directly targeting HMGA2. Int J Oncol, 44(6), 2050-2058. doi: 10.3892/ijo.2014.2360*

Zhu, A.X., Meyerhardt, J.A., Blaszkowsky, L.S., Kambadakone, A.R., Muzikansky, A., Zheng, H., Clark, J.W., Abrams, T.A., Chan, J.A., Enzinger, P.C., Bhargava, P., Kwak, E.L., Allen, J.N., Jain, S.R., Stuart, K., Horgan, K., Sheehan, S., Fuchs, C.S., Ryan, D.P., Sahani, D.V. (2010). Efficacy and safety of gemcitabine, oxaliplatin, and bevacizumab in advanced biliary-tract cancers and correlation of changes in 18-fluorodeoxyglucose PET with clinical outcome: a phase 2 study. Lancet Oncol, 11(1), 48-54.

Zoller, M. (2009). Tetraspanins: push and pull in suppressing and promoting metastasis. Nat Rev Cancer, 9(1), 40-55. doi: 10.1038/nrc2543

Zou, Q., Xiong, L., Yang, Z., Lv, F., Yang, L., & Miao, X. (2012). Expression levels of HMGA2 and CD9 and its clinicopathological significances in the benign and malignant lesions of the gallbladder. World J Surg Oncol, 10, 92. doi: 10.1186/1477-7819-10-92

Diagnostic Values and Molecular-targeted of Oncofetal Glypican-3 for Hepatocellular Carcinoma

Dengfu Yao[*], Min Yao[†], Li Wang[‡], Zhizhen Dong[§]

1 Introduction

Hepatocellular carcinoma (HCC) is one of the most common and rapidly fatal malignancies worldwide (Yang JD, *et al.*, 2012; El-Serag HB, *et al.*, 2011) with a multi-factorial, multistep, complex process, and poor prognosis, which is associated with a background of chronic and persistent infection of hepatitis B virus (HBV) or hepatitis C virus (HCV) along with alcohol and aflatoxin B1 intake are widely recognized etiological agents in HCC (Bruix J, *et al.*, 2014; Jain S, *et al.*, 2010). Most of HCC patients died quickly because of the rapid tumor progression, and hepatic resection or transplantation is the only potential curative treatment for HCC patients, the treatment options are rather limited with insensitive to radiotherapy or chemotherapy (Welzel TM, *et al.*, 2013; Tyson GL, et al), high rate of recurrence after surgery, and metastasis, lead to a poor prognosis of HCC patients. Therefore, improving the early diagnosis and looking for a more effective treatment for HCC become an urgent problem (Jemal A, *et al.*, 2011; Maluccio M, *et al.*, 2012).

Recently, microRNA (miRNA) is a small non-coding RNA molecule, which functions in transcriptional and post-transcriptional regulation of gene expression as endogenous silencers of numerous target genes, and some miRNAs are involved in inhibiting etoposide-induced apoptosis of hepatoma cells, which may contribute to facilitating chronic HBV infection and HCC development (Qu KZ, *et al.*, 2011). Glypicans are a family of heparan sulfate proteoglycans that are linked to the exocytoplasmic surface of the plasma membrane through a glycosylphosphatidy- linositol anchor. Six glypicans have been identified in mammals (GPC-1 to 6), and two in Drosophila (Dally and Dally-like protein). Glypicans are expressed predominantly during development, in a stage- and tissue-specific manner, suggesting that they play a role in morphogenesis. Genetic and functional studies demonstrated that glypicans regulate the signaling activity of various morphogens, including Wnts, Hedgehogs (Hhs), bone morphogenic proteins, and fibroblast growth factors (Filmus J, *et al.*, 2008; Capurro M, *et al.*, 2003).

Glypican-3 (GPC-3) as a molecule that links to cell membrane surface with a glycosylphosphatidy-linositol anchor is closely associated with HCC (Capurro M, *et al.*, 2003). Oncofetal GPC-3 is a specific marker during hepatocyte malignant transformation and HCC diagno-

[*] Research Center of Clinical Medicine, Affiliated Hospital of Nantong University, Nantong, China

[†] Department of Immunology, Nantong University, Nantong, China

[‡] Department of Medical Informatics, Nantong University, Nantong, China

[§] Department of Diagnostic, Affiliated Hospital of Nantong University, Nantong, Nantong, China

sis (Yao M, *et al.*, 2011). GPC-3 promotes HCC growth and metastasis through stimulating multiple signaling pathways, and the suppression of its activation was significantly inhibited hepatoma cell proliferation. This paper reviewed on the oncofetal GPC-3 as a specific biomarker for HCC diagnosis and a valuable target for HCC gene therapy through the Wnt/β-catenin and hedgehog (HH) singling pathways.

2   GPC-3 in HCC Tissues

GPC-3 links to the cellular membrane through a glycosylphosphatidylinositol anchor and plays an important role in regulating cells growth and is closely related to HCC (Libbrecht L, *et al.*, 2006). The two subunits are produced by cleavage between Arg^{358} and Ser^{359}, which generates an N-terminal fragment of 40 kD (soluble) and a C-terminal fragment of 30 kD (combined with membrane) (Cheng W, *et al.*, 2008; Libbrecht L, *et al.*, 2006). Recently, it has been suggested that GPC-3 can induce oncogenesis through activation of insulin-like growth factor–II (IGF-II) signaling pathway. Its expression with carcinoembryonic nature was brown, nested distribution and deep stained in HCC tissues, present in the cytoplasm and cell membrane. The incidence of hepatic GPC-3 was 80.6 % in HCC-, 41.7 % in its surrounding-, and no expression in distal cancerous- tissues (Figure 1). The intensity of GPC-3 expression in HCC tissues was significantly higher than that in their surrounding or distal cancerous tissues (Yao M, *et al.*, 2013). The significant difference of GPC-3 expression indicated that GPC-3 derived from HCC tissues is a specific tumor biomarker.

3   GPC-3 Expression in Hepatocyte Malignant Transformation

HCC is characterized by a multi-cause, multi-stage and multi-focus process of tumor progression (Wang HL, *et al.*, 2008; Filmus J, *et al.*, 2008) with poor prognosis and hard to early diagnosis (Yao DF, *et al.*, 2007). The dynamic expression of oncofetal antigen GPC-3 and GPC-3 mRNA were investigated in hepatocarcinogenesis for exploring their early diagnostic value for HCC. A hepatoma model was induced in male Sprague-Dawley rats with 0.05% 2-fluorenyl acetamide and confirmed by hematoxylin and eosin staining and γ-glutamyl transferase (GGT) expression (Yao DF, *et al.*, 2000). The positive GPC-3 expression showed as brown granule-like staining localized in the cytoplasm during morphological stages of granule-like degeneration, atypical hyperplasia (precancerous), and cancer formation, with a progressive increase of liver total RNA and GGT expression. The incidence of liver GPC-3 mRNA, GPC-3, and serum GPC-3 was 100%, 100% and 77.8% in HCC group, 100%, 100%, and 66.7% in precancerous group, 83.3%, 83.3%, and 38.9% in degeneration group, and no expression in liver tissues or blood of normal group, respectively (ure 2). There was a close positive correlation between liver GPC-3 mRNA and total RNA level ($r = 0.475$, $P < 0.05$) or hepatic GPC-3 ($r = 1.0$, $P < 0.001$) or serum GPC-3 ($r = 0.994$, $P < 0.001$), indicated that abnormal circulating oncofetal antigen GPC-3 and GPC-3 mRNA expression in rat hepatocarcinogenesis might be promising molecular markers for early diagnosis of HCC (Wang L, *et al.*, 2014; Morford LA, *et al.*, 2007).

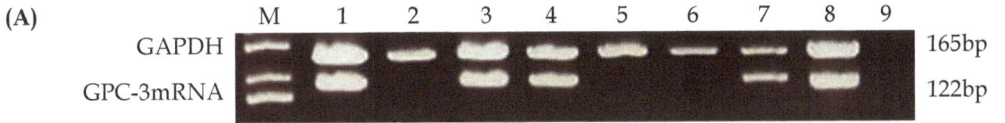

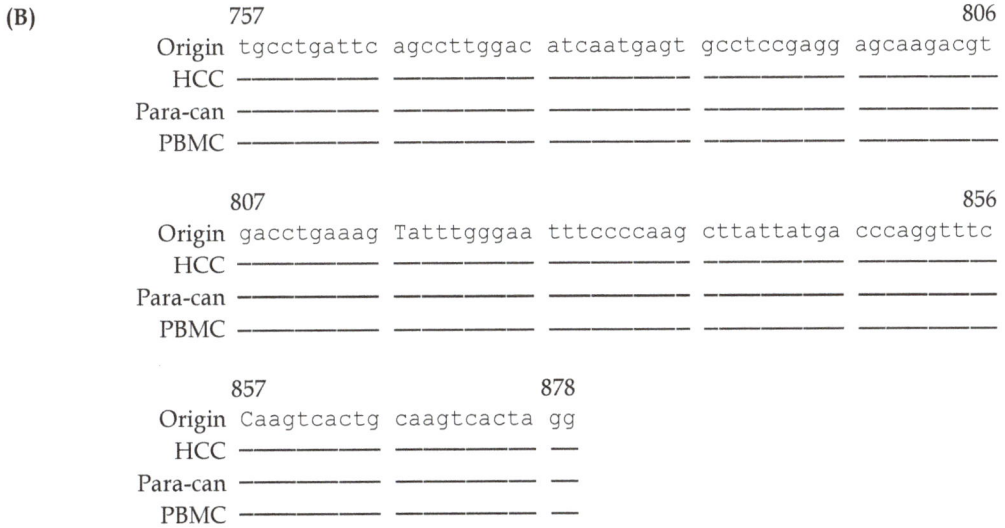

(B)

```
       757                                                              806
Origin tgcctgattc agccttggac atcaatgagt gcctccgagg agcaagacgt
HCC    ————————— ————————— ————————— ————————— —————————
Para-can ——————— ————————— ————————— ————————— —————————
PBMC   ————————— ————————— ————————— ————————— —————————

       807                                                              856
Origin gacctgaaag Tatttgggaa tttccccaag cttattatga cccaggtttc
HCC    ————————— ————————— ————————— ————————— —————————
Para-can ——————— ————————— ————————— ————————— —————————
PBMC   ————————— ————————— ————————— ————————— —————————

       857                   878
Origin Caagtcactg caagtcacta gg
HCC    ————————— ————————— ——
Para-can ——————— ————————— ——
PBMC   ————————— ————————— ——
```

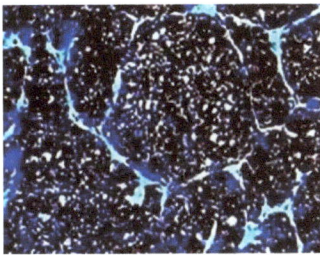
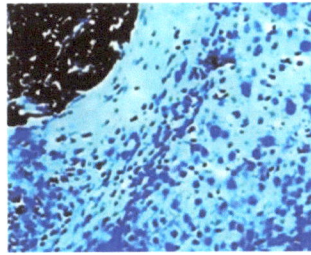
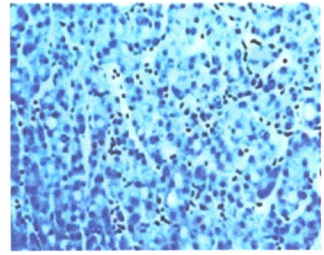

(C1)   (C2)   (C3)

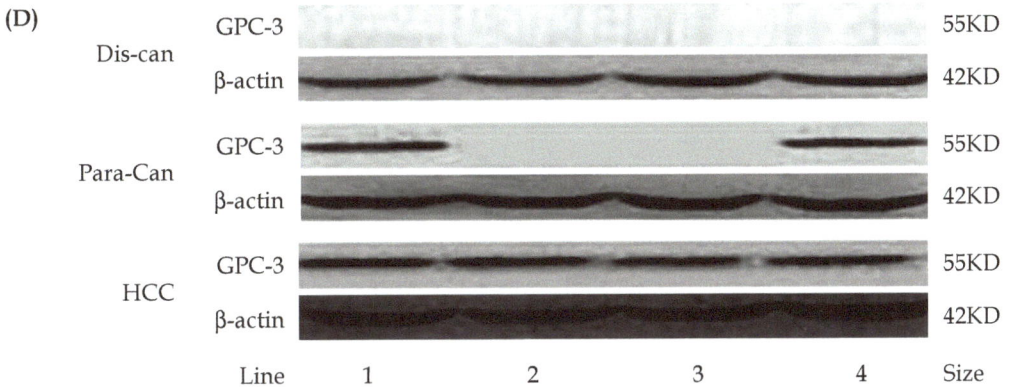

Figure 1: Analysis of hepatic GPC-3 expression in human HCC tissues and circulating PBMC. **A:** The fragment (122 bp) of GPC-3 mRNA was amplified by RT-PCR, separated on 1.5% agarose gel, and stained with ethidium bromide; glyceroldehyde-3-phosphate dehydrogenase (GAPDH) as control gene (165 bp); M: DNA molecular marker. Lane 1-5: amplification of GPC-3 mRNA

Continued on next page...

...Continued from previous page

fragment from PBMC, Lane 1, 3 and 4: HCC; Lane 2: chronic hepatitis; Lane 5: liver cirrhosis; Lane 6-9: amplification of GPC-3 mRNA fragment from liver tissues: Lane 6, 7 and 8 were distal cancerous-, paracancerous-, and HCC tissues, respectively. Lane 9: blank control. **B**: Alignment of nucleotide sequences of amplified GPC-3 gene fragments. GPC-3: original sequence (nt 757 ~ 878, 122 bp) of human GPC-3 from GenBank (NM_001164617); HCC: cancerous tissues; Para-can: para-cancerous tissues: PBMC: peripheral blood mononuclear cells. **C1**: GPC-3 positive in cytoplasm in HCC focus tissues analyzed by immunohistochemical staining with anti-GPC-3 antibody (S-P, original magnification × 200) from HCC patients; **C2**: Comparative analysis of GPC-3 expression in cancerous (positive staining) or paracancerous (negative staining) tissues from HCC patients; **C3**: No GPC-3 expression in distal cancerous tissues from HCC patients; **D**: The analysis of hepatic GPC-3 expression in different parts of HCC tissues by Western blotting, GPC-3 expression in cytoplasm of liver analyzed in different parts of HCC. Lanes 1-4, liver tissues from different HCC patients. HCC: the cancerous tissues; Para-can: their paracancerous tissues, and Dis-can: their distal cancerous tissues. GPC-3, GPC-3 protein, 55 KD; and β-actin, 42 KD as the control protein.

4   Circulating GPC-3 in HCC Diagnosis

Specific diagnosis of HCC at early stage is utmost importance. Appropriate screening patients at risk for HCC might be an appropriate way to achieve early diagnosis and improve the treatment outcome. Although AFP is a useful marker for HCC that greatly affects diagnosis and the evaluations of therapy and therapeutic policy. However, it is sometimes very difficult to make the distinction between tumors and falsely elevated AFP levels due to benign liver diseases (Kwack MH, *et al.*, 2006; Shafizadeh N, *et al.*, 2008). The level of circulating GPC-3 expression in values of diagnosis and monitoring metastasis of HCC was analyzed in sera of patients with liver diseases (Yamauchi N, *et al.*, 2005; Cheng W, *et al.*, 2008). Serum GPC-3 was detected only in HCC (52.8 %, Table 1) and significant difference was found between GPC-3 and tumor size ($\chi^2 = 6.318$,   P = 0.012) or HBV infection ($\chi^2 = 23.362$, P < 0.001). GPC-3 over-expression was associated closely with HCC and could be a specific marker for HCC diagnosis and monitoring metastasis.

5   Circulating GPC-3 mRNA in HCC Metastasis

GPC-3 gene transcription from liver tissues and circulating peripheral blood mononuclear cells (PBMC) was associated with extra-hepatic metastasis of HCC. Metastasis is the final stage in tumor progression and is thought to be responsible for up to 90% of HCC deaths associated with cancerous cells enter the circulation, eventually grow into lethal tumor in distal organs, and reflect inherent differences within the disseminating cells of distinct tumors (Qian J, *et al.*, 2010; Llovet JM, *et al.*, 2008). It could be examined in the majority of cancerous tissues or circulating PBMC from HCC patients that GPC-3 gene fragments were amplified and confirmed by sequencing (Figure 1B), and not in distal cancerous liver tissues or the cells from benign liver diseases.

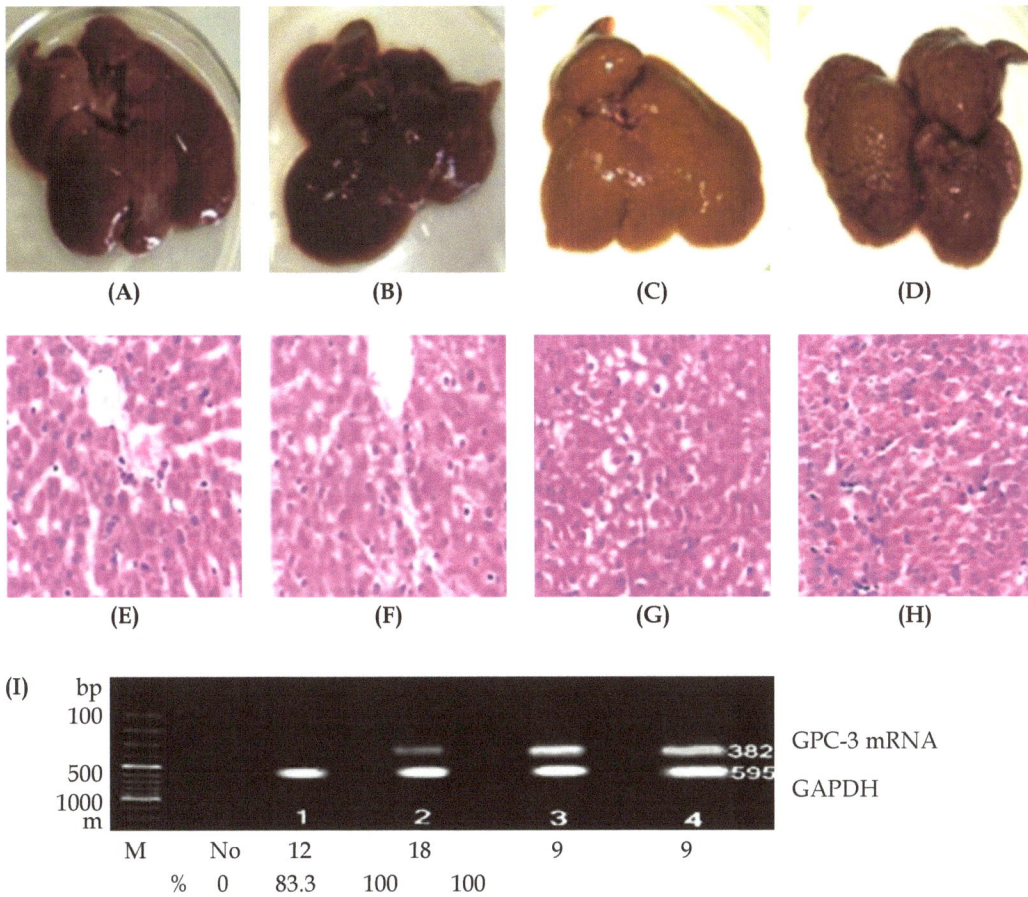

Figure 2: Malignant transformations of rat hepatocytes and GPC-3 expression. Hepatoma models were made in SD rats inducing with 2-FAA. **A**, control rat livers; **B**, rat livers at the early stage; **C**, rat livers at the medial stage; and **D**, rat livers at the end stage; **E ~ H**, the pathological examination of the correspondence to **A ~ D**; **I**, the fragment (372 bp) of rat GPC-3 mRNA was amplified by RT-PCR, separated on 1.5% agarose gel, and stained with ethidium bromide; GAPDH as control gene (595 bp); **M**: DNA molecular marker. **Lane 1 ~ 4**: amplification of rat GPC-3 mRNA fragments from rat livers of normal, hepatocyte degeneration, precancerous, and cancer, respectively.

Group	No. of Cases	GPC-3 (ng/mL)				AFP (ng/mL)	
		Range	Pos.(%)	Z value	P value	Pos.(%)	P value
HCC	123	0.0~4000	65(52.8)		-	87(70.7)	-
LC	70	0.0~95.1*	2(1.4)*	6.989	<0.001	14(20.0)*	<0.001
CH	70	0.0~0.0*	0(0.0)*	7.246	<0.001	12(17.1)*	<0.001
AH	56	0.0~0.0*	0(0.0)*	6.575	<0.001	8(14.3)*	<0.001
NT	50	0.0~128.4*	1(2.0)*	4.573	<0.001	0(0.0)*	<0.001
NC	30	0.0~0.0*	0(0.0)*	4.979	<0.001	0(0.0)*	<0.001

*$P < 0.001$, compared with the HCC group. LC: liver cirrhosis; CH: chronic hepatitis; AH: acute hepatitis; NT: non-hepatic tumors; NC: normal controls; Pos. (%): positive rate.

Table 1: Comparative analysis of serum GPC-3 and AFP levels for HCC diagnosis.

GPC-3 mRNA from circulating PBMC from 123 HCC patients or 246 patients with other diseases or 36 HCC tissues was amplified by quantitative real-time PCR, and confirmed by DNA sequencing. Hepatic GPC-3 mRNA increased dynamically during HCC formation. Circulating GPC-3 mRNA (Table 2) was detected in 70.7 % of HCC, with related to TNM stage, periportal cancerous embolus, and extra-hepatic metastasis ($P < 0.001$, Table 3). The combination of circulating GPC-3, GPC-3 mRNA and AFP had complementary values (94.3 %, Table 4) for HCC diagnosis. The higher incidence was found in HCC patients with I ~ II staging, HBV infection, and small size tumor, especially in HCC patients with periportal cancer embolus or extra-hepatic metastasis group, suggesting that the up-regulation of circulating GPC-3 mRNA is a more sensitive and specific biomarker for monitoring metastasis of HCC (Yao M, *et al.,* 2013; Saffroy R, *et al.,* 2007; Saleh HA, *et al.,* 2009).

6   Molecular Mechanism of GPC-3 Stimulating Hepatoma Growth

GPC-3 stimulates proliferation of HCC cells through activation of multiple related signaling pathway such as Wnt, HH, and IGF (Stigliano I, *et al.,* 2009; Rehem RN, *et al.,* 2011), especially in the canonical Wnt/β-catenin pathway that is closely associated with occurrence and development of HCC. GPC-3 has been shown to mediate activation of the canonical Wnt/β-catenin pathway (Figure 3) by acting as co-receptors for β-catenin or p-GSK3β expression which play critical roles in HCC development or hepatocyte malignant transformation. Both are the key signaling molecules in the canonical Wnt/β-catenin pathway, and involved in turning off a protein complex dedicated to respond cells and to enter the nucleus. After silencing GPC-3 gene expression of HepG2 or Hep3B cells, the cellular localization of β-catenin was almost disappeared from nucleus and cytoplasm, and even induced cell apoptosis, and the key molecules of Wnt/β-catenin pathway were significantly down-regulated, suggesting that silencing GPC-3 through the Wnt/β- catenin pathway inhibiting hepatoma cell proliferation or promoting cell apoptosis should be one of molecular mechanisms (Pang RW, *et al.,* 2008; Clevers H, *et al.,* 2012).

Group	No. of Cases	C_T (GPC-3) Positive (%)	C_T (GPC-3) Mean	C_T (GAPDH) Positive (%)	C_T (GAPDH) Mean	ΔC_T
HCC	123	87 (70.7)	28.6	13.8 – 19.2	16.8	11.8
LC	70	2 (1.4)	0.0*	13.6 – 18.8	16.6	0.0*
CH	70	0 (0)	0.0*	14.2 – 19.0	16.4	0.0*
AH	56	0 (0)	0.0*	14.1 – 17.6	16.8	0.0*
NT	50	1 (2)	0.2*	13.8 – 18.6	16.7	0.0*
NC	30	0 (0)	0.0*	14.6 – 19.0	16.9	0.0*

*$P < 0.001$, compared with HCC group.
ΔC_T = the C_T value of GPC-3 minus the C_T value of GAPDH.
LC: liver cirrhosis; CH: chronic hepatitis; AH: acute hepatitis.
NT: non-hepatic tumor; NC: normal control.

Table 2: Relative quantity of GPC-3 mRNA from peripheral blood mononuclear cells in patients with liver diseases or non-liver tumors.

Group		No.of Cases	GPC-3 Positive	GPC-3 Negative	χ^2	P
Sex	Male	103	74	29	0.379	0.538
	Female	20	13	7		
Age	≥ 60 yr	56	39	17	0.059	0.808
	<60 yr	67	48	19		
TNM staging	I ~ II	47	39	8	5.551	0.019
	III ~ IV	76	48	28		
Tumor size	≥ 3.0cm	98	65	33	4.520	0.034
	<3.0cm	25	22	3		
AFP (ng/mL)	≥ 400	52	36	16	0.098	0.754
	<400	71	51	20		
HBsAg	Positive	89	79	10	50.571	<0.001
	Negative	34	8	26		
Tumor number	Single	58	40	18	0.165	0.685
	Multiple	65	47	18		
Child-pugh	A	60	40	20	1.005	0.605
	B	45	34	11		
	C	18	13	5		
Periportal cancer embolus	With	44	44	0	28.347	<0.001
	Without	79	43	36		
Extra-hepatic metastasis	With	65	65	0	57.019	<0.001
	Without	58	22	36		

Table 3: The pathological characteristics of circulating GPC-3 mRNA in peripheral blood mononuclear cells from HCC patients.

GPC-3	GPC-3	mRNA	AFP*	Total
Sensitivity (%)	52.8	70.7	70.7	94.3
Specificity (%)	98.8	99.8	86.2	85.8
Diagnostic accuracy (%)	83.5	89.4	81.0	88.6
Positive predictive value (%)	95.6	96.7	71.9	76.8
Negative predictive value (%)	80.7	87.1	85.5	96.8

*Serum AFP level > 20 ng/ml.

Table 4: Combining diagnostic values of circulating GPC-3, GPC-3 mRNA and AFP levels for HCC.

7 Silencing GPC-3 Promoting Hepatoma Cell Apoptosis

HCC is a highly chemoresistant cancer with no effective systemic therapy (Imbeaud S, *et al.*, 2010; Hayashi E, *et al.*, 2005). Despite of surgical or locoregional therapies, prognosis remains poor because of high tumor recurrence or progression, and currently there are no well-established effective adjuvant therapies. Continued increasing of HCC incidence has been attached importance to many years because of majority of patients with incurable disease, difficulties of early diagnosis and lack of effective systemic therapies. Recently, molecular targeted therapy offers an effective option for non-surgical HCC patient management, but the

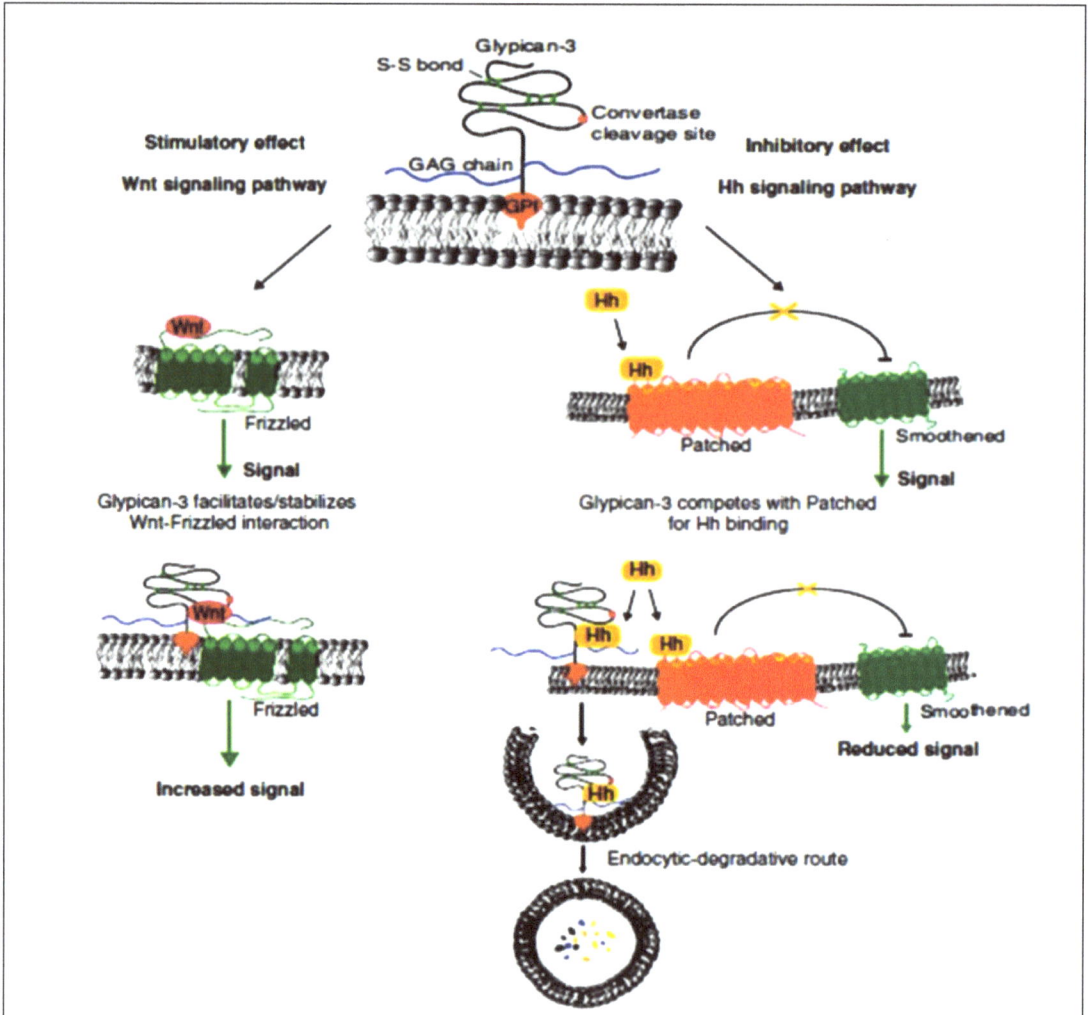

Figure 3: GPC-3 and the canonical Wnt or HH signaling pathway. The Wnt or HH signal transduction cascade controls myriad biological phenomena throughout hepatoma development. In parallel, aberrant Wnt or HH signaling underlies a wide range of pathologies in human hepatoma. Active Wnt or HH signaling rearranges these complexes, the former with stimulatory effect and latter with inhibitory effect. In the inactive state, β-catenin levels are kept low through interactions with the protein kinases GSK-3 and the scaffolding protein axin. β-catenin is degraded after phosphorylation by GSK-3 through the ubiquitin pathway.

response of most patients to this treatment is very limited, and it remains a chanllenge mainly due to a lack of specific targets (El-Serag HB, *et al.,* 2012; Tang YH, *et al.,* 2012; Cao H, *et al.,* 2012).

The expressions of GPC-3 were checked among the hepatoma SMMC-7721, MHCC-97H, Bel-7402, PLC/PRF/5, HepG2, Hep3B, and Bel-7404 cells, and the HepG2 or Hep3B cells not only with predominant GPC-3 but also higher effectively miRNA transfection After the HepG2 or Hep3B cells transfected with four kinds of different miRNA (Figure 4), the remarkably down-regulation of GPC-3 at the level of mRNA or protein, and the proliferations of HepG2 or Hep3B cells *in intro* were obviously inhibited by the most effective miRNA$_1$ in a

(A)

(B)

(C)

(C1)

(C2)

(C3)

(C4)

(D1)

(D2)

(D3)

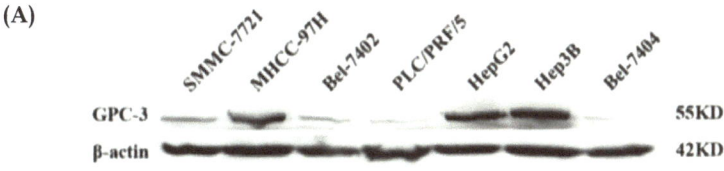

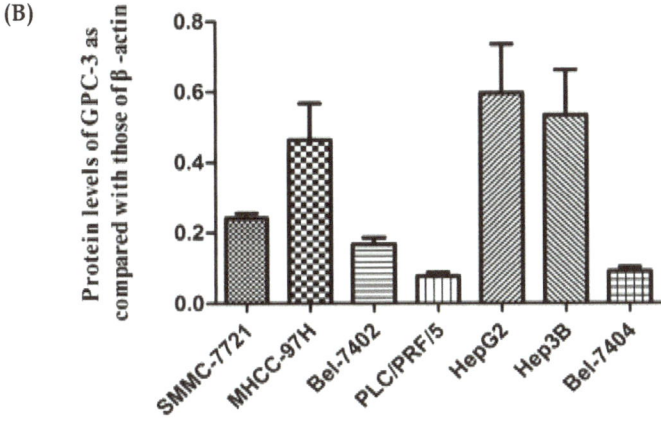

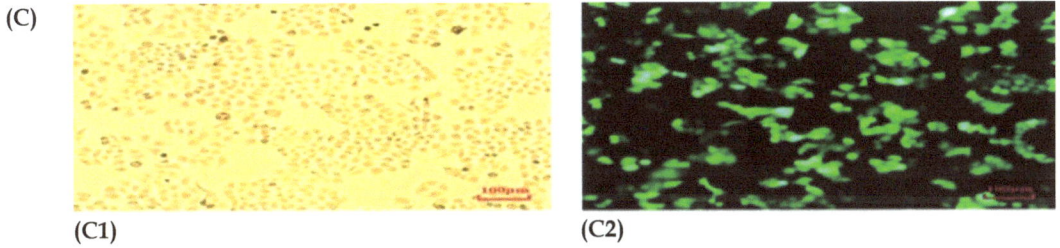

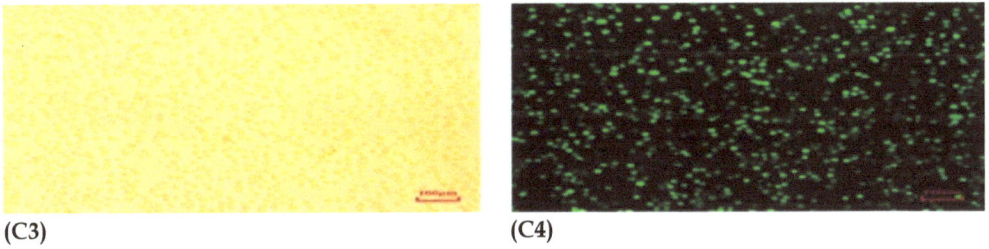

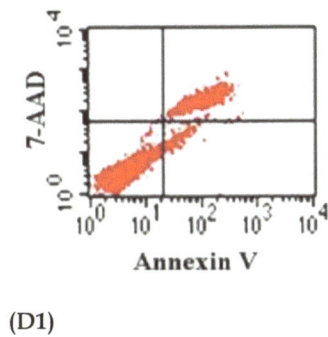

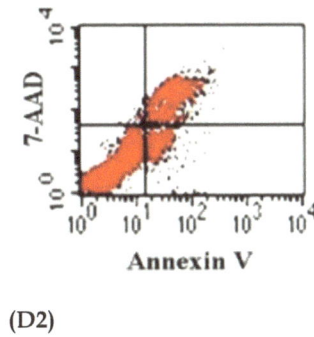

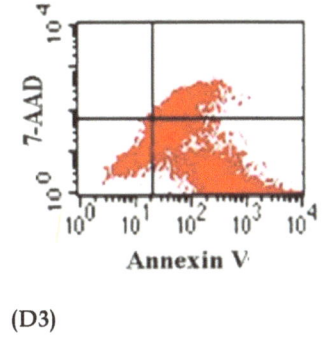

Continued on next page…

...continued from previous page

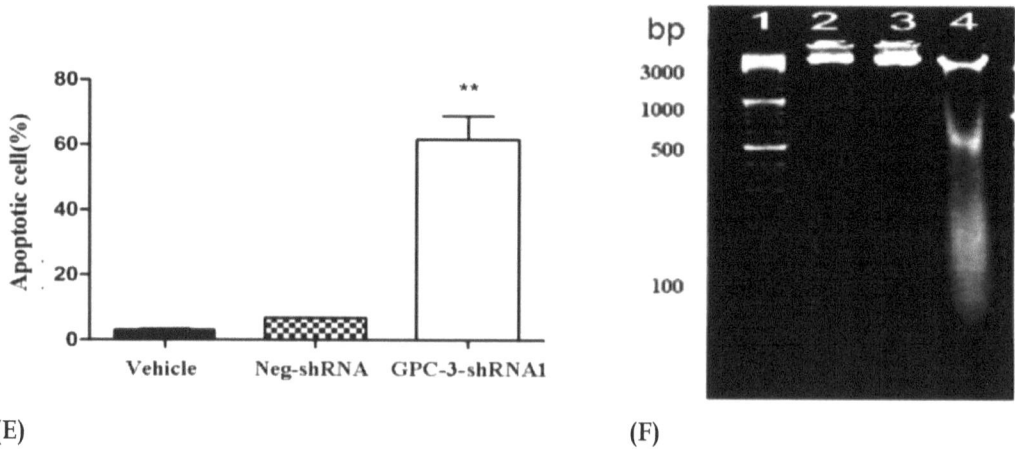

(E)   (F)

Figure 4: GPC-3 expressions among hepatoma cells, miRNA transfection and hepatoma apoptosis. A: the GPC-3 expression among 7 kinds of hepatoma cells at protein level; **B**: the ratio of GPC-3 to correspondence β-actin, the relative level of the band intensities were estimated by the Quantity One Program (Bio-Rad, USA) with the results were expressed as mean ± SD values (n = 3); **C1 & C2**: the phase contrast or fluorescence photomicrographs in the same vision field of the HepG2 cells transfected with GPC-3-miRNA at 48 h; **C3 & C4**: the phase contrast or fluorescence photo- micrographs in the same vision field of the Hep3B cells transfected with GPC-3- miRNA at 48 h; Scale bar, 100 μm. **D**: apoptosis increasing after HepG2 cells transfected with shRNA$_1$. the number of apoptotic cells of the knockdown group (**D3**) was significantly higher than the negative (**D2**) or control group (**D1**); **E:** the number of cells with nuclear morphological features of apoptosis was counted after staining with Hoechest 33342. Data are expressed as percentage of apoptotic cells based on counting 100 cells in randomly selected fields. Data are from three separate experiments (mean ± SD). **F**: DNA was extracted and DNA-ladder electrophoresis assay was used to detect the apoptosis.*1*, DNA marker; *2*, the control group; *3*, the negative-shRNA; and *4*, the shRNA1 group. When the cells were apoptosis, the DNA was degaradated and the DNA-ladder would be detected on the agarose gel electrophoresis. **$P<0.01$.

time-dependent manner, especially enhancing inhibitory effects in serum-free culture. Specific Specific GPC-3shRNA might intervene effectively GPC-3 gene transcription and inhibit HCC cell proliferation by promoting apoptosis mechanism, suggesting that GPC-3 should be a po tential molecular target for HCC gene therapy (Finn RS, *et al.*, 2009; Wang L, *et al.*, 2014; Yu DD, *et al.*, 2013).

The alterations of cell cycle in the miRNA group at the G$_1$ phase arrest with the occurrence of cell apoptosis in Hep3B cells. The expressions of cell cycle regulators CyclinD1 was also significantly down-regulated, the silencing GPC-3 could mediate the cell cycle progression through modulation of CyclinD1, caused G$_1$ arrest, thereby contributing to cell proliferation inhibition. The aggressive viability of HCC is generally viewed as one of the most essential factors during metastasis process, and results in recurrence or poor prognosis of HCC. the ability of hepatoma cells to survive was observed in an anchorage-independent manner is critical after transfected with miRNA$_1$, the colony-forming capacities of HepG2 or Hep3B cells were significantly inhibited not only in plates but also in soft agar anchorage- independent manner, indicted that intervening *GPC-3* gene transcription *in vitro* could suppress hepatoma cell migration and invasion (Broderick JA, *et al.*, 2011; Xu C, *et al.*, 2011).

8 Down-regulating GPC-3 Inhibiting Hepatoma Growth

GPC-3 is specifically over-expressed in hepatoma and a valuable molecular target for HCC. The percentage of the transfected cell proliferation inhibition was 71.1% in the shRNA group, and 80.1% in the shRNA plus sorafenib (100 μM/L) group, respectively (Yu DD, *et al.*, 2013; Capurro MI, *et al.*, 2005; Nakano K, *et al.*, 2009).

The cell cycles were arrested in the G_1 phase from 42.4% up to 65.6%, and its apoptosis rate was increasing from 6.92% to 66.75% in the neg-shRNA group compared with in the shRNA1 group. The xenograft models are commonly used in the tumor researches, because of its convenient operation, high success rate, short latent period, and easy to dynamic monitoring tumor angiogenesis. After the nude mice injected with the stable HepG2 cells with miR-NA1, the average time or volumes of tumor-forming in the miRNA group were significantly longer or smaller ($P < 0.01$) than those in the untreated or miRNA-neg group, and no significant difference was found between the neg-miRNA and the untreated group.

Silencing *GPC-3* in HepG2 cells effected the pathological alteration and tumor growth with β-catenin, p-GSK3β, and CyclinD1 expressions significantly decreased, and consistent with *in vitro* studies. Immunohistochemical analysis confirmed that down-regulating GPC-3 with miRNA could significantly decrease ($P < 0.01$) the β-catenin, p-GSK3β, and CyclinD1 expressions (Figure 5) compared with that in the miRNA-neg or untreated group. The β-catenin and GSK3β not only plays the important roles in regulating metabolism, transcription, embryonic development, and other processes, but also served the key roles in the Wnt/β-catenin inducing GSK3β phosphorylation results in the dissolution of the complex responsible for the degradation of β-catenin; Consequently, β-catenin accumulates in cytosol and is subsequently translocated into nucleus, increasing Tcf/Lef transcription and up-regulating CyclinD1 and c-Myc genes should promote cell cycle progression and stimulating cell proliferation.

9 Conclusions

In conclusion, the specific miRNA was successfully used to interfering GPC-3 expression in hepatoma cells with the viability alteration, proliferation inhibition, decreasing migration or invasion, and promoting apoptosis. As an oncofetal antigen GPC-3 promotes the HCC development through the up-regulation of Wnt/β-catenin signaling pathway that should provide new mechanism insight into molecular-targeted therapy for HCC. The up-regulations of the key molecules, CyclinD1, β-catenin and GSK3β, stimulate hepatoma cell proliferation. The present data confirmed that intervening GPC-3 gene by miRNA should inhibit HCC cell proliferation *in vitro* or hepatoma growth *in vivo* through the Wnt/β-catenin pathway, suggesting that GPC-3 gene should be a novel therapeutic target for HCC (Gailhouste L, *et al.*, 2013; Berger F, *et al.*, 2013). Further work should be explored combination of miRNA plus multi-targeting strategies for HCC effective therapy.

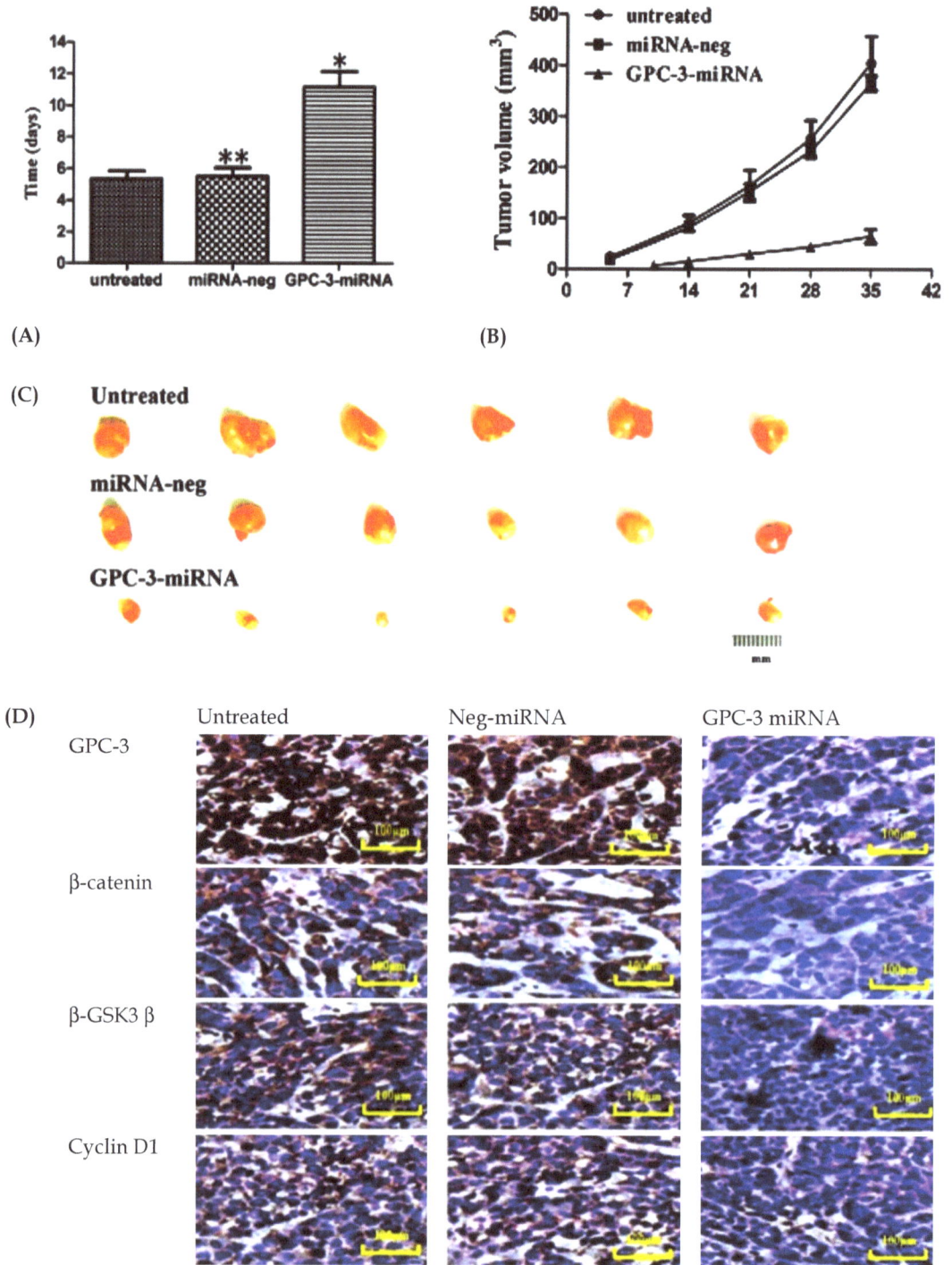

Figure 5: Silencing *GPC-3* inhibited the growth of nude mice xenograft tumors. A: the forming times of the xenograft tumors after nude mice injected the stable HepG2 cells with miRNA plasmids; **B:** the comparative analysis of the nude mice xenograft tumor volumes and the forming cause in the

continued on next page…

...continued from previous page

different group, and the data were expressed as mean ± SD (n = 6); **C:** the dissected hepatoma xenograft tumors and the actual tumor sizes in the different group; **D:** The immunohistochemical analysis of the related molecules (GPC-3, β-catenin, p-GSK3β and cyclinD1) in the Wnt/β-catenin pathway or cell proliferation *in vivo*. Representative images are shown. Scale bar, 100 μm. **GPC-3-miRNA**: the HepG2 cells stable transfected with miRNA$_1$; **miRNA-neg**: the HepG2 cells stable transfected with miRNA-neg plasmid; and **untreated**: the HepG2 cells without any transfected as a control. Compared with the untreated group, * $P < 0.01$, ** $P > 0.05$.

Abbreviations

FQ-RT-PCR, fluorescence quantitative reverse transcriptase-polymerase chain reaction; **GGT**, γ-glutamyl transferase; **GPC-3**, glypican-3; **HCC**, hepatocellular carcinoma; **HH**, hedgehog signaling pathway; **miRNA**, microRNA; **PBMC**, peripheral blood mononuclear cells; **shRNA**, short hairpin RNA; **VEGF**, vascular endothelial growth factor; and **Wnt**, Wnt/β-catenin signaling pathway.

Acknowledgments

This work was supported in part by the Grants from the Projects of Jiangsu Medical Science (2013-WSW-011, 2014-YY-028, and Qinglan Program), the Nantong Undertaking and Technological Innovation (H2014078), the Post-doctor Scientific Funds (2013M53139, JS2012- 468), and the International S&T Cooperation Program (2013DFA32150) of China.

References

Berger, F., & Reiser, M. F., (2013). *Micro-RNAs as potential new molecular biomarkers in oncology: have they reached relevance for the clinical imaging sciences? Theranostics, 3: 943-952 [PMID: 24396505]*

Broderick, J. A., & Zamore, P. D. (2011). *MicroRNA therapeutics. Gene therapy, 18: 1104 -1110 [PMID: 21525952]*

Bruix, J., Gores, G. J., & Mazzaferro, V. (2014). *Hepatocellular carcinoma: clinical frontiers and perspectives. Gut, 63(5): 844-885 [PMID: 24531850]*

Cao, H., Phan, H., & Yang, L. X. (2012). *Improved chemotherapy for hepatocellular carcinoma. Anticancer Res, 32: 1379-1386 [PMID: 22493374]*

Capurro, M., Wanless, I. R., Sherman, M., Deboer, G., Shi, W., Miyoshi, E., & Filmus, J. (2003). *Glypican-3: a novel serum and histochemical marker for hepatocellular carcinoma. Gastroenterology, 125: 89-97 [PMID: 12851874]*

Capurro, M. I., Xiang, Y. Y., Lobe, C., & Filmus, J. (2005). *Glypican-3 promotes the growth of hepatocellular carcinoma by stimulating canonical Wnt-signaling. Cancer Res, 65: 6245-6254. [PMID: 16024626]*

Cheng, W., Tseng, C. J., Lin, T. T., Cheng, I., Pan, H. W., Hsu, H. C., et al., (2008). *Glypican-3-mediated oncogenesis involves the insulin-like growth factor- signaling pathway. Carcinogenesis, 29: 1319-1326. [PMID: 18413366]*

Clevers, H., & Nusse, R. (2012). *Wnt/β-catenin signaling and disease. Cell, 149: 1192- 1205[PMID: 22682243]*

El-Serag, H. B. (2012). *Epidemiology of viral hepatitis and hepatocellular carcinoma. Gastroenterology, 142: 1264-1273[PMID: 22537432]*

El-Serag, H.B. (2011). *Hepatocellular carcinoma. N Engl J Med, 365(12): 1118– 1127 [PMID: 21992124]*

Filmus, J., & Capurro, M. (2008). *The role of glypican-3 in the regulation of body size and cancers Cell Cycle, 7: 2787-2790. [PMID: 18787398]*

Finn, R. S., & Zhu, A. X. (2009). *Targeting angiogenesis in hepatocellular carcinoma: focus on VEGF and bevacizumab. Expert Rev Anticancer Ther, 9: 503-509 [PMID: 19374603]*

Gailhouste, L., & Ochiya, T. (2013). *Cancer-related microRNAs and their role as tumor suppressors and oncogenes in hepatocellular carcinoma. Histol Histopathol, 28: 437-451 [PMID: 23224781]*

Hayashi, E., Kuramitsu, Y., Okada, F., Fujimoto, M., Zhang, X., Kobayashi, M., et al., (2005). *Protoemics profiling for cancer progression differential display analysis for the expression of intracellular proteins between regressive and progressive cancer cell lines. Proteomics, 5: 1024-1032. [PMID: 15712240]*

Imbeaud, S., Ladeiro, Y., & Zucman-Rossi, J. (2010). *Identification of novel oncogenes and tumor suppressors in hepatocellular carcinoma. Semin Liver Dis, 30: 75-86. [PMID: 20175035]*

Jain, S., Singhal, S., Lee, P., & Xu, R. (2010). *Molecular genetics of hepatocellular neoplasia. Am J Transl Res, 2: 105-118. [PMID: 20182587]*

Jemal, A., Bray, F., Center, M.M., Ferlay, J., Ward, E., & Forman, D. (2011). *Global cancer statistics. CA Cancer J Clin, 61: 69-90 [PMID: 21296855]*

Kwack, M. H., Choi, B. Y., & Sung, Y. K. (2006). *Cellular changes resulting from forced expression of glypican-3 in hepatocellular carcinoma cells. Mol Cells, 21: 224-228. [PMID: 16682817]*

Libbrecht, L., Severi, T., Cassiman, D., Vander, Borght, S., Pirenne, J., Nevens, F., et al., (2006). *Glypican-3 expression distinguishes small hepatocellular carcinomas from cirrhosis, dysplastic nodules, and focal nodular hyperplasia-like nodules. Am J Surg Pathol, 30: 1405-1411. [PMID: 17063081]*

Llovet, J. M., & Bruix, J. (2008). *Molecular targeted therapies in hepatocellular carcinoma. Hepatology, 48: 1312-1317. [PMID: 18821591]*

Maluccio, M., & Covey, A. (2012). *Recent progress in understanding, diagnosing, and treating hepatocellular carcinoma CA Cancer J Clin, 62(6): 394-399 [PMID: 23070690]*

Morford, L. A., Davis, C., Jin, L., Dobierzewska, A., Peterson, M. L., & Spear, B. T. (2007). *The oncofetal gene glypican-3 is regulated in the postnatal liver by zine fingers and homeoboxes 2 and in the regenerating liver by alpha-fetoprotein regulator 2. Hepatology, 46: 1541-1547. [PMID: 17668883]*

Nakano, K., Orita, T., Nezu, J., Yoshino, T., Ohizumi, I., Sugimoto, M., et al., (2009). *Anti- glypican 3 antibodies cause ADCC against human hepatocellular carcinoma cells. Biochem Biophy Res Commun, 378: 279-284. [PMID: 19022220]*

Pang, R. W., Joh, J. W., Johnson, P. J., Monden, M., Pawlik, T. M., & Poon, R. T. (2008). *Biology of hepatocellular carcinoma. Ann Surg Oncol, 15: 962-971. [PMID: 18236113]*

Qian, J., Yao, D., Dong, Z., Wu, W., Qiu, L., Yao, N., et al., (2010). *Characteristics of hepatic igf-ii expression and monitored levels of circulating igf-ii mRNA in metastasis of hepatocellular carcinoma. Am J Clin Pathol, 134: 799-806. [PMID: 20959664]*

Qu, K. Z., Zhang, K., Li, H., Afdhal, N. H., & Albitar, M. (2011). *Circulating microRNAs as biomarkers for hepatocellular carcinoma. J Clin Gastroenterol, 45(4): 355-360 [PMID: 21278583]*

Rehem, R. N., & El-Shikh, W. M. (2011). *Serum IGF-1, IGF-2 and IGFBP-3 as parameters in the assessment of liver dysfunction in patients with hepatic cirrhosis and in the diagnosis of hepatocellular carcinoma. Hepatogastroenterology, 58: 949-954. [PMID: 21830422]*

Saffroy, R., Pham, P., Reffas, M., Takka, M., Lemoine, A., & Debuire, B. (2007). *New perspectives and strategy research biomarkers for hepatocellular carcinoma. Clin Chem Lab Med, 45: 1169-1179. [PMID: 17635075]*

Saleh, H. A., Aulicino, M., Zaidi, S. Y., Khan, A. Z., & Masood, S. (2009). *Discriminating hepato- cellular carcinoma from metastatic carcinoma on fine-needle aspiration biopsy of the liver: the utility of immunocytochemical panel. Diagn Cytopathol, 37: 184-190. [PMID: 19170172]*

Shafizadeh, N., Ferrell, L. D., & Kakar, S. (2008). *Utility and limitations of glypican-3 expression for the diagnosis of hepatocellular carcinoma at both ends of the differentiation spectrum. Mod Pathol, 21: 1011-1018. [PMID: 18536657]*

Stigliano, I., Puricelli, L., Filmus, J., Sogayar, M. C., Balde, Kier, Joffé, E., & Peters, M. G. (2009). Glypican-3 regulates migration, adhesion, and actin cytoskeleton organization in mammary cells through Wnt signaling modulation. Breast Cancer Res Treat, 114: 251-262. [PMID: 18404367]

Tang, Y. H., Wen, T. F., & Chen, X. (2012). Resection margin in hepatectomy for hepatocellular carcinoma: a systematic review. Hepatogastroenterology, 59: 1393-1397 [PMID: 22683956]

Tyson, G. L., Duan, Z., Kramer, J. R., Davila. J. A., Richardson, P. A., & El-Serag, H. B. (2011). Level of α-fetoprotein predicts mortality among patients with hepatitis C-related hepatocellular carcinoma.Clin Gastroenterol Hepatol, 9: 989-894 [PMID: 21820396]

Wang, H. L., Anatelli, F., Zhai, Q. J., Adley, B., Chuang, S. T., & Yang, X. J. (2008). Glypican-3 as a useful diagnostic marker that distinguishes hepatocellular carcinoma from benign hepatocellular mass lesions. Arch Pathol Lab Med, 132: 1723-1728. [PMID: 18976006]

Wang, L., Yao, M., Dong, Z., Zhang, Y., & Yao, D. (2014). Circulating specific biomarkers in diagnosis of hepatocellular carcinoma and its metastasis monitoring. Tumor Biol, 35: 9-20. [PMID: 24006223]

Welzel, T. M., Graubard, B. I., Quraishi, S., Zeuzem, S., Davila, J. A., El-Serag, H. B., & McGlynn, K. A. (2013). Population-attributable fractions of risk factors for hepatocellular carcinoma in the United States Am J Gastroenterol, 108: 1314-1321. [PMID: 23752878]

Xu, C., Lee, S. A., & Chen, X. (2011). RNA interference as therapeutics for hepatocellular carcinoma. Recent Pat Anticancer Drug Discov, 6: 106-115[PMID: 21110827]

Yao, M., Yao, D. F., Bian, Y. Z., Zhang, C. G., Qiu, L. W., Wu, W., Sai, W. L., Yang, J. L., & Zhang, H. J. (2011). Oncofetal antigen glypican-3 as a promising early diagnostic marker for hepatocellular carcinoma Hepatobiliary Pancreat Dis Int, 10: 289-294 [PMID: 21669573]

Yao, M., Yao, D. F., Bian, Y. Z., Wu, W., Yan, X. D., Yu, D. D., Qiu, L. W., Yang, J. L., Zhang, H. J., Sai, W. L., & Chen, J. (2013). Values of circulating GPC-3 mRNA and alpha-fetoprotein in detecting patients with hepatocellular carcinoma Hepatobiliary Pancreat Dis Int, 12(2): 171-179.

Yu, D. D., Dong, Z. Z., Yao, M., Wu, W., Yan, M. J., Yan, X. D., Qiu, L. W., Chen, J., Sai, W. L., & Yao, D. F. (2013). Targeted glypican-3 gene transcription inhibited the proliferation of human hepatoma cells by specific short hairpin RNA. Tumor Biol, 34: 661-668. [PMID: 23192642]

Yamauchi, N., Watanabe, A., Hishinuma, M., Ohashi, K., Midorikawa, Y., Morishita, Y., et al., (2005). The glypican 3 oncofetal protein is a promising diagnostic marker for hepatocellular carcinoma. Mod Pathol, 18: 1591-1598. [PMID: 15920546]

Yang, J. D., & Roberts, L. R. (2012). Hepatocellular carcinoma: a global view. Nat Rev Gastroenterol Hepatol, 7: 449-458. [PMID: 20628345]

Yao, D. F., Dong, Z. Z., & Yao, M. (2007). Specific molecular markers in hepatocellular carcinoma. Hepatobiliary Pancreatic Dis Int, 6: 220-226. [PMID: 17548245]

Yao, D. F,, Jiang, D. R., Huang, Z. W., Lu, J. X., Tao, Q. Y., Yu, Z. J,, et al., (2000). Abnormal expression of hepatoma specific gamma-glutamyl transferase and alteration of gamma-glutamyl transferase gene methylation status in patients with hepatocellular carcinoma. Cancer, 88:761-769. [PMID: 10679644]

Oral Cavity Cancer:
Literature Review and Current Management

Rodrigo Arrangoiz*, Fernando Cordera*, Manuel Munoz-Juarez*,
Eduardo Moreno Paquetin* and Enrique Luque-de-Leon*

1 Introduction

In 2014, it is estimated that about 55,070 new cases of head and neck cancers will occur, which represent approximately 3% to 5% of all cancers in the United States (Society, 2014; Siegel R *et al.*, 2014). During the same time period it is estimated that there will be approximately 12,000 deaths (Society, 2014; Siegel R *et al.*, 2014). Incidence rates are more than twice as high in men as in women (Society, 2014). From 2006 to 2010 incidence rates remained stable in men and have decreased by 0.9% per year in women (Society, 2014). Death rates have been decreasing over the past three decades; from 2006 to 2010, rates decreased by 1.2% per year in men and by 2.1% per year in women (Society, 2014).

Most head and neck cancers present with metastatic disease at the time of diagnosis, with regional nodal involvement and distant metastatic disease in 43% and 10% of the cases, respectively (Ridge, 2013). It is estimated that there will be 42,440 new cases of cancer of the oral cavity and pharynx (30,220 men, 12,220 women) (Table 1) in 2014 (Society, 2014).

	Estimated New Cases	Estimated Deaths
Oral Cavity and Pharynx	42,440 (M: 30,220; F: 12,220)	8390 (M: 5,730; F: 2,660)
Tongue	13,590 (M: 9,720; F: 3,870)	2,150 (M: 1,450; F: 700)
Floor of the Mouth	11,920 (M: 7,150; F: 4,770)	2,070 (M: 1,130; F: 940)
Other site of the oral cavity	2,520 (M: 1,800; F: 720)	1,630 (M: 1,250; F: 380)

Table 1: Estimated New Cases and Mortality for the Year 2014 in the United States.

Patients with head and neck cancers often develop second primary tumors, this is because they share common risk factors (Day and Blot, 1992). These tumors develop at an annual rate of 3% to 7% and 50% to 75% of these new cancers are located in upper aero digestive tract or lungs (Ridge, 2013).

The boundaries of the oral cavity are:

- Superior border - from the vermillion border to the junction of the hard and soft palates.
- Inferior border - from the vermillion border to the circumvallate papillae of the oral tongue.
- The lateral border - is the mucosa of the mouth up to the anterior tonsilar pillars.

* Surgical Oncology Department, American British Cowdray Medical Center, Mexico

The oral cavity includes the lips, buccal mucosa, upper and lower alveolar ridges, gingiva, retromolar trigone, floor of mouth, hard palate and the anterior two thirds of the tongue ("oral tongue"). The main lymphatic drainage is to level IA (submental triangle), IB (submandibular triangle) and II (upper deep jugular nodes) (Lindberg, 1972).

The oral cavity is continuously been exposed to inhaled and consumed carcinogens, and thus it is the most common site for the origin of malignant epithelial neoplasms in the head and neck region. Known carcinogens in the oral cavity include those present in tobacco, alcohol, and betel nuts. The association of human papilloma virus (HPV) with oral cancer is not as well established as in oropharyngeal cancers. Primary tumors of the oral cavity may arise from the surface epithelium, minor salivary glands, submucosal soft tissue, and tumors of dento-alveolar origin. More than 90% of cancers in the oral cavity are squamous cell in origin and we will be focusing our review on these neoplasms.

2   Epidemiology

Cancer of the oral cavity is by far more common in men than in women (66% to 95% of cases) (Society, 2014). The incidence by gender varies depending on the anatomic location and has been changing due to the increase in the number of women who smoke. The male to female ratio is currently 3:1 (Society, 2014). The incidence of oral cavity cancer increases with age, especially after age 50. Most patients are between 50 and 70 years but can also occur in younger patients (Ridge, 2013).

There are large differences in the incidence of oral cavity cancer among different geographical regions. The highest incidence of this disease is found in Asia and is believed to reflect the prevalence of certain risk factors, such as chewing betel nut (Ho *et al.*, 2002) and the use of smokeless tobacco (snuff) (Boffetta *et al.*, 2008). In the United States, in urban areas the high incidence among men is thought to reflect exposure to snuff and alcohol. Among women in rural areas in the United States the increase risk of oral cavity cancer is associated with the use of smokeless tobacco (snuff) (Society, 2014).

3   Etiology and Risk Factors

One of the most important risk factors for the development of squamous cell carcinoma (SCC) of the oral cavity is tobacco. Smoking cigarettes, cigars, or pipes; chewing tobacco; and using snuff are the single largest risk factors for head and neck cancer. Eighty-five percent (85%) of head and neck cancers are linked to tobacco use (Secretan *et al.*, 2009; Gandini *et al.*, 2008). Secondhand smoke may also increase a person's risk of developing a head and neck cancer (Program *et al.*, 2005).

Patients often make the mistake to think that cigar smoking is less of a risk factor to ones health than smoking cigarettes. This is not true, based on epidemiologic studies, cigar smoking is important risk factors for oral cavity tumors and the only difference between cigarette smoking and cigar smoking is that it instigates a change in the usual anatomic location for these tumors (Society, 2014; Shapiro *et al.*, 2000). The use of smokeless tobacco is also associated with an increased incidence of cancer of the oral cavity (Siegel R *et al.*, 2014; Society,

2014). Chewing snuff is the leading cause of SCC of the oral cavity and oropharynx in India, part of Southeast Asia, China, and Taiwan, especially when consumed with betel containing areca nut (Znaor *et al.*, 2003). Users of smokeless snuff frequently develop premalignant lesions such as oral leukoplakia. Over time, these lesions may progress to invasive carcinomas. The prevalence of active smoking is associated with a significant increase in the risk of developing a second primary tumor (compared with former smokers or people who have never smoked) (Browman *et al.*, 1993).

Alcohol by itself is a risk factor for the development of oral cavity cancer, although it is less potent carcinogen than tobacco (Hashibe *et al.*, 2006, 2007). For people who use tobacco and alcohol, these risk factors appear to be synergistic and result in a multiplicative increase in risk, 30 to 36 times higher for people who smoke and drink heavily (Hashibe *et al.*, 2009).

Poor oral hygiene and edentulous patients can be risk factors for cancer of the oral cavity (Graham *et al.*, 1977; Guha *et al.*, 2007). The use of mouthwashes that have high alcohol content could be a risk factor for oral cavity SCC (but has not been proven) (Guha *et al.*, 2007; Wynder *et al.*, 1983). The consumption of mate, a tea beverage usually consumed by South Americans, has been associated with an increased risk of cancer of the oral cavity (Barnes, 2005) .

Epidemiologic studies suggest that the intake of vitamin A, -carotene, and -tocopherol may reduce the risk of developing oral cavity cancers (Benner *et al.*, 1993; Contreras Vidaurre *et al.*, 2001; Goldenberg *et al.*, 2003; Hong *et al.*, 1986; Lippman *et al.*, 1994; Smith *et al.*, 1992). Exposure to ultraviolet (UV) light is a risk factor for the development of cancer of the lip (Abreu *et al.*, 2009; Lindqvist & Teppo, 1978). Approximately 33 % of patients with lip cancer have outdoor occupations (Abreu *et al.*, 2009). Research suggests that people who have used marijuana may be at higher risk for head and neck cancer (Rosenblatt *et al.*, 2004), but the degree of risk is unknown (Rosenblatt *et al.*, 2004).

People with certain syndromes caused by inherited defects (mutations) in certain genes have a very high risk of developing cancer of the oral cavity and pharynx. Fanconi anemia is a disease that can be caused by inherited defects in several genes that contribute to DNA repair. People with this syndrome often have hematologic problems an early age, which can lead to leukemia or aplastic anemia. They also have a risk of developing cancer of the oral cavity (Gasparini *et al.*, 2006; Lustig *et al.*, 1995). Dyskeratosis congenita is a genetic syndrome that can cause aplastic anemia, skin rashes, and nail abnormalities of the hands and feet; they also increase the risk of developing oral cavity cancer (Alter *et al.*, 2009; Greer & Goldman, 1974).

4   Mechanism of Carcinogenesis

The development of oral cavity SCC is a multistep progression that involves changes related to specific genes, epigenetic events, and signal transduction within the cell (Tanaka *et al.*, 2011). Tobacco smoke contains agents that may act as mutagens. Also, tobacco smoke extract has been shown to activate the epidermal growth factor receptor (EGFR) in vitro and EGFR activation has been shown, in turn, to increase the production of prostaglandins, including PGE2 which may act in a positive feedback fashion by increasing EGFR signal transduction. Cyclin-D1 is frequently overexpressed in head and neck cancer and increased cyclin-D1 activity is a downstream event triggered by EGFR activation (Sasahira *et al.*, 2014).

Genetic alterations that are present early in the course of carcinogenesis are mutations or deletions of chromosome 3p and 9p. Telomerase activation also occurs early in carcinogenesis. Mutations or deletions at chromosome 17p (involving the p53 tumor suppressor gene), and chromosome 13q and chromosome 18q generally are seen later in the process. Patients whose tumors contain HPV mRNA have a significantly lower rate of deletions of chromosomes 3p, 9p, and 17p, suggesting an alternate molecular mechanism in these patients. The viral proteins E6 and E7 have been shown to cause deregulation of the cell cycle by inactivating p53 and retinoblastoma protein, which may be the mechanism of HPV-mediated carcinogenesis (Tornesello *et al.*, 2014).

An important epigenetic event in the progression to cancer is the silencing of gene promoter regions through hypermethylation (Arantes *et al.*, 2014), which has been shown to affect the tumor suppressor's p16, DAP-kinase, and E-cadherin. Also, the gene for retinoic acid receptor-beta (RAR-beta) is silenced by methylation of its promoter (Olasz *et al.*, 2007).

In addition to deletions or mutations of individual genes, evidence exists demonstrating that numeric chromosomal imbalances, known as aneuploidy, may be a cause rather than a consequence of malignant transformation (Garcia Martinez *et al.*, 2014). Aneuploidy may occur as a result of mutations in genes controlling chromosome segregation during mitosis and centrosome abnormalities.

5   Diagnosis

The need for a rapid diagnosis and referral of patients to a skilled physician with expertise in the management of tumors of the head and neck is very important because early diagnosis can lead to a reduction in mortality (Ridge *et al.*, 2013). The risk factors mention on the etiology section of this paper, including history of tobacco and alcohol use should be interrogated. Any adult patient with symptoms attributable to the upper aero digestive tract lasting more than 2 weeks or an asymptomatic cervical (neck) tumor should undergo a full examination with a high index of suspicion for malignancy (Ridge *et al.*, 2013).

The physical examination is the best way to detect lesions of the upper aero digestive tract. Often the initial assessment also indicates the severity and chronicity of the disease. Due to the frequent occurrence of synchronous primary tumors in patients with head and neck cancers (approximately 5%), a careful evaluation of the entire upper aero digestive tract is required at the time of diagnosis (Erkal *et al.*, 2001).

Oral cavity cancers usually cause symptoms related to the upper aero digestive tract, including changes in swallowing, speech, hearing and breathing: During the interrogation the physician must give emphasis to the following symptoms: epiphora, dysphagia, odynophagia, globus sensation, dysphonia (hoarseness), changes in the ability to form words, epistaxis, ear pain, hemoptysis, otic fullness, and trismus (Table 2). A complete physical examination should be performed on every patient with specific emphasis on the head and neck exam (inspection, palpation, otoscopic exam, indirect laryngoscopy, and when indicated nasopharyngolaryngoscopy) and a neurological exam with emphasis on cranial nerves V, through XII.

The most common presenting complaint of patients with oral cavity tumors is a sore in the mouth or on the lips. Bleeding from the surface of the lesion is a characteristic of malignancy and immediately raises suspicion for a neoplastic process. When patients present with nasal obstruction we should suspect of a lesion originating in the hard palate that has extended to involve the maxillary antrum or nasal cavity. Mal occlusion or trismus is another symptom and sign that is usually seen when an oral cavity tumor has extended to involve structures of the oropharynx or has invaded the pterygoid muscles. Middle ear effusion is usually seen when a tumor has invaded the nasopharynx or has invaded the tensor veli palatini muscle. Absence of corneal reflex is seen when the lesion invades the maxillary division of the trigeminal nerve (CN V). Atrophy of the masseter or temporalis muscle is seen when the tumor involves the mandibular division of the trigeminal nerve (CN V) (Ridge *et al.*, 2013).

Epiphora	Oral cavity pain
Sialorrhea	Non-healing ulcerated lesion
Xerophthalmia	Halitosis
Xerostomia	Ill-fitting dentures
Dysphagia	Nasal Obstruction
Odynophagia	Middle ear effusion
Globus sensation	Mal occlusion
Dysphonia	Atrophy of the masseter muscle
Difficulty articulating words	Atrophy of the temporalis muscle
Epistaxis	Decrease tongue mobility
Hemoptysis	Absence of corneal reflex
Otalgia	

Table 2: Symptoms and Signs of Head and Neck Cancer.

Approximately one third of the patients come in to the office with a neck lump (de Braud & al-Sarraf, 1993). Cancer of the oral mucosa may present as an indurated ulcer with raised edges (Figure 1) or as an exophytic growth (Figure 2). SCC of the floor of the mouth may manifest as a red or ulcerated lesion or as a papillary growth (Figure 3). Gingival cancer usually presents as an ulcer or proliferative growth. Tongue cancer may appear as an infiltrating ulcer and may haves decreased mobility. Cancer of the hard palate often presents as an exophytic papillary growth.

The differential diagnosis of SCC of the oral cavity includes other malignant tumors such as minor salivary gland neoplasms (Figure 4), mesenchymal tumors (sarcomas), melanoma, and lymphoma. Systemic diseases like, pyogenic granuloma, tuberculosis, aphthous ulcers, canker sores, and other benign tumors of the oral cavity may mimic a SCC of the oral cavity. Benign lesions include papilloma's (Figure 5) and keratoacanthomas, which can be exophytic or infiltrative. The exophytic lesions are less aggressive, the infiltrative papillomas and keratoacanthomas are associated with destruction of adjacent tissues and may progress to malignancy.

Biopsy of the primary tumor can often be performed in the office or as an outpatient surgery depending on the anatomic site and patient preference. One can perform the biopsy in the office setting using a punch biopsy or using biopsy forceps (Figure 6). The biopsy should be obtained from the edge of the lesion, away from areas of obvious necrosis or excess keratinization.

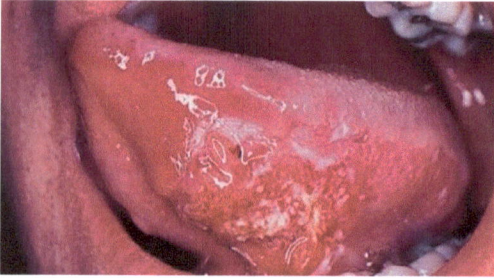

Figure 1: Ulcerated Lesion of the Tongue.

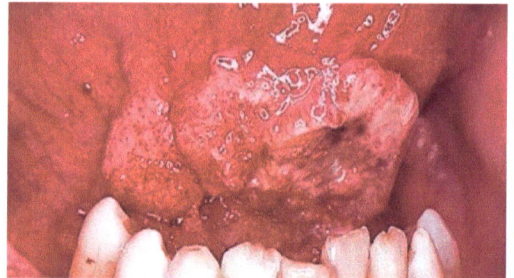

Figure 2: Exophytic Lesion of the Floor of the Mouth.

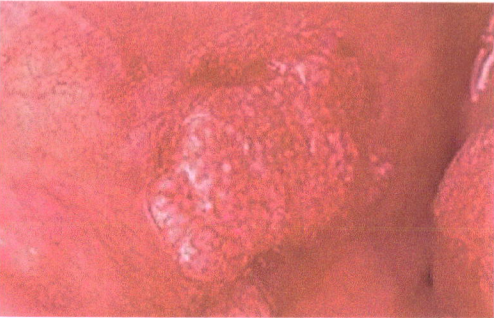

Figure 3: Exophytic Papillary Carcinoma of the Buccal Mucosa.

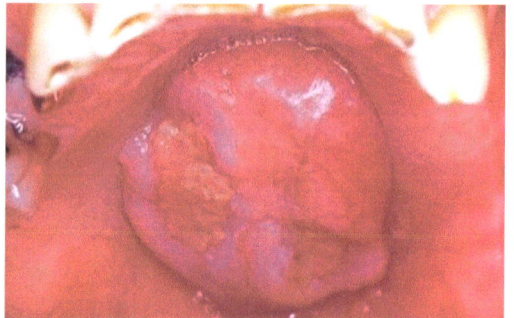

Figure 4: Mucoepidermoid carcinoma of the Palate.

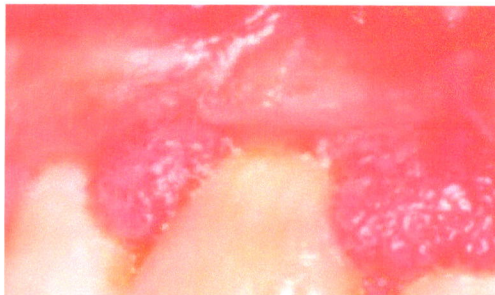

Figure 5: Papilloma.

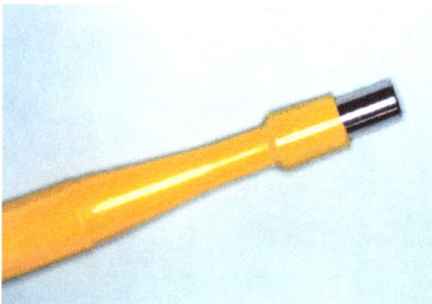

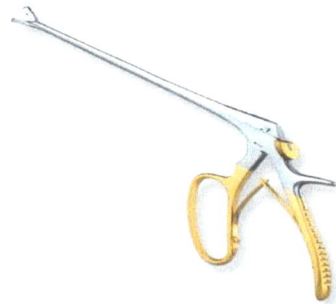

Figure 6: Punch Biopsy and Forceps to Perform the Biopsy.

Fine needle aspiration (FNA) is a useful diagnostic modality (Layfield, 1996; Shaha *et al.*, 1986; Tatomirovic *et al.*, 2009) for differentiating benign from malignant lymph nodes in the neck. A fine gauge needle (#23 gauge) makes multiple passes over the lesion while continues suction is applied. Suction must be released before removing the needle of the lesion. This procedure has a false negative rate of 7% (Tatomirovic *et al.*, 2009). Cytology is particularly useful to distinguish metastatic SCC from other malignant histology's. However, a negative result should not be interpreted as "absence of disease" when the clinical scenario is highly suspicions for malignancy. A core needle biopsy should not be performed in a lump in the neck, with the exception of an already diagnosed lymphoma. Martin Hayes in a communication to the medical profession in general stated "not only to the needlessness but also to the possible harmfulness of excisional lymph node biopsy as the first or even as an early step in the diagnosis of cancer" (Martin, 1961). Open biopsies should be done only when the diagnosis has not been made after extensive clinical evaluation and after at least two non-diagnostic FNA's. The surgeon performing the open biopsy should be prepared to perform a definitive surgical treatment at that moment in time, which may involve a formal neck dissection, if the diagnosis turns out to be a SCC.

Computed tomography (CT) is probably the most informative test in the evaluation of tumors of the oral cavity (Brown & Langdon, 1995). It can help define the extent of disease and the presence and extent of lymph node involvement. CT provides high spatial resolution, can discriminate between fat, muscle, bone and other soft tissues. CT outperforms magnetic resonance imaging (MRI) in detecting bone erosion (Figure 7) (Mukherji *et al.*, 2001), has a sensitivity of 100% and specificity of 85% (Steinkamp *et al.*, 1993). MRI can provide accurate information on the size, location and extent of the tumor involvement of the soft tissues. It is not very reliable to provide information regarding bone extension, unless there is full involvement of the medullary cavity. The MRI has a relatively higher sensitivity than CT but has lower specificity (Brown & Langdon, 1995; Mukherji *et al.*, 2001; Steinkamp *et al.*, 1993; Hao & Ng, 2000). PET has been evaluated in primary and recurrent carcinomas of the head and neck. In a multicenter, prospective study of patients newly diagnosed with a tumor of the head and neck region the results were discrepant when PET was compared with CT in 43% of cases, and the therapeutic plan was altered in 14 % of patients (Lonneux *et al.*, 2010). PET should not be routinely used in the diagnosis or evaluation of patients with early tumors of the oral cavity.

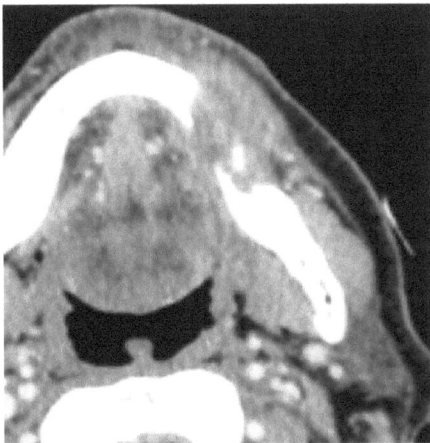

Figure 7: CT of the Head and Neck Showing Bone Erosion.

6   Pathology and Histologic grade of Oral Cavity Tumors

Over 90% of head and neck cancers (including the oral cavity tumors) are SCC. The World Health Organization classifies squamous tumors of the head and neck in different histologic subtypes (Slootweg & Eveson, 2014; Thompson, 2003): conventional, verrucous, basaloid, papillary, spindle cell (sarcomatoid), acantholytic, adenosquamous and cuniculatum.

Each of these variants can develop in any of the different regions of the head and neck with the exception of the Cuniculatum subtype that only develops in the lining of the oral cavity (Massano *et al.*, 2006). Variants of SCC frequently arise within the mucosa of the upper aero digestive tract, accounting for up to 15% of SCCs in these areas. The most common variants include verrucous, exophytic or papillary, spindle-cell (sarcomatoid), basaloid and adenosquamous carcinoma. Each of these variants has a unique histomorphologic appearance, which raises a number of different differential diagnostic considerations, with the attendant clinically relevant management decisions. Stage for stage each one of these different subtypes of SCC has the same prognosis and is management identically.

Broder's grading system was the first of the systems, which initiated quantitative grading of cancer. This classification system was based on the estimated ratio of differentiated to undifferentiated elements in the tumor. There are four histologic grades based on the amount of keratinization (Massano *et al.*, 2006; Bansberg *et al.*, 1989):

Well-differentiated tumor - > 75% keratinization.
Moderately differentiated tumor - 50% to 75% keratinization.
Poorly differentiated tumor - 25% to 50% keratinization.
Anaplastic or undifferentiated tumor - < 25% keratinization.

Histologic grade is not a consistent predictor of clinical behavior. The characteristics that predict aggressive behavior include perineural infiltration, lymphatic invasion, and tumor extension beyond the capsule of the lymph nodes (Close *et al.*, 1989; Massano *et al.*, 2006).

Immunohistochemical studies may be useful in poorly differentiated lesions to help make the diagnosis because SCC's express epithelial markers such as cytokeratin's. Squamous cells are immune - positive for certain cytokeratin's such as AE1/AE3 and pancytokeratin's. CK5/CK6 and p63 are also excellent markers for squamous differentiation (Dabbs, 2006).

7   Precursor Lesions of the Oral Cavity Cancer

There is a sequence of disease progression from atypia / dysplasia, to in situ carcinoma, to invasive cancer. Leukoplakia and erythroplakia are terms given to clinically identifiable lesions that may harbor invasive cancer or undergo malignant transformation. Precursor lesions may present as small patches or as a large verrucous plaques. The surface can be brown to red (erythroplakia) or may have circumscribed whitish plaques (leukoplakia). White spots may ulcerate.

Leukoplakia (Figure 8) develops as a result of chronic irritation of the mucous membranes by carcinogens; this irritation stimulates proliferation of epithelial and connective tissue. Histopathologic examination reveals underlying hyperkeratosis associated with epithelial hyperplasia. In the absence of underlying dysplasia, leukoplakia rarely (<5 %) is associated with progression to malignancy (Ridge, 2013; Massano *et al.*, 2006; Thompson, 2003).

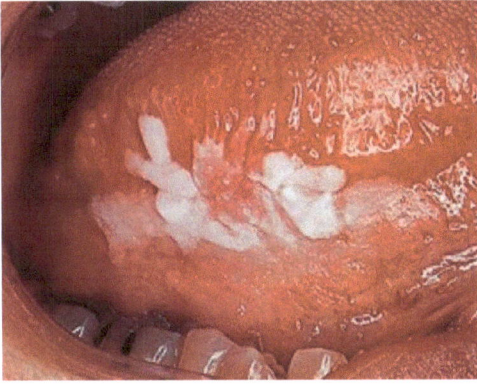

Figure 8: Leukoplakia.

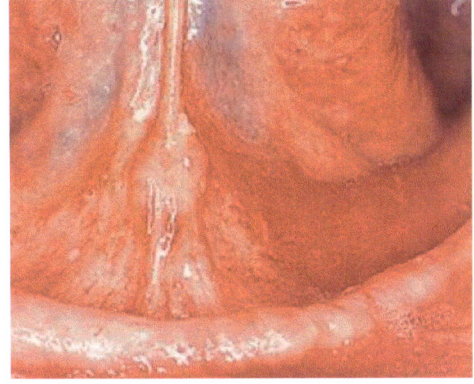

Figure 9: Erythroplakia.

Red spots, friable adjacent normal mucosa, characterize erythroplakia (Figure 9). It is associated with underlying epithelial dysplasia and has a much greater potential for malignancy than leukoplakia. Carcinoma is found in nearly 40 % of cases of erythroplakia (Ridge, 2013).

The classification of the world health organization (WHO) of precursor lesions is as follows (Barnes, 2005):

Squamous cell hyperplasia;

Hyperplasia describes an increase in the number of cells;

This can be in the spinous layer (acanthosis), and / or in the layers of basal / parabasal cells (progenitor compartment) called basal cell hyperplasia.

Dysplasia - is characterized by cellular atypia, loss of normal cellular maturation, and loss of epithelial stratification:

Mild dysplasia (squamous intraepithelial neoplasia 1)

Moderate dysplasia (squamous intraepithelial neoplasia 2)

Severe dysplasia or carcinoma in situ (squamous intraepithelial neoplastic 3)

The probability of developing a carcinoma depends on the degree of dysplasia. In the case of severe dysplasia, up to 24% of patients may have an occult invasive squamous cell cancer (Ridge, 2013).

8   Concept of Field Cancerization (Field Defect)

It is an important concept related to the natural history of oral cavity cancer. This term describes diffuse injury of the epithelium of the head and neck region, lung and esophagus resulting from chronic exposure to carcinogens (Slaughter *et al.*, 1953). Clinically field cancerization manifests by the frequent occurrence of abnormalities of the mucosa, such as leukoplakia and dysplasia, beyond the margins of an oral cavity cancer or second primary tumors in this field. The lifetime risk of a patient with oral cavity cancer to develop a new cancer is 20% to 40% (Speight, 2007).

9   TNM Classification of Tumors of the Head and Neck

The TNM staging system of the AJCC maintains uniformity in the staging of head and neck tumors, and is based on the best estimate of the extent of disease prior to treatment (Table 3 to Table 6). Assessment of the primary tumor is based on inspection and palpation when possible, by indirect mirror examination and direct endoscopy when necessary (Edge *et al.*, 2010).

The prognosis is strongly correlated with the stage of the disease at diagnosis. Survival of patients with stage I disease exceeds 80% (Siegel R et al, 2014). For patients with locally advanced disease at the time of diagnosis (i.e., stage III and IV), survival drops below 40% (Edge *et al.*, 2010). The development of metastases in lymph nodes reduces the survival of a patient with a small primary tumor by 50% (Ridge, 2013; Siegel R et al, 2014). Most patients with head and neck cancers at the time of diagnosis are found to be stage III or IV (Edge *et al.*, 2010; Wallner *et al.*, 1986).

TX	Primary tumor cannot be assessed
T0	No evidence of primary tumor
Tis	Carcinoma in situ
T1	Tumor ≤ 2 cm in greatest dimension
T2	Tumor > 2 cm but ≤ 4 cm in greatest dimension
T3	Tumor > 4 cm in greatest dimension
T4a	Local disease moderately advanced: (Lips) - Tumor invades cortical bone cortical, inferior alveolar nerve, floor of the mouth or skin of the face (chin) (Oral cavity) - Tumor invades only adjacent structures (for example, cortical bone cortical, [mandible or maxilla], extrinsic muscle of the tongue, maxillary sinus or skin of the face)
T4b	Local disease very advanced: Tumor invades masticator space, pterygoid plates, base or the skull and / or encases internal carotid artery

Table 3: TNM Classification of Oral Cavity Cancer - Primary tumor (T) (Edge *et al.*, 2010).

NX	Region lymph nodes cannot be assessed
N0	No region lymph nodes metastasis
N1	Metastasis in single ipsilateral lymph, ≤ 3 cm in greatest dimension
N2	Metastasis in single ipsilateral lymph, > 3 cm, but ≤ 6 cm in greatest dimension Metastasis in multiple ipsilateral lymph nodes, none > 6 cm in greatest dimension Metastasis in bilateral o contralateral lymph nodes, none > 6 cm in greatest dimension
N2a	Metastasis in single ipsilateral lymph, > 3 cm, but ≤ 6 cm in greatest dimension
N2b	Metastasis in multiple ipsilateral lymph nodes, none > 6 cm in greatest dimension
N2c	Metastasis in bilateral o contralateral lymph nodes, none > 6 cm in greatest dimension
N3	Metastasis in a lymph node > 6 cm in greatest dimension

Table 4: TNM Classification of Oral Cavity Cancer - Lymph Nodes (N) (Edge *et al.*, 2010).

M0	No distant metastasis
M1	Distant metastasis

Table 5: TNM Classification of Oral Cavity Cancer - Distance metastasis (M) (Edge *et al.*, 2010).

Staging	T	N	M
0	Tis	N0	M0
I	T1	N0	M0
II	T2	N0	M0
III	T3	N0	M0
	T1	N1	M0
	T2	N1	M0
	T3	N1	M0
IVA	T4a	N0	M0
	T4a	N1	M0
	T1	N2	M0
	T2	N2	M0
	T3	N2	M0
	T4a	N1	M0
IVB	Any T	N3	M0
	T4b	Any N	M0
IVC	Any T	Any N	M1

Table 6: Anatomical staging and prognostic groups (Edge *et al.*, 2010).

10   Patterns of Relapse

Despite aggressive treatment of the primary most relapses occur within the same region of the primary oral cavity tumor. Local and regional recurrences represent approximately 80% of primary treatment failures (Wong *et al.*, 2003). Distant metastases increase as the disease progresses and more frequently include the lungs, and to a lesser extent, bone and liver. This is a reason to use PET/CT for assessing the distant spread of the cancer in patients with disease recurrence of progression. In 10% to 30% of patients distant metastases are detected at the time of death (Harrison LB & Hong, 2009).

11   Treatment Options

Management of oral cavity cancers requires a multidisciplinary team made up of a surgical oncologist specialized in head and neck cancers, dentist, prosthodontist, plastic reconstructive surgeons, medical oncologist, radiation oncologist, speech therapist, fiscal rehabilitation therapist, social worker, and psychologist. The diagnostic and management algorithm is outlined in Figure 10.

The treatment depends on the site, the extent of the primary tumor, and lymph node status, and may include (Brown & Langdon, 1995; Harrison LB & Hong, 2009; Wang, 1997):

1.   Surgery alone.

2.   Radiation therapy alone.

3.   A combination of the above.

Possible Oral Cavity Malignancy

Complete History and Physical Exam
(Head and Neck Exam, Mirror and Fiberoptic Examination as Clinically Indicated)

Biopsy

HNSCC Confirmed by Pathologist

Staging

CT with Contrast and/or MRI of Primary and Neck

PET/CT in very Selected Cases of Locally Advanced HNSCC

Exam Under Anesthesia (EUA) with Endoscopy, if Indicated

Dental/Prosthodontic Evaluation, Including Jaw Imagining as Clinically Indicated

Nutrition, Speech and Swallowing Evaluation / Therapy as Indicated

Present in a Multidisciplinary Tumor Board

Manage According to Staging and Consensus of the Tumor Board

T1, T2, N0

T3, N0

T1-3, N1-3

T4a, Any T

T4b, Any N, or Unresectable Nodal Disease or Unfit for Surgery

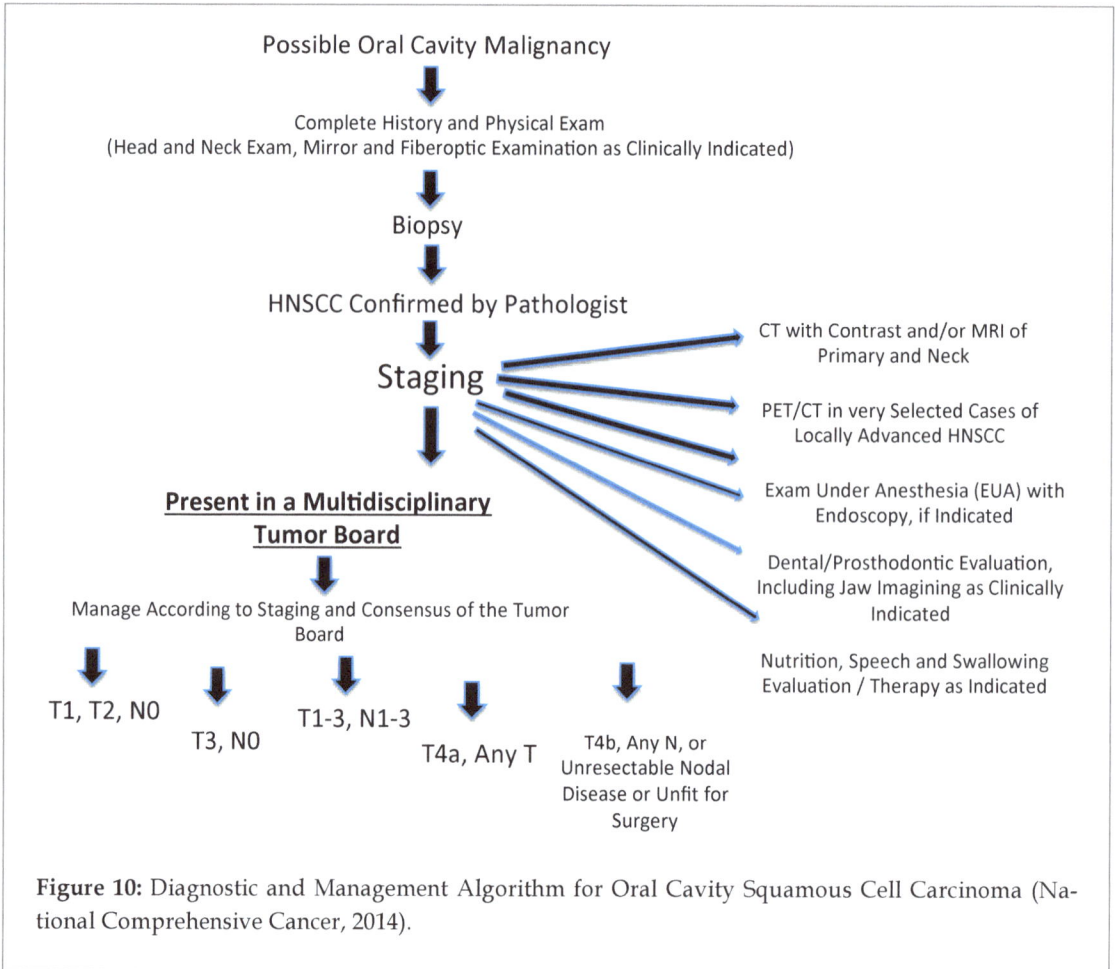

Figure 10: Diagnostic and Management Algorithm for Oral Cavity Squamous Cell Carcinoma (National Comprehensive Cancer, 2014).

The best therapeutic approach for the primary tumor depends on the anatomic site. Most early cancers of the head and neck can be treated equally well with surgery or radiation therapy, therefore the method chosen to treat the neck is based on the mode that has been selected for the primary tumor. When the primary tumor is treated with radiation, regional lymph nodes "at risk" are incorporated into the field of treatment (Ridge, 2013). Patient factors and experience should influence the choice of treatment. Due to the lower morbidity of primary surgical resection of oral cavity tumors compared to primary radiation therapy most international guidelines recommend surgery as the primary modality for oral cavity lesions (National Comprehensive Cancer, 2014). Larger cancers may require composite resections with reconstruction of the defect by pedicle flaps and often require adjuvant therapy with radiation and chemotherapy (Kramer *et al.*, 1987; Peters *et al.*, 1993).

The classical surgical principles of oncology are applied to oral cavity cancers. Complete en bloc resection is necessary. Ensuring adequate margins can be challenging due to the important structures in this area (Looser *et al.*, 1978). The reconstruction after surgery is complex after resection of tumors of the oral cavity because the surgical procedure may have an important impact on appearance, speech and swallowing. Experienced surgeons should perform the decisions regarding the extent of resection. Prosthodontic rehabilitation is important, especially in the early stages of cancer, to ensure better quality of life.

For lesions of the oral cavity, surgery should resect all macroscopic evidence of the disease keeping in mind the possibility of microscopic extension. If regional nodes are positive, cervical lymph node dissection is usually done in the same procedure. Neck dissection must be standardized (i.e. complete anatomical dissections, instead of random biopsies) in these situations to prevent incomplete surgery. Elective neck dissection is recommended for patients who have a oral cavity tumors with a minimum thickness of 4 mm (Ridge, 2013), although some researchers believe that tumor thickness of 2-3 mm would be a more appropriate cut off (McGuirt *et al.*, 1995; Spiro *et al.*, 1986) (Table 7).

Tumor Thickness	5 y Overall Survival	Treatment Failure
< 2 mm	97 %	2 %
2 – 8 mm	83%	
> 8 mm	65%	45%

Table 7: Thickness of oral cancer predicts survival and failure (Spiro *et al.*, 1986).

The management algorithms of early stage and locally advanced oral cavity cancers are depicted in Figures 11 and 12.

Supraomohyoid neck dissection is recommended in patients with a clinical stage N0 who are treated surgically. There is evidence of skip metastases through the levels of the neck (Byers *et al.*, 1997) and in some cases just involving level IV without involving the first levels. Therefore some authors recommend extended supraomohyoid neck dissection (Byers *et al.*, 1997). Bilateral neck dissection is performed if the tumor is close to or abutting the midline (Figure 13).

Sentinel lymph node (SLN) biopsy is another new option to standard elective neck dissection for identifying an occult cervical metastasis in patients with an early (T1 or T2) oral cavity cancer in centers where expertise for this procedure exists (Civantos *et al.*, 2010; Govers *et al.*, 2013). Patients who are found to have metastatic disease in their SLN's must undergo a completion neck dissection while those without a positive SLN can be observed with close follow up. The precision of the SLN biopsy for staging of the neck in early oral cavity cancer has been tested at length in multiple single-center trials and in two mutli-institutional studies against the reference standard of elective neck dissection with a pooled estimated sensitivity of 0.93 and negative predictive value ranging from 0.88 to 1 (Alkureishi *et al.*, 2010; Broglie *et al.*, 2013; Civantos *et al.*, 2010; Govers *et al.*, 2013; Pezier *et al.*, 2012; Samant, 2014). This is a technically demanding procedure that has a steep learning curve in which the success rate is dependent on the experience and expertise of the surgeon. Up to know a direct comparison with the policy of elective neck dissection is lacking (Samant, 2014), so we recommend using this procedure very selectively. For example, very early carcinomas of the oral cavity (T1 or may be T2), excluding floor of the mouth tumors because the accuracy in the studies we have up to date is inferior to other anatomical sites within the oral cavity such as the tongue (Alkureishi *et al.*, 2010; Civantos *et al.*, 2010), that have a tumor thickness less than 4 mm.

Although the different surgical techniques available to the head and neck surgeon are beyond the scope of this review we will be talking about some of the general principals such as the different surgical approaches available to gain access to the tumors. Various surgical approaches are available to the surgeon and include the peroral approach for small (T1, T2), anteriorly located tumors of oral cavity, mandibulotomy approach to gain access to larger

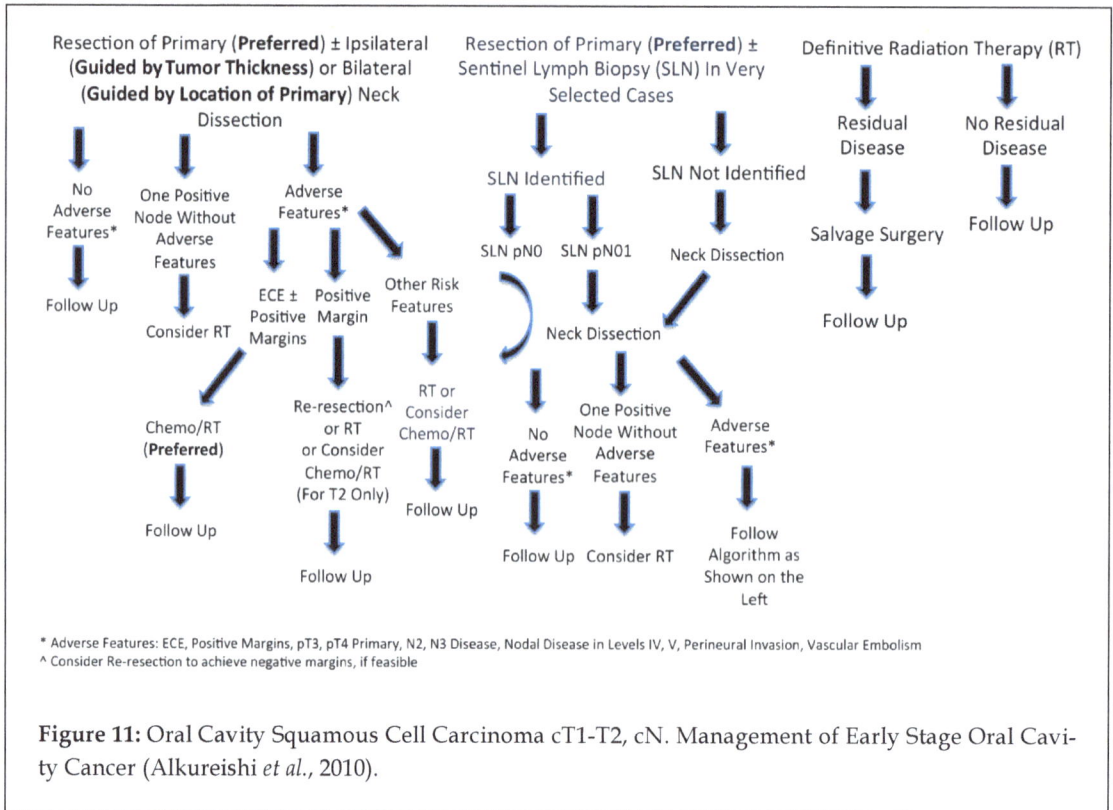

Figure 11: Oral Cavity Squamous Cell Carcinoma cT1-T2, cN. Management of Early Stage Oral Cavity Cancer (Alkureishi *et al.*, 2010).

lesions located more posteriorly in the oral cavity, a lower cheek flap, a visor flap, and an upper cheek flap. The lower cheek flap requires a midline lip splitting incision that may be continued laterally into the neck for exposure and neck dissections. This approach can be used for most oral cavity tumors with the exception of upper gum and hard palate tumors. Mandibular resection (marginal or segmental) and reconstruction require a lower cheek flap in most instances. A visor flap is used for anteriorly located lesions, for posterior lesions it is not appropriate due to the poor exposure. The benefits of a visor flap are that it avoids lower lip splitting incision but it produces permanent loss of sensation on the chin because the mental nerve is sacrificed for adequate mobilization. Lower lip sagging and drooling is another complication because of loss of sensation and support. The upper cheek flap, such as the Weber Ferguson incision and its modifications are used for large upper gum and hard palate lesions (Jatin *et al.*, 2012).

To gain access to large tumors (especially those close to the base of the tongue) that are not involving the mandible a mandible sparing incision, called a mandibulotomy, needs to be performed. The three most common types of madibulotomy are lateral, medial and paramedian. The lateral mandibulotomy has several drawbacks. First, the muscular pull on the two segments of the mandible is uneven, putting the mandibulotomy site under substantial stress causing a holdup in healing (for this reason, intermaxillary fixation may be needed). Second, the ability to gain access to the suture line to maintain hygiene following surgery in the oral cavity is hindered as a result of the intermaxillary fixation, leading to poor oral hygiene and the potential risk for sepsis of the suture line. Furthermore, a lateral mandibuloto-

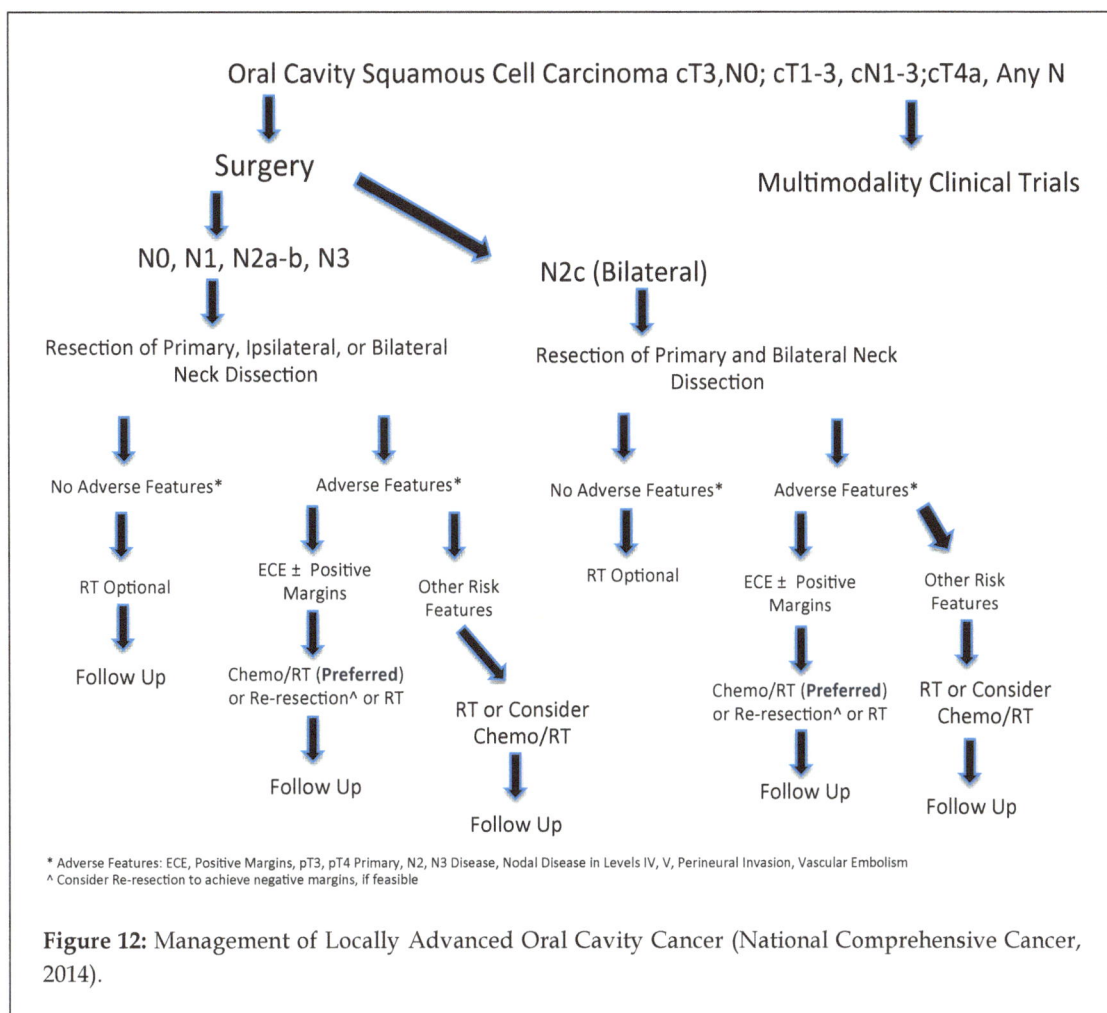

Figure 12: Management of Locally Advanced Oral Cavity Cancer (National Comprehensive Cancer, 2014).

my poses several anatomic shortcomings leading to denervation of the teeth distal to the mandibulotomy site and the skin of the chin as a result of transection of the inferior alveolar nerve. A lateral mandibulotomy also causes devascularization of the distal teeth and the distal segment of the mandible from its endosteal blood supply. Another weakness of this procedures is that the exposure provided by a is inadequate and if the patient needs postoperative radiation, the mandibulotomy site is directly within the lateral portal of the radiation field, leading to delayed healing and complications (Jatin *et al.*, 2012).

By placing the site of the mandibulotomy on the anterior midline, medial mandibulotomy, all the detriments of a lateral mandibulotomy are prevented. However, splitting the mandible in the midline requires extraction of the central incisor tooth to avoid exposure of the both roots of the central incisor teeth, which are at risk of extrusion. Removal of one central incisor tooth to avoid this situation modifies the aesthetic appearance of the lower dentition. In addition, a midline mandibulotomy requires division of the muscles arising from the genial tubercle, (geniohyoid and genioglossus), leading to a delayed recovery of the functions of mastication and swallowing. Consequently a median mandibulotomy is also not the preferred technique (Jatin *et al.*, 2012).

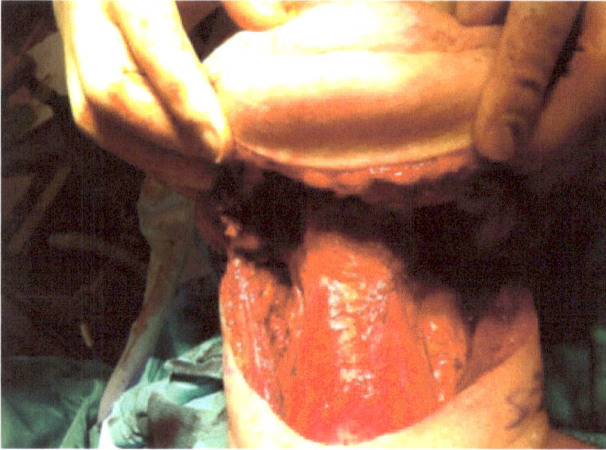

Figure 13: Bilateral Supraomohyoid Neck Dissection for a Tongue Cancer > 4 mm in Thickness.

On the other hand, paramedian mandibulotomy avoids all the disadvantages of a lateral mandibulotomy and the sequelae of a midline mandibulotomy. It offers important benefits, such as wide exposure and preservation of the geniohyoid and genioglossus muscles, leading to preservation of the hyomandibular complex. The only muscle requiring division is the mylohyoid muscle, which leads to negligible swallowing difficulties. A paramedian mandibulotomy does not cause denervation or devascularization of the skin of the chin or the teeth and mandible. Fixation at the mandibulotomy site is simple, and the site of the mandibulotomy does not fall within the lateral portal field of radiation if the patient requires adjuvant therapy (Jatin *et al.*, 2012).

The surgeon operating on head and neck tumors must understand the potential routes of spread of the primary malignancy in order to decide what surgical procedure to perform. McGregor *et al.* (1987) have reported that the major route of invasion of squamous cell cancers of the oral cavity depends on whether the patient is dentulous or edentulous. In the edentulous mandible the route of spread is through paucities in the occlusal of the cortical bone. The route of propagation in the dentulous mandible that has not been irradiated is through the site of insertion of the teeth, and the presence of the teeth is a barrier for tumor infiltration. Furthermore, the toothed jaw has a greater height from the floor of the mouth, making tumor invasion more difficult, as compared to the edentulous jaw, due to alveolar ridge resorption after tooth loss.

Radiation therapy for cancer of the oral cavity may be administered as external beam radiotherapy (EBRT) or interstitial implantation alone. It is difficult getting enough dose to primary with brachytherapy while still delivering adequate dose to the regional nodes, so for many sites using both modalities produces better control and better functional outcomes (Wendt *et al.*, 1990). Small superficial cancers can be treated very successfully by local implantation using any of the various radioactive sources (intraoral cone therapy, or electrons) (de Visscher *et al.*, 1999). Larger lesions are frequently managed using external beam radiotherapy, which includes the primary site and regional lymph nodes (even if not clinically affected) (Harrison LB & Hong, 2009). Supplementation with interstitial radiation sources may be required to achieve adequate doses for bulky large primary tumors and / or lymph node metastases. A review of published clinical results of radical radiation therapy for head and neck tumors suggests a significant loss of local control when the administration of radiation therapy was prolonged, therefore, lengthening of standard treatment programs should be avoided whenever possible (Fowler & Lindstrom, 1992; Langendijk *et al.*, 2003).

Radiation therapy with curative intent usually involves daily treatment for 6 to 7 weeks (total dose: 60-70 Gy) (National Comprehensive Cancer, 2014). Although there is no loss of tissue with radiation therapy as with surgery, potential complications include dry mouth, tissue fibrosis, trismus, bone necrosis, hypothyroidism, and dysphagia (Dirix *et al.*, 2008; Cooper *et al.*, 1995; Trotti *et al.*, 2003). Some of these problems are common and debilitating enough to require significant attention during treatment planning. Surgery often results in less morbidity in the oral cavity, while radiation therapy causes less morbidity in other regions such as the oropharynx, larynx and nasopharynx.

The definitive indications for postoperative radiotherapy are positive margins, multiple positive nodes with metastatic disease, and extra capsular nodal extension (Yuen *et al.*, 2002). Less certain indications include lymphovascular space invasion, perineural spread, single encapsulated positive lymph node, and thick tumors (Yuen *et al.*, 2002). Tumors with a thickness between 3 to 9 mm have 44% subclinical node positivity and a 7% local recurrence rate and tumors with a thickness greater than 9 mm thickness have 53% subclinical node positivity and a 24% local recurrence rate (Yuen *et al.*, 2002).

One of the reasons why radiation therapy is recommended after surgery is based on the results of the RTOG 73-03 (Kramer *et al.*, 1987). This study was performed in patients with locally advanced head and necks cancers (supraglottic larynx, hypopharynx, oral cavity, and oropharynx). The patients were randomized to receive either preoperative (50 Gy) versus postoperative radiation therapy (60 Gy). The study recruited 277 patients and with a 10-year follow it showed improved local and regional control in the postoperative radiation arm (65%) compared to the radiation arm (48%), which was statistically significant (p=0.04). It also showed a trend toward improved overall survival 38% versus 33% (p=0.10) (Tupchong *et al.*, 1991). The surgical and radiation complications were very similar. The RTOG 73-03 established 60 Gy as the postoperative radiation dose (Tupchong *et al.*, 1991).

MD Anderson performed a prospective randomized trial evaluating the radiation dose for 240 patients with resected stage III/IV cancers of oral cavity, oropharynx, hypopharynx, and larynx (Peters *et al.*, 1993). Patients receiving $\leq$ 54 Gy had significantly higher failure rate than those receiving $\geq$ 57.6 Gy (p = 0.02). No dose response beyond 57.6 Gy was seen with the exception of patients with extra-capsular nodal spread (ECE). Positive ECE needed to be treated with at least 63 Gy. "Clusters" of two or more of the following also predicted increased risk of failure and need for 63 Gy: oral cavity primary, positive/close margins, nerve invasion, $\geq$ 2 positive nodes, largest node > 3 cm, treatment delay > 6 weeks, Zubrod performance status $\geq$ 2 (Peters *et al.*, 1993). Moderate to severe complications were seen in 7.1% of the cases, more if the radiation dose was $\geq$ 63 Gy. Dose escalation above 63 Gy did not appear to improve the therapeutic ratio.

In conclusion postoperative radiotherapy (60-70 Gy in 6-7 weeks) reduces the rate of local and regional recurrence from 50% to 15% for tumors with pathologic features that predict high local and regional failure rates (de Visscher *et al.*, 1999; Cooper *et al.*, 2004; Yorozu *et al.*, 2001). The indications for postoperative radiotherapy are well established and are outlined in Table 8.

Close or positive margins
An affected lymph node > 3 cm
Multiple lymph nodes involved
Extra capsular extension (ECE)
Patients who had an open biopsy of a suspicious neck node and did not undergo neck dissection at the time
Perineural invasion, lymphovascular space invasion, invasion of cartilage, bone or deep soft tissues
Recommendation of the surgeon due to intraoperative findings

Table 8: Possible Indications for postoperative radiotherapy.

Two randomized clinical trials were conducted to determine whether adding chemotherapy to radiation therapy improves local /regional control and survival in high-risk patients with head and neck cancers after definitive surgical resection. The results of these trials were published in 2004 (Bernier *et al.*, 2004; Cooper *et al.*, 2004). Patients with high-risk features (two or more lymph nodes, extra capsular extension or positive margins after definitive surgical resection) were randomized to receive 60-66 Gy of postoperative radiation with or without cisplatin (100 mg / m² administered on days 1, 22, and 43) in the RTOG 95-01/Intergroup trial (Cooper *et al.*, 2004). With a median follow up of 45.9 months, the rate of local and regional control in two years was 82% in the combined therapy group versus 72% in the radiotherapy group (P = 0.01). The disease-free interval (p = .04) but not in overall survival time (P = .19) was significantly higher in the combined treatment group, although the study was conducted to demonstrate a difference in local and regional recurrence, it was not designed to demonstrate a survival advantage. The incidence of acute adverse effects (grade 3 or higher) was higher in the combination group (77% vs. 34 %, P < 0.001) (Cooper *et al.*, 2004).

The EORTC 22931 had similar findings (Bernier *et al.*, 2004). This study included patients with T3 or T4 disease, perineural invasion and lymphovascular space involvement, in addition to positive margins and extracapsular extension. The overall survival rate was significantly improved in the combination therapy group compared with the radiotherapy alone group. After an average of 60 months, the overall survival of 334 randomized patients was 53% in the combined treatment group versus 40% in the group treated with radiation alone (P = 0.02) group. The discrepancy in overall survival between the two studies is believed to be associated to the different entry criteria used in the RTOG and EORTC studies (Table 9).

End Point	EORTC 22931			RTOG 9501		
	RT	RT + CT	P Value	RT	RT + CT	P Value
5 y Disease Free Survival	36%	47%	0.04	61%	78%	0.004
LR Control	69%	82%	0.007	72%	82%	0.01
OS	40%	53%	0.002	57%	63%	0.19

Table 9: Results from the EORTC 22931 and RTOG 9501 Studies.

In a comparative analysis of the two trials, the presence of extracapsular extension and/or microscopically involved surgical margins were the only risk factors for the positive impact that chemo radiation had over improved survival (Bernier *et al.*, 2005). The adjuvant treatment for patients with oral cavity cancers is summarized in table 10.

Risk Based on Factors for Treatment Failure	Management
Low Risk	No adjuvant radiation
Intermediate Risk (- Margin, - ECE)	Radiation therapy (60 Gy)
High Risk (+ Margin and/or + ECE)	Chemo radiation (60-66 Gy) with Cisplatin

Table 10: Summary of Adjuvant Treatment of Oral Cavity Cancers.

Recently the results of the RTOG-0234 examining concurrent chemoradiotherapy and cetuximab in the postoperative treatment of patients head and neck squamous cell carcinoma (HNSCC) with high-risk pathologic features was published (Harari *et al.*, 2014). The study recruited 238 patients were with stage III to IV HNSCC with gross total resection showing positive margins and/or extracapsular nodal extension and/or two or more nodal metastases. Patients were randomly assigned to 60 Gy radiation with cetuximab once per week plus either cisplatin 30 mg/m2 or docetaxel 15 mg/m2 once per week. With a median follow-up of 4.4 years, 2-year overall survival (OS) was 69% for the cisplatin arm and 79% for the docetaxel arm; 2-year disease-free survival (DFS) was 57% and 66%, respectively. DFS in this study was compared with that in the chemoradiotherapy arm of the RTOG-9501 trial, which had a hazard ratio of 0.76 for the cisplatin arm versus control (P=0.05) and 0.69 for the docetaxel arm versus control (P=0.01), reflecting absolute improvement in 2-year DFS of 2.5% and 11.1%, respectively. The delivery of postoperative chemoradiotherapy and cetuximab to patients with HNSCC is possible and tolerated with predictable toxicity. The docetaxel regimen shows favorable outcome with improved DFS and OS relative to historical controls and has commenced formal testing in a phase II/III trial (RTOG 1216).

The recommendations for follow-up are based on the risk of relapse, second primaries, treatment sequelae, and toxicities includes a history and physical (including a complete head and neck exam; mirror and fiberoptic examinations as clinically indicated every 1 to 3 months for the first year, every 2-6 months for the second year, every 4 to 8 months years 3 to 5, and every 12 months after 5 years. To facilitate this our group sees the patient every three moths for the first five years. Post-treatment baseline imaging of the primary (and neck, if treated) is recommended within 6 months of treatment, further imaging is indicated based on signs and symptoms (but is not routinely recommended without worrisome manifestations). Chest imaging as clinically indicated for patients with a smoking history. If the neck was radiated, the NCCN guidelines recommend thyroid stimulating hormone (TSH) testing every 6 to 12 months. Smoking and alcohol counseling as clinically indicated (National Comprehensive Cancer, 2014).

For recurrent lesions of the mouth, anterior tongue, buccal mucosa, floor of mouth, retromolar trigone, upper gingiva and hard palate, treatment will be dictated by the location and size of the recurrent lesion and pretreatment (Harrison LB & Hong, 2009 Vikram *et al.*, 1985). The options available to treat recurrent tumors are:

- Surgery is the preferred treatment, if radiation therapy was used as initial therapy (Wong *et al.*, 2003).

- Surgery, radiation therapy, or a combination of these may be considered for treatment if surgery is was used to treat the initial lesion (Wong *et al.*, 2003).

- Although chemotherapy has been shown to induce responses, it does not increase survival.

Treatment options that are currently under consideration include clinical trials testing new chemotherapy drugs, chemotherapy and re-irradiation or hyperthermia should be considered because the clinical response to a salvage surgery after primary treatment with radiation or primary surgery followed by radiation have poor results (Hong & Bromer, 1983; Janot *et al.*, 2008; Vokes & Athanasiadis, 1996).

12   Conclusion

Cancer of the oral cavity comprises a diverse group of rare tumors that are often aggressive in their biologic behavior that require a multidisciplinary team approach to their management that includes a surgical oncologist, medical oncologist, radiation oncologist, dentist, oral maxillary surgeon, prosthodontist, rehabilitation therapists, rehabilitation speech therapist, as well as of emotional support by psychologists or social workers. Early referral to a center that has the expertise in the management of these complex tumors has been shown to improve outcomes and is highly encouraged.

References

Abreu, L., Kruger, E. and Tennant, M. Lip cancer in Western Australia, 1982-2006: a 25-year retrospective epidemiological study. Aust Dent J, 2009. 54(2): p. 130-5.

Alkureishi, L.W., et al., Sentinel node biopsy in head and neck squamous cell cancer: 5-year follow-up of a European multicenter trial. Ann Surg Oncol, 2010. 17(9): p. 2459-64.

Alter, B.P., et al., Cancer in dyskeratosis congenita. Blood, 2009. 113(26): p. 6549-57.

Arantes, L.M., et al., Methylation as a biomarker for head and neck cancer. Oral Oncol, 2014. 50(6): p. 587-92.

Bansberg, S.F., Olsen, K.D. and Gaffey, T.A. High-grade carcinoma of the oral cavity. Otolaryngol Head Neck Surg, 1989. 100(1): p. 41-8.

Barnes, L., Pathology and Genetics. 2005: W.H. Organization 2005: IARC Press, Lyon.

Benner, S.E., et al., Regression of oral leukoplakia with alpha-tocopherol: a community clinical oncology program chemoprevention study. J Natl Cancer Inst, 1993. 85(1): p. 44-7.

Bernier, J., et al., Defining risk levels in locally advanced head and neck cancers: a comparative analysis of concurrent postoperative radiation plus chemotherapy trials of the EORTC (#22931) and RTOG (# 9501). Head Neck, 2005. 27(10): p. 843-50.

Bernier, J., et al., Postoperative irradiation with or without concomitant chemotherapy for locally advanced head and neck cancer. N Engl J Med, 2004. 350(19): p. 1945-52.

Boffetta, P., et al., Smokeless tobacco and cancer. Lancet Oncol, 2008. 9(7): p. 667-75.

Broglie, M.A., et al., Occult metastases detected by sentinel node biopsy in patients with early oral and oropharyngeal squamous cell carcinomas: impact on survival. Head Neck, 2013. 35(5): p. 660-6.

Browman, G.P., et al., Influence of cigarette smoking on the efficacy of radiation therapy in head and neck cancer. N Engl J Med, 1993. 328(3): p. 159-63.

Brown, A.E. and J.D. Langdon, Management of oral cancer. Ann R Coll Surg Engl, 1995. 77(6): p. 404-8.

Byers, R.M., et al., Frequency and therapeutic implications of "skip metastases" in the neck from squamous carcinoma of the oral tongue. Head Neck, 1997. 19(1): p. 14-9.

Civantos, F.J., et al., Sentinel lymph node biopsy accurately stages the regional lymph nodes for T1-T2 oral squamous cell carcinomas: results of a prospective multi-institutional trial. J Clin Oncol, 2010. 28(8): p. 1395-400.

Close, L.G., et al., Microvascular invasion and survival in cancer of the oral cavity and oropharynx. Arch Otolaryngol Head Neck Surg, 1989. 115(11): p. 1304-9.

Contreras Vidaurre, E.G., et al., Retinoids: application in premalignant lesions and oral cancer. Med Oral, 2001. 6(2): p. 114-23.

Cooper, J.S., et al., Late effects of radiation therapy in the head and neck region. Int J Radiat Oncol Biol Phys, 1995. 31(5): p. 1141-64.

Cooper, J.S., et al., Postoperative concurrent radiotherapy and chemotherapy for high-risk squamous-cell carcinoma of the head and neck. N Engl J Med, 2004. 350(19): p. 1937-44.

Dabbs, D.J., Diagnostic Immunohistochemestry: Theranostic and Genomic Applications. Fourth Edition ed. 2006, 1600 John F. Kennedy Blvd. Philadelphia: Elsevier.

Day, G.L. and Blot, W.J. Second primary tumors in patients with oral cancer. Cancer, 1992. 70(1): p. 14-9.

de Braud, F. and al-Sarraf, M. Diagnosis and management of squamous cell carcinoma of unknown primary tumor site of the neck. Semin Oncol, 1993. 20(3): p. 273-8.

de Visscher, J.G., et al., A comparison of results after radiotherapy and surgery for stage I squamous cell carcinoma of the lower lip. Head Neck, 1999. 21(6): p. 526-30.

Dirix, P., et al., The influence of xerostomia after radiotherapy on quality of life: results of a questionnaire in head and neck cancer. Support Care Cancer, 2008. 16(2): p. 171-9.

Edge, S., Byrd, D.R., Comptom, C.C., et al., AJCC Cancer Staging Manual. 7th. ed. Lip and oral cavity cancer. 2010, New York, NY: Springer. 29-40.

Erkal, H.S., et al., Synchronous and metachronous squamous cell carcinomas of the head and neck mucosal sites. J Clin Oncol, 2001. 19(5): p. 1358-62.

Fowler, J.F. and Lindstrom, M.J. Loss of local control with prolongation in radiotherapy. Int J Radiat Oncol Biol Phys, 1992. 23(2): p. 457-67.

Gandini, S., et al., Tobacco smoking and cancer: a meta-analysis. Int J Cancer, 2008. 122(1): p. 155-64.

Garcia Martinez, J., et al., DNA aneuploidy-specific therapy for head and neck squamous cell carcinoma. Head Neck, 2014.

Gasparini, G., et al., Fanconi anemia manifesting as a squamous cell carcinoma of the hard palate: a case report. Head Face Med, 2006. 2: p. 1.

Goldenberg, D., Golz, A. and Joachims, H.Z. The beverage mate: a risk factor for cancer of the head and neck. Head Neck, 2003. 25(7): p. 595-601.

Goldenberg, D., et al., Habitual risk factors for head and neck cancer. Otolaryngol Head Neck Surg, 2004. 131(6): p. 986-93.

Govers, T.M., et al., Sentinel node biopsy for squamous cell carcinoma of the oral cavity and oropharynx: a diagnostic meta-analysis. Oral Oncol, 2013. 49(8): p. 726-32.

Graham, S., et al., Dentition, diet, tobacco, and alcohol in the epidemiology of oral cancer. J Natl Cancer Inst, 1977. 59(6): p. 1611-8.

Greer, R.O. and Goldman, H.M. Oral papillomas. Clinicopathologic evaluation and retrospective examination for dyskeratosis in 110 lesions. Oral Surg Oral Med Oral Pathol, 1974. 38(3): p. 435-40.

Guha, N., et al., Oral health and risk of squamous cell carcinoma of the head and neck and esophagus: results of two multicentric case-control studies. Am J Epidemiol, 2007. 166(10): p. 1159-73.

Hao, S.P. and Ng, S.H. Magnetic resonance imaging versus clinical palpation in evaluating cervical metastasis from head and neck cancer. Otolaryngol Head Neck Surg, 2000. 123(3): p. 324-7.

Harari, P.M., et al., Postoperative Chemoradiotherapy and Cetuximab for High-Risk Squamous Cell Carcinoma of the Head and Neck: Radiation Therapy Oncology Group RTOG-0234. J Clin Oncol, 2014.

Harrison LB, S.R., Hong W.K., eds., Head and Neck Cancer: A Multidisciplinary Approach. 3rd ed. ed. 2009, Philadelphia, PA.: Lippincott, William and Wilkins 2009.

Hashibe, M., et al., Alcohol drinking in never users of tobacco, cigarette smoking in never drinkers, and the risk of head and neck cancer: pooled analysis in the International Head and Neck Cancer Epidemiology Consortium. J Natl Cancer Inst, 2007. 99(10): p. 777-89.

Hashibe, M., et al., Evidence for an important role of alcohol- and aldehyde-metabolizing genes in cancers of the upper aerodigestive tract. Cancer Epidemiol Biomarkers Prev, 2006. 15(4): p. 696-703.

Hashibe, M., et al., Interaction between tobacco and alcohol use and the risk of head and neck cancer: pooled analysis in the International Head and Neck Cancer Epidemiology Consortium. Cancer Epidemiol Biomarkers Prev, 2009. 18(2): p. 541-50.

Ho, P.S., et al., The incidence of oropharyngeal cancer in Taiwan: an endemic betel quid chewing area. J Oral Pathol Med, 2002. 31(4): p. 213-9.

Hong, W.K. and Bromer, R. Chemotherapy in head and neck cancer. N Engl J Med, 1983. 308(2): p. 75-9.

Hong, W.K., et al., 13-cis-retinoic acid in the treatment of oral leukoplakia. N Engl J Med, 1986. 315(24): p. 1501-5.

Janot, F., et al., Randomized trial of postoperative reirradiation combined with chemotherapy after salvage surgery compared with salvage surgery alone in head and neck carcinoma. J Clin Oncol, 2008. 26(34): p. 5518-23.

Jatin, P., Shah, S.G.P., Bhuvanesh Singh, Jatin Shah's Head and Neck Surgery and Oncology. 4th Edition ed. 2012, Philadelphia: Elsevier.

Kramer, S., et al., Combined radiation therapy and surgery in the management of advanced head and neck cancer: final report of study 73-03 of the Radiation Therapy Oncology Group. Head Neck Surg, 1987. 10(1): p. 19-30.

Langendijk, J.A., et al., Postoperative radiotherapy in squamous cell carcinoma of the oral cavity: the importance of the overall treatment time. Int J Radiat Oncol Biol Phys, 2003. 57(3): p. 693-700.

Layfield, L.J., Fine-needle aspiration of the head and neck. Pathology (Phila), 1996. 4(2): p. 409-38.

Lindberg, R., Distribution of cervical lymph node metastases from squamous cell carcinoma of the upper respiratory and digestive tracts. Cancer, 1972. 29(6): p. 1446-9.

Lindqvist, C. and Teppo, L. Epidemiological evaluation of sunlight as a risk factor of lip cancer. Br J Cancer, 1978. 37(6): p. 983-9.

Lippman, S.M., Benner, S.E. and Hong, W.K. Cancer chemoprevention. J Clin Oncol, 1994. 12(4): p. 851-73.

Lonneux, M., et al., Positron emission tomography with [18F]fluorodeoxyglucose improves staging and patient management in patients with head and neck squamous cell carcinoma: a multicenter prospective study. J Clin Oncol, 2010. 28(7): p. 1190-5.

Looser, K.G., Shah, J.P. and Strong, E.W. The significance of "positive" margins in surgically resected epidermoid carcinomas. Head Neck Surg, 1978. 1(2): p. 107-11.

Lustig, J.P., et al., Head and neck carcinoma in Fanconi's anaemia--report of a case and review of the literature. Eur J Cancer B Oral Oncol, 1995. 31B(1): p. 68-72.

Martin, H., Untimely lymph node biopsy. Am J Surg, 1961. 102: p. 17-8.

Massano, J., et al., Oral squamous cell carcinoma: review of prognostic and predictive factors. Oral Surg Oral Med Oral Pathol Oral Radiol Endod, 2006. 102(1): p. 67-76.

McGregor, I.A. and MacDonald, D.G. Spread of squamous cell carcinoma to the nonirradiated edentulous mandible--a preliminary report. Head Neck Surg, 1987. 9(3): p. 157-61.

McGuirt, W.F., Jr., et al., Floor of mouth carcinoma. The management of the clinically negative neck. Arch Otolaryngol Head Neck Surg, 1995. 121(3): p. 278-82.

Mukherji, S.K., et al., CT detection of mandibular invasion by squamous cell carcinoma of the oral cavity. AJR Am J Roentgenol, 2001. 177(1): p. 237-43.

National Comprehensive Cancer, N., Head and Neck Cancer. 2014.

Olasz, J., et al., RAR beta2 suppression in head and neck squamous cell carcinoma correlates with site, histology and age. Oncol Rep, 2007. 18(1): p. 105-12.

Peters, L.J., et al., Evaluation of the dose for postoperative radiation therapy of head and neck cancer: first report of a prospective randomized trial. Int J Radiat Oncol Biol Phys, 1993. 26(1): p. 3-11.

Pezier, T., et al., Sentinel lymph node biopsy for T1/T2 oral cavity squamous cell carcinoma--a prospective case series. Ann Surg Oncol, 2012. 19(11): p. 3528-33.

Yuen, P.W.A., et al., Prognostic factors of clinically stage I and II oral tongue carcinoma-A comparative study of stage, thickness, shape, growth pattern, invasive front malignancy grading, Martinez-Gimeno score, and pathologic features. Head Neck, 2002. 24(6): p. 513-20.

Program, N.T., Report on Carcinogens, Eleventh Edition, P.H.S. US Department of Health and Human Services, National Toxicology Program, 2005., Editor. 2005.

Ridge, J.A., Cancer Management: A Multidisciplinary Approach Medical, Surgical, and Radiation Oncology. Head and Neck Tumors, ed. L.D.W. Damiel G. Haller, Kevin A, CAmphausen, William J, Hoskins. 2013, Cancer Network Home of the Journal Oncology: Cancer Network.

Rosenblatt, K.A., et al., Marijuana use and risk of oral squamous cell carcinoma. Cancer Res, 2004. 64(11): p. 4049-54.

Samant, S., Sentinel node biopsy as an alternative to elective neck dissection for staging of early oral carcinoma. Head Neck, 2014. 36(2): p. 241-6.

Sasahira, T., Kirita, T. and Kuniyasu, H. Update of molecular pathobiology in oral cancer: a review. Int J Clin Oncol, 2014. 19(3): p. 431-6.

Secretan, B., et al., A review of human carcinogens--Part E: tobacco, areca nut, alcohol, coal smoke, and salted fish. Lancet Oncol, 2009. 10(11): p. 1033-4.

Shaha, A., Webber, C. and Marti, J. Fine-needle aspiration in the diagnosis of cervical lymphadenopathy. Am J Surg, 1986. 152(4): p. 420-3.

Shapiro, J.A., Jacobs, E.J. and Thun, M.J. Cigar smoking in men and risk of death from tobacco-related cancers. J Natl Cancer Inst, 2000. 92(4): p. 333-7.

Siegel R, M.J., Zou, Z, Jemal, A., Cancer statistics, 2014. Cancer J Clin, 2014. 64: p. 9-29.

Slaughter, D.P., Southwick, H.W. and Smejkal, W. Field cancerization in oral stratified squamous epithelium; clinical implications of multicentric origin. Cancer, 1953. 6(5): p. 963-8.

Slootweg, P.J., Eveson, J.W. Tumours of the Oral Cavity and Oropharynx, I.A.f.R.o. Cancer, Editor. 2014. p. 163-208.

Smith, M.A., et al. Retinoids in cancer therapy. J Clin Oncol, 1992. 10(5): p. 839-64.

Society, A.C. Cancer Facts and Figures 2014. Atlanta: American Cancer Society; 2014, 2014.

Speight, P.M. Update on oral epithelial dysplasia and progression to cancer. Head Neck Pathol, 2007. 1(1): p. 61-6.

Spiro, R.H., et al. Predictive value of tumor thickness in squamous carcinoma confined to the tongue and floor of the mouth. Am J Surg, 1986. 152(4): p. 345-50.

Steinkamp, H.J., et al. Magnetic resonance tomography and computerized tomography in tumor staging of mouth and oropharyngeal cancer. HNO, 1993. 41(11): p. 519-25.

Tanaka, T., Tanaka, M. and Tanaka, T. Oral carcinogenesis and oral cancer chemoprevention: a review. Patholog Res Int, 2011. 2011: p. 431246.

Tatomirovic, Z., et al. Fine needle aspiration cytology in the diagnosis of head and neck masses: accuracy and diagnostic problems. J BUON, 2009. 14(4): p. 653-9.

Thompson, L.D.R. Squamous Cell Carcinoma Variants of the Head and Neck. Current Diagnostic Pathology, 2003. 9: p. 384-396.

Tornesello, M.L., et al. HPV-related oropharyngeal cancers: From pathogenesis to new therapeutic approaches. Cancer Lett, 2014. 351(2): p. 198-205.

Trotti, A., et al. Mucositis incidence, severity and associated outcomes in patients with head and neck cancer receiving radiotherapy with or without chemotherapy: a systematic literature review. Radiother Oncol, 2003. 66(3): p. 253-62.

Tupchong, L., et al. Randomized study of preoperative versus postoperative radiation therapy in advanced head and neck carcinoma: long-term follow-up of RTOG study 73-03. Int J Radiat Oncol Biol Phys, 1991. 20(1): p. 21-8.

Vikram, B., et al. Intraoperative radiotherapy in patients with recurrent head and neck cancer. Am J Surg, 1985. 150(4): p. 485-7.

Vokes, E.E. and Athanasiadis, I. *Chemotherapy of squamous cell carcinoma of head and neck: the future is now.* Ann Oncol, 1996. 7(1): p. 15-29.

Wallner, P.E., et al. *Patterns of Care Study. Analysis of outcome survey data-anterior two-thirds of tongue and floor of mouth.* Am J Clin Oncol, 1986. 9(1): p. 50-7.

Wang, C. *Radiation Therapy for Head and Neck Cancers.* 1997, New York: Wiley-Liss.

Wendt, C.D., et al. *Primary radiotherapy in the treatment of stage I and II oral tongue cancers: importance of the proportion of therapy delivered with interstitial therapy.* Int J Radiat Oncol Biol Phys, 1990. 18(6): p. 1287-92.

Wong, L.Y., et al. *Salvage of recurrent head and neck squamous cell carcinoma after primary curative surgery.* Head Neck, 2003. 25(11): p. 953-9.

Wynder, E.L., et al. *Oral cancer and mouthwash use.* J Natl Cancer Inst, 1983. 70(2): p. 255-60.

Yorozu, A., Sykes, A.J. and Slevin, N.J. *Carcinoma of the hard palate treated with radiotherapy: a retrospective review of 31 cases.* Oral Oncol, 2001. 37(6): p. 493-7.

Znaor, A., et al. *Independent and combined effects of tobacco smoking, chewing and alcohol drinking on the risk of oral, pharyngeal and esophageal cancers in Indian men.* Int J Cancer, 2003. 105(5): p. 681-6.

Morbidity of Inguinofemoral Lymphadenectomy in Vulvar Cancer and Evolution of Operative Treatment

Amr A. Soliman[*], Basel Refky[†] and Eduard Malik[*]

1 Epidemiology

Vulvar cancer is the fourth most common gynecologic malignancy, accounting for 5 to 8% of all female genital tract malignancies (Stehman, 2007). It affects 4850 new patients annually in the United States (Siegel, Ma, Zou, & Jemal, 2014) and 3190 new patients in Germany (Kaatsch et al., 2013), with an annual estimated death rate of 1030 and 750, respectively, in the two countries (Kaatsch et al., 2013; Siegel et al., 2014). The incidence of the disease is on the rise, and has almost doubled in the last 10 years (Kaatsch et al., 2013), with a bimodal age distribution of a first peak at 45 to 50 years of age and a second peak at 70 to 75 years of age(Jones, Baranyai, & Stables, 1997).

The main risk factor for developing vulvar cancer is human papilloma virus (HPV) infection, whereas 40 to 60% of vulval cancers and 90% of vulvar intraepithelial neoplasia (VIN) are related to HPV infection (Hampl, Deckers-Figiel, Hampl, Rein, & Bender, 2008). HPV subtypes 6, 16, 18, 31, and 33 are most related to the development of vulvar cancer, especially type 16, which has the largest share, approaching 50% of all the affected cases (Insinga, Liaw, Johnson, & Madeleine, 2008). The role of high risk HPV infections was thoroughly studied in cervical dysplasia as a precancerous lesion(Saccardi et al., 2014) that makes us convinced that there is much to be explored in the field of vulvar cancer. The role of HPV vaccination is well established in cervical cancer and its precancerous lesions(Gizzo, Noventa, & Nardelli, 2013) but still needs to be further explored in vulvar cancer. Moreover, the role of antiretroviral medications was explored in precancerous lesions of cervical cancer(Patrelli et al., 2013) while its role in the field of vulvar cancer is still unclear. Other possible risk factors of vulvar cancer are smoking and immune deficiency, whether inherited or acquired.

The mainstay of treatment has always been operative, unless the tumor has already reached beyond local clearance so that palliative radiation therapy or combined radiochemotherapy remains the only possible option. Figure 1 shows a locally advanced vulvar cancer before (a) and after (b) a radical vulvectomy with bilateral inguinofemoral lymphadenectomy using a triple incision and abdominal wall flap to cover the resulting defect.

2 En Bloc Resection of the Vulva and Inguinofemoral Lymph Nodes as a Primary Operative Treatment

[*] University Women's Hospital of Oldenburg, University of Oldenburg, Germany
[†] Department of Surgical Oncology, Oncology Center, University of Mansoura, Egypt

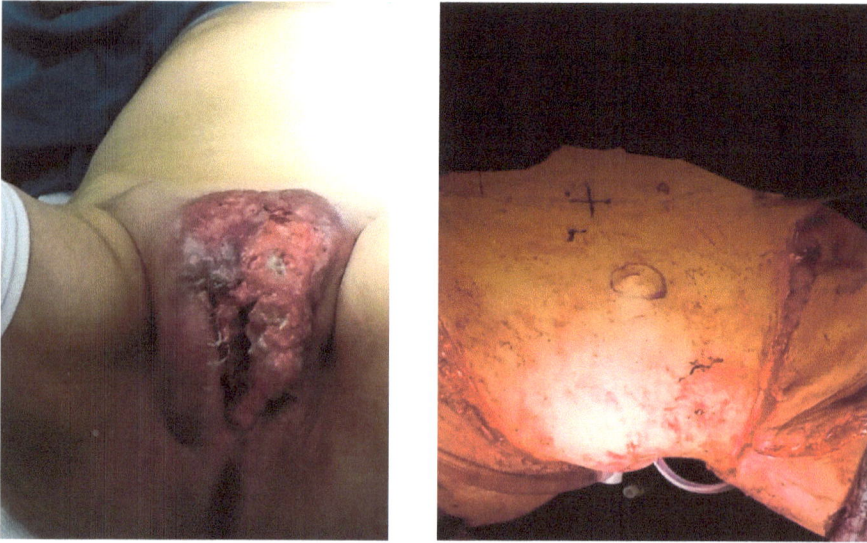

Figure 1: (a) A locally advanced vulvar cancer. (b) A local radical excision with bilateral inguinofemoral lymphadenectomy via a triple incision with an abdominal flap to cover the defect.

Operative therapy has been the primary treatment of choice for vulvar cancer for decades, providing complete resection of the primary tumor and removal of the draining locoregional lymph node groups, namely the inguinofemoral lymph nodes. Primary radio(chemo)therapy is reserved for locally advanced tumors, where a complete resection of the tumor does not seem achievable or for multi-morbid patients whose general condition does not allow such a radical procedure to be performed without grave consequences.

2.1   The Operative Technique

Since its introduction by Taussig in the 1940s (Taussig, 1940) and up to the 1990s, en bloc radical vulvectomy with bilateral inguinofemoral lymphadenectomy, the 'butterfly resection', has been the standard therapy for vulvar cancer. The aim of radical en bloc resection is to remove all tissue possibly involved in vulvar cancer, including the skin bridge between the vulva and the groins (Magrina *et al.*, 1998; Taussig, 1940). However, the severe morbidity of this mutilating procedure as well as the consecutive psychosexual impairment are a very high price for the treatment.

In butterfly incision, a single incision is made, starting from 2 cm medial and about 2 cm caudal to the anterior superior iliac spine, curving downwards, above the superior border of the inguinal ligament, to the inguinal ring including the mons pubis, and extends to meet the same starting point on the contralateral side. Through this incision, bilateral inguinofemoral lymphadenectomy can be performed. The same incisions are continued at their lateral edge, across the groin skin, downwards along the labiocrural folds on each side and across the perineum, where they meet. Through this part of the incision, the radical vulvectomy is performed. A medial mucosal incision is made along the introitus, extending through the anterior vestibule and around the urethral meatus. Attempts are made to attain at least a 2 cm margin of normal specimen, as a safety margin. The removed specimen then includes the tumor, the surrounding vulvar tissues till the fascia in the depth, the clitoris, the labia minora and possibly majora, according to the tumor location and size, and variable areas from the vaginal mucosa according to the location of the primary tumor. The wound is then copiously irrigated, hemostasis is secured, and groin wounds are closed in layers. Drains are inserted through separate incisions bilaterally. The vulvar wound is closed with delayed absorbable sutures (Byron RL, 1962; Lin, DuBeshter, Angel, & Dvoretsky, 1992). One step towards further radicality was introduced by (Way, 1978), who reported an improvement in survival in vulvar cancer patients by integrating pelvic lymphadenectomy into the procedure, which was advocated to be the standard operative therapy for some time (Way, 1978). A study from MD Anderson Hospital showed that of 191 patients, only nine (4.7%) had positive deep pelvic nodes, and all nine patients also had metastatic disease in the groin nodes (Curry, Wharton, & Rutledge, 1980). This study has demonstrated that the pelvic lymph nodes are only involved when the inguinal lymph nodes are already involved, an observation that suggests pelvic lymphadenectomy should be reserved for patients with involved inguinal lymph nodes (Stehman, 2007).

2.2   Morbidity of en Bloc Butterfly Resection

Although the en bloc resection resulted in reported cure rates of 80 to 90% for patients with stage I disease and exceeding 90% in cases without lymph node involvement (Hacker, Berek, Lagasse, Leuchter, & Moore, 1983; Podratz, Symmonds, Taylor, & Williams, 1983), the technique had high reported morbidity rates. The reported morbidities after en bloc resection included wound breakdown and/or infection (18 to 91%), chronic leg edema (8 to 70%), lymphocyst formation (0 to 31%), genital prolapse (0 to 14%), stress incontinence (0 to 12%), thrombophlebitis (0 to 9%), grafting skin flaps (0 to 24%), inguinal or femoral hernia (0 to 5%), pulmonary embolism (0 to 3%), ruptured femoral artery (0 to 5%), and hospital deaths (0 to 12%) (C. Morrow & Townsend, 1987), with the overall morbidity of 85% in the treated patients (Sultana & Naz, 2007).

3   The Triple Incision Technique as a Primary Operative Treatment

As a result of the aggressive nature of en bloc butterfly resection of the vulva and the inguino-femoral lymph nodes, with the very high reported primary morbidity rates, a modification of the technique was suggested (DiSaia, Creasman, & Rich, 1979). The aim of this modification is to remove the primary tumor, and as radically as is required, to remove the inguinal lymph nodes superficial to the cribriform fascia through a separate incision, preserving vulval and inguinal tissues as much as possible. If the superficial lymph nodes are involved, the group of lymph nodes deeper than the cribrifom fascia are then removed. The outcome and survival, as reported, are comparable to the more radical en bloc resection (DiSaia et al., 1979; Helm et al., 1992). Hence, the triple incision technique offers a less radical approach without sacrificing outcome, with less reported morbidity.

3.1   The Operative Technique

As originally described, the operative technique comprises three incisions, one for each groin and a separate incision for the radical vulvectomy. The superficial group of inguinal lymph nodes is removed first and sent for frozen section examination. If it is not involved, the procedure then comes to an end. If the superficial group of lymph nodes is involved, the deep group of lymph nodes along the femoral vessels should also be removed. No intentional attempts are made to preserve the great saphenous vein even if the cribriform fascia is not opened or removed (Berman, Soper, Creasman, Olt, & Disaia, 1989; DiSaia *et al.*, 1979; Hacker, Leuchter, Berek, Castaldo, & Lagasse, 1981). Some authors reported, however, a complete inguinofemoral lymphadenectomy, removing both the superficial and the deep group of lymph nodes, as a part of the standard technique, not employing the superficial group of lymph nodes as a sentinel for the deep group (Gaarenstroom *et al.*, 2003; Soliman, Heubner, Kimmig, & Wimberger, 2012). Figure 2 shows the boundaries of the superficial inguinofemoral lymphadenectomy as presented by (Stehman, 2007).

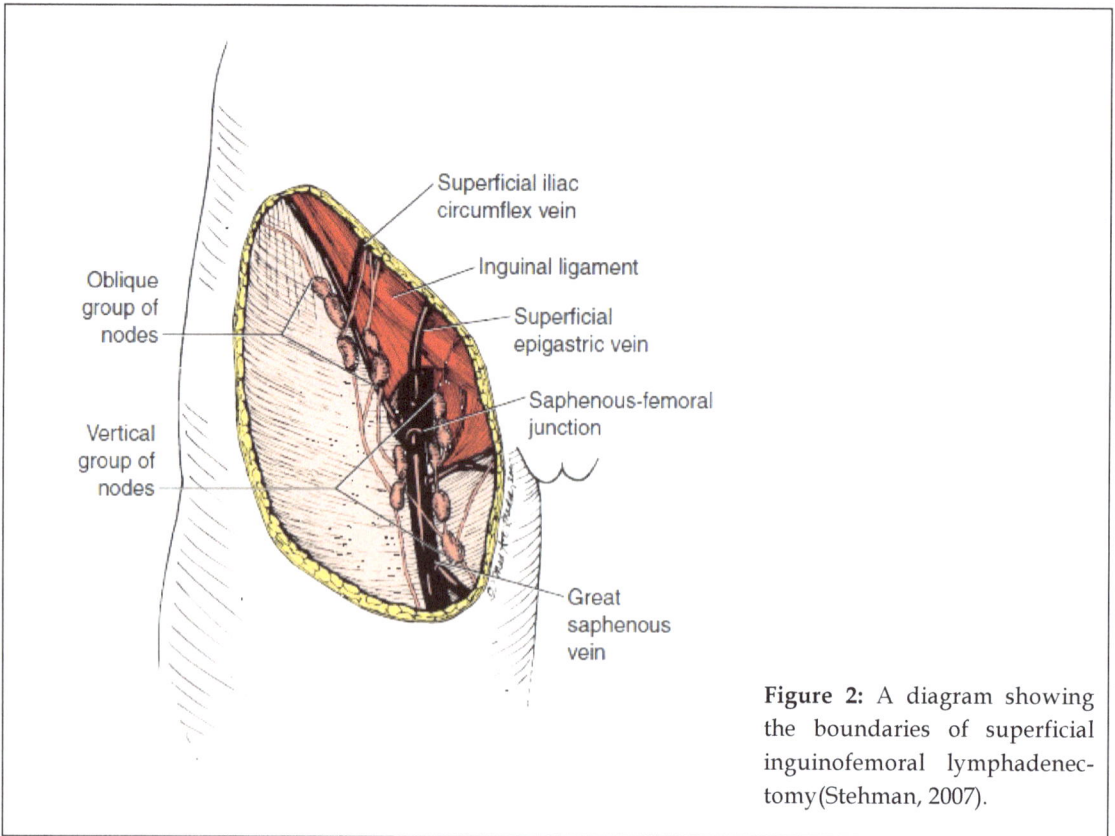

Figure 2: A diagram showing the boundaries of superficial inguinofemoral lymphadenectomy(Stehman, 2007).

Inguinofemoral lymphadenectomy is performed through a skin incision between the anterior superior iliac spine and the pubic tubercle, parallel to the inguinal ligament and with a length of 8 to 10 cm. The superficial part of the lymphadenectomy involves removal of the superficial inguinal lymph nodes that lie within the superficial fascial compartment of the groin and surround the branches of the saphenous vein. The anatomic boundaries of the superficial lymphatic dissection are the inguinal ligament superiorly, the border of the sartorius muscle laterally, the border of the adductor longus muscle medially, and the superficial subcutaneous fascia anteriorly. The deep femoral nodes are approached by opening the cribriform fascia along the sartorius muscle and mobilizing the fascia medially as a part of the specimen or by splitting the fascia lata longitudinally over the proximal femoral vessels. Once the femoral vein is identified and dissected free, the deep nodes that lie mainly medial to the femoral vein beneath the cribriform fascia are removed. These tissues are removed along with the cribriform fascia just below the inguinal ligament till about 2 cm proximal to the beginning of Hunter's canal when the femoral vessels are crossed by the Sartorius muscle. At the conclusion of the groin dissection, a suction drain is left in situ and the wound is closed in two layers (Soliman *et al.*, 2012).

Radical vulvectomy in the triple incision technique commences on the mons and extends posteriorly along the labial crural folds to the perineum. The medial incision extends around the vaginal mucosa at the introitus and anterior to the urethra. The vulva is resected to the level of the fascia overlying the urogeniral diaghragm (total deep vulvectomy) (Siller *et al.*, 1995). Table 1 shows a scheme of the operative management of vulvar cancer according to its stage.

Vulvar cancer stage	Management
T1a	Wide local excision
T1b	Vulvectomy, Lymph node dissection Ipsilateral, contralateral if < 1 cm from midline (triple incision). Sentinel lymph node procedure could be offered.
Locally advanced	Patient tailored according to the infiltrated organ

Table 1: Operative management of vulvar cancer according to stage.

Modification of the vulvar dissection to radical local excision or heimvulvectomy, according to the size and site of the presenting tumor, reduces local morbidity, with no increase in local recurrence (Burrell, Franklin, Campion, Crozier, & Stacy, 1988; Leminen, Forss, & Paavonen, 2000; Lin *et al.*, 1992). From the 1990s and till now, modified radical vulvectomy and bilateral inguinofemoral lymphadenectomy using separate incisions is the most appropriate form of surgical management for the majority of patients presenting with early stage vulvar cancer (Griffiths, Silverstone, Tobias, & Benjamin, 1997). Regardless of which surgical procedure is adopted for the vulvar lesion, i.e., radical vulvectomy or wide local excision, a minimal intraoperative macroscopic safety margin of 10 mm should be achieved, in order to ensure that the 8 mm margins required for the pathological examination to assign the specimen margins as tumor-free are still reachable even after artifacts from shrinkage during specimen fixation (Heaps, Fu, Montz, Hacker, & Berek, 1990).

In a Cochrane review comparing en bloc radical resection to the triple incision technique, the authors concluded that radical local excision, ipsilateral lymph node dissection for lateral tumors, and the triple incision technique with bilateral lymph node dissection for midline tumors are safe treatment options for early vulvar cancer (Ansink & van der Velden, 2000). However, superficial groin node dissection resulted in an excess of groin recurrences compared with a full inguinofemoral lymphadenectomy.

3.2   Morbidity of the Triple Incision Technique

Despite modifications of the technique, the triple incision technique still has high morbidity rates. The morbidity rates are much lower than those reported after en bloc resection, but they are high enough to affect the quality of life of the patients in the long term. The morbidity rates of this technique and the possible factors affecting their development have been reported by many groups. In a report concerning the complications of inguinofemoral lymphadenectomy and the predictors of their development, the authors demonstrated a variety of postoperative problems but could not highlight a single factor as a predictor of occurrence of complications (Gould et al.,2001). In this retrospective cohort of 67 vulvar cancer patients who received triple incision as primary operative treatment, early postoperative cellulitis developed in 35.4% while late cellulitis developed in 22.2%. Early wound breakdown occurred in 19.4%, late wound breakdown developed in 3.2%, early lymphedema occurred in 4.8%, and 29.5% developed late lymphedema. A total of 13.1% of patients developed early lymphocysts while 5% developed late lymphocysts. Patients who developed early cellulitis were more likely to have early wound breakdown ($p < 0.001$) or early lymphocyst formation ($p < 0.02$). The type of procedure, postoperative prophylactic antibiotic use, need for adjuvant therapy, and duration of suction drainage did not significantly influence the incidence of early cellulitis. Late cellulitis was unaffected by early cellulitis, early wound breakdown, type of procedure, use of prophylactic antibiotics, duration of suction drainage, and need for adjuvant therapy (Gould et al., 2001). These results are summarized in Table 2.

Wound cellulitis	35.4%
Wound breakdown	19.4%
Wound seroma	13.1%
Early lower limb lymphedema formation	4.8%

Table 2: Frequency of complications after inguinofemoral lymphadenectomy(Gould et al., 2001).

In a retrospective cohort of 194 patients, another report concluded that preservation of the fascia lata and saphenous vein in inguinofemoral lymphadenectomy was associated with a decreased risk of postoperative morbidity, without jeopardizing outcomes (Rouzier, Haddad, Dubernard, Dubois, & Paniel, 2003). Table 3 shows the frequency of distribution of cellulitis, wound breakdown, and lymphedema in this cohort and the correlation with possible factors affecting their development.

A recent retrospective cohort of 67 operated groins showed an incidence of wound cellulitis of 24.2%, while 9.7% developed wound breakdown, 12.5% developed wound seroma, and 3.2% developed wound infection; 4.8% developed early limb lymphoedema while on long-term follow-up and 21.4% showed lower limb lymphedema (Soliman et al., 2012). Table 4 shows the frequency of occurrence of simultaneous complications in the same groin (Soliman et al., 2012).

Another report studying the same issue reported retrospectively from a cohort of 101 patients that as many as 66% of the patients suffered one or more complications following groin dissection (Gaarenstroom et al., 2003). Wound breakdown of the groin, lymphocyst formation, infection, and lymphedema were noted in 17%, 40%, 39%, and 28% of the patients,

		Cellulitis		Wound Breakdown		Lymphedema	
Age	< or = 70	25.3%		21.1%		43.4%	
	> 70	25.4%	p = 0.98	36.0%	p = 0.002*	30.1%	p = 0.01*
Obesity	Yes	32.1%		33.6%		37.2%	
	No	21.1%	p = 0.02	26.1%	p = 0.13	37.2%	p = 0.99
Sartorius transposition	Yes	28.4%		43.3%		55.2%	
	No	29.5%	p = 0.87	36%	p = 0.31	21.6%	p < 0.001*
Saphenous vein preservation	Yes	29.8%		36.4%		45.3%	
	No	17.7%	p = 0.01*	16.2%	p < 0.001*	23.1%	p < 0.001*
Number of lymph nodes removed	< or = 8	22.5%		28.9%		34.8%	
	> 8	31.2%	p = 0.16	31.2%	p = 0.96	40.4%	p = 0.28

Table 3: Frequency of occurrence of complications and factors affecting their development. p < 0.05 is statistically significant (Rouzier *et al.*, 2003).

	Wound cellulitis	Wound breakdown	Wound seroma formation	Wound infection	Early leg lymphedema
Wound cellulitis		5 (p < 0.001)*	3	1	1
Wound breakdown	5 (p < 0.001)*		1	0	0
Wound seroma formation	3	1		0	0
Wound infection	1	0	0		0
Early leg lymphedema	1	0	0	0	

Table 4: Frequency (n) of simultaneous complications in the same groin. p < 0.05 is statistically significant (Soliman *et al.*, 2012).

respectively. Regarding the rate of complications per groin, the incidence was 11%, 27%, 27%, and 21%, respectively. The study also reported that the occurrence of early complications after groin dissection such as wound breakdown, lymphocyst formation, and infection was significantly related to the occurrence of late lymphedema (p = 0.002). Of the 187 complete inguinofemoral lymph node dissections reported in this study, the great saphenous vein was ligated in 150 groins, preserved in 19 groins, and the status was unknown in 18 groins. The overall complication rate of the groin dissection was not significantly related to removal of the saphenous vein. In particular, the development of lymphedema showed no relationship with ligation or removal of the vein. Table 5 shows a comparison of the three relatively recent case series reporting on the incidence of wound complications of the triple incision technique for vulvar cancer.

The above-mentioned reports studied, in addition to the rates of development of morbidities after inguinofemoral lymphadenectomies, factors that may lead to the development of inguinal wound and lower limb morbidities. Unfortunately, no single factor was found to be directly related to the development of complications; thus, the practice cannot be selectively changed in order to avoid the development of wound morbidity. The studied factors were cardiovascular disorders, diabetes, amount of intraoperative blood loss, number of infiltrated lymph nodes, saphenous vein ligation, number of removed lymph nodes, duration of suction drainage, and amount of exudate accumulated in the drains (Gaarenstroom *et al.*, 2003;

	Soliman *et al.*	Gaarstroom *et al.*	Gould *et al.*
Wound cellulitis	24.2% (n = 15)	Not studied	35.4%
Wound breakdown	9.7% (n = 6)	11% (n = 21)	19.4%
Wound seroma	12.5% (n = 8)	27% (n = 50)	13.1%
Wound infection	3.2% (n = 2)	27% (n = 51)	Not studied
Early lower limb lymphedema formation	4.8% (n = 3)	21% (n = 40)	4.8%

Table 5: Comparison of the incidence of wound complications in the published case series of the triple incision technique for vulvar cancer (Gaarenstroom *et al.*, 2003; Gould *et al.*, 2001; Soliman *et al.*, 2012).

Soliman *et al.*, 2012). However, development of early lower limb edema was related to development of long-term lower limb edema (Gaarenstroom *et al.*, 2003; Gould *et al.*, 2001; Soliman *et al.*, 2012).

3.3   Modifications of the Triple Incision Technique Aimed at Decreasing Morbidity

Modifications have been introduced in an attempt to decrease the morbidity of the triple incision. One of these modifications is preservation of the great saphenous vein during the groin operation. In a prospective study on 64 patients, 31 of them received a vein-sparing groin operation while in 33 patients, the vein was ligated or excised. The key process of the saphenous vein-sparing technique is to dissect the saphenous vein trunk in its way to the saphenofemoral junction during superficial inguinal lymphovascular fat tissue removal and then to spare it. When the saphenous vein affects exposure of the operative area during deep inguinal node excision, it should be pulled aside using a vein retractor rather than being severed or excised (Zhang *et al.*, 2007). The reported complications from this study are summarized in Table 6.

	Postoperative fever	Acute cellulitis	Seroma	Acute low extremity phlebitis	Lymphocele	Acute lymphedema
Sparing	96.8%	67.7%	30.6%	11.3%	25.8%	43.5%
Excision	93.9%	72.7%	37.9%	25.8%	31.8%	66.7%
p value	>0.05	>0.05	>0.05	<0.05*	>0.05	<0.01*

Table 6: Comparing the incidence of complications in the saphenous vein-sparing and saphenous vein excision groups. *$p < 0.05$ is statistically significant (Zhang *et al.*, 2007).

The findings of this report, however, contradict the findings of two reports that studied retrospectively the morbidity of inguinofemoral lymphadenectomy and the factors that might affect its development and found no correlation between saphenous vein ligation/preservation and the development of any type of groin complications (Gaarenstroom *et al.*, 2003; Soliman *et al.*, 2012). Another operative modification aimed at decreasing groin wound complications was addressed through a randomized controlled trial that assessed whether different cutaneous skin flap dissection above or below the inguinal ligament would reduce groin wound complications (Manci *et al.*, 2009). This prospective randomized clinical trial of 62 consecutive patients affected by vulvar carcinoma requiring inguinal lymphadenectomy compared skin inguinal incision carried out 3 to 4 cm above the inguinal ligament (group A) and that carried out below it (group B). Inguinal dehiscence was present in 32.1% of patients in group B and in 16.7% of patients in group A (p = 0.10). Lymphocele was observed in 18.9% of lymphadenectomies in group B and in 5.6% of dissections in group A (p = 0.07). Upper incision allows more precise identification of the Camper's fascia, is less painful, and gives better cosmetic results. Moreover, there may be other advantages, albeit not statistically significant, regarding wound dehiscence rate and speed of wound healing. The study concluded that there was no difference in chronic leg edema, number of nodes removed, or hospital stay when adopting the new incision site.

In an attempt to decrease morbidity, Bell *et al.* (2000) performed the lymphadenectomy with preservation of the fascia lata and cribriform fascia superficial to the femoral vessels. The main aim was to assess the recurrence rates after this procedure. They reported low incidence rates of lymphedema (13%) and lymphocyst (15%) in their retrospective cohort of 60 patients. The groin recurrence rate was, however, 7.6% in patients with fewer than three involved lymph nodes. The study concluded that the zero groin recurrence rate in patients with negative nodes and the low rate of recurrence in patients with positive nodes indicated that groin lymphadenectomy with preservation of the fascia lata was complete, therapeutic, and comparable to radical techniques of lymphadenectomy involving skeletonization of femoral vessels, resection of the fascia lata, and muscle transposition.

Another modification to the operative technique was studied in a randomized controlled prospective trial in 61 patients and 99 operated groins, comparing transposition of the sartorius muscle versus non-transposition in an attempt to decrease postoperative groin morbidity (Judson *et al.*, 2004). The results revealed, however, that there were no statistically significant differences in the incidence of wound cellulitis, wound breakdown, lymphedema, or re-hospitalization. The incidence of lymphocyst formation was increased in the sartorius transposition group. After adjusting for age, however, the groups appeared similar. The study concluded that sartorius transposition after inguinofemoral lymphadenectomy did not reduce postoperative wound morbidity.

Modifications to the triple incision technique were not only limited to the operative steps. A randomized gynecologic oncology group (GOG) trial used a fibrin sealant in order to decrease the incidence of lower extremity edema following inguinofemoral lymphadenectomy (Carlson *et al.*, 2008). A total of 150 patients were enrolled into the study and randomized to receive standard closure (SC) of the wound using sutures or the VH fibrin sealant (FS) (Tisseel®, Baxter Healthcare Corporation, Glendale, CA, USA) followed by suture closure. The incidence of grade 2 and 3 lymphedema was 67% in the SC arm and 60% in the FS arm (p = 0.478). At the 6-week assessment, 48% of the patients demonstrated grade 2 or worse lymphedema. The frequency of grade 2 or 3 lymphedema increased to 57% at 3 months and 63.5% at 6 months. Among those patients who developed a grade 2 or 3 lymphedema, 75.9% had done so by 6-week follow-up and 90.8% by the 3-month follow-up. The overall complication rate was 59% for patients in the SC arm and 61% for those in the FS arm. The overall incidence of inguinal infections was 35% in the SC arm and 36% in the FS arm. The incidence of inguinal wound breakdown was 13% in both treatment arms. The number of patients who had either a grade 3 or grade 4 inguinal infection was also similar between the SC (n = 8) and FS (n = 7) arms. The incidence of either a grade 3 or grade 4 vulvar infection was the same (n = 3) in both arms. The study concluded that postoperative lymphedema at 6 months was not affected by utilization of a fibrin sealant in the inguinal wound.

Madhuri *et al.* used a Plasmajet® hand piece to seal the groin lymphatics after inguino-femoral lymphadenectomy with saphenous vein preservation, and suggested this method could promise decreasing the rate of postoperative wound complications(Madhuri, Tailor, & Butler-Manuel, 2011).

Moreover, the laparoscopic approach to inguinofemoral lymphadenectomy, which is reported for managing penile carcinoma, may provide an acceptable treatment modality with lower complications rate(Pompeo *et al.*, 2013; Tobias-Machado *et al.*, 2007; Yuan *et al.*, 2014). The data as regard this technique is however not yet mature to consider it a standard proce-dure.

As demonstrated above, many modifications have been introduced to the technique of triple incision. However, they have failed to improve the morbidity rates. Nevertheless, the technique remains, to date, the recommended standard operative therapy. Despite these failed attempts to decrease the morbidity, further trials were conducted to find a better thera-peutic option for patients suffering early vulvar cancer. These trials and new modalities are discussed in the next section.

4   The Sentinel Lymph Node Technique in Vulvar Cancer: Lower Morbidity without Compromising the Oncological Outcome

The triple incision technique as introduced by (DiSaia *et al.*, 1979) considered the superficial inguinal group of lymph nodes as a 'sentinel' group of nodes for the whole groin. When this group is involved, a full inguinofemoral clearance is necessary. The aim of introducing this surgical technique was less radicality, with consequently less morbidity without sacrificing oncological outcome. Based on the reports about the sentinel lymph node technique in cuta-neous melanoma, (Levenback *et al.*, 1994) published the results of their pilot study examining the feasibility of sentinel lymph node examination for vulvar cancer patients. They recruited nine patients in whom 12 groins were examined. They used blue dye and succeeded in identi-fying seven of 12 sentinel lymph nodes. Moreover, one positive non-sentinel lymph node was identified in a sentinel-negative patient. They concluded that intraoperative lymphatic map-ping was technically feasible in patients with vulvar cancer, particularly those with unilateral disease. They recommended further studies be designed to gain more experience with this technique. Since then, the technique has been applied in breast cancer with high accuracy (Mansel *et al.*, 2006) and improved quality of life of patients (Lucci *et al.*, 2007; Purushotham *et al.*, 2005). Many study groups are interested in examining the sentinel technique in vulvar cancer in order to improve the morbidity rates after a formal inguinofemoral lymphadenec-tomy and hence the quality of life of the patients. The motive for these studies, besides the high rate of postoperative complications for a systematic inguinofemoral lymphadenectomy, is that only 25 to 35% of patients with early stage disease will have lymph node metastases, and the remaining 65 to 75% of patients are unlikely to benefit from elective inguinofemoral lymphadenectomy but will be at risk for its significant morbidity (Bell, Lea, & Reid, 2000; Hacker *et al.*, 1981).

Although some early reports about this new technique were very promising, with a 100% success rate in detecting sentinel lymph nodes and 0% false negative rates (De Cicco *et al.*, 2000), some authors were skeptical about it. In a prospective trial of the GOG in 121 patients with early stage vulvar cancer (Stehman, Bundy, Dvoretsky, & Creasman, 1992), the authors questioned the benefit of the sentinel procedure concerning recurrence in the groins that did not receive a formal inguinofemoral lymphadenectomy based on a negative sentinel lymph node procedure, as originally described by (DiSaia *et al.*, 1979). The groin recurrence in this report was almost always fatal; five of the seven patients with groin recurrence passed away.

In their study in 37 patients with a total of 55 operated groins, (De Cicco *et al.*, 2000) aimed to verify the predictive value of the sentinel lymph node status in a larger series of patients. They used technetium-99m-labeled colloid human albumin administered perilesionally 1 day before surgery to perform lymphoscintigraphy of the groin, and used a gamma-detecting probe intraoperatively to find sentinel lymph nodes. An inguinofemoral lymphadenectomy was performed regardless of the results of the sentinel mapping. As mentioned above, they reported a 100% detection rate of sentinel lymph nodes and a 0% false negative rate. They concluded that this technique was an easy and reliable method for the detection of sentinel nodes in early vulvar cancer. This technique may represent a true advance in the direction of less aggressive treatments in patients with vulvar cancer. The high accuracy and negative predictive value are attributed to using lymphoscintigraphy, applying strict quality control steps while performing the sentinel procedure, and using step section and immuno-histochemistry in the examination of the sentinel lymph nodes by the pathologist.

In 51 patients in which blue dye was used to identify sentinel lymph nodes, (Ansink *et al.*, 1999) reported a very low detection rate of only 56%, with a relatively high false negative rate (two false negative sentinels), rendering the technique unreliable. There is no consensus on which technique is better to use. Some authors advocate the use of blue dye alone (M. Morrow *et al.*, 1999), while others advocate the use of radioactive isotope alone (Levenback *et al.*, 2001) or a combination of both (de Hullu *et al.*, 2004).

The detection rate and false negative rate of the sentinel procedure remain controversial. In a multicenter prospective study, Hampl *et al.* recruited 127 patients suffering T1 to T3 vulvar cancers, performed a sentinel lymph node biopsy uni- or bilaterally, according to the tumor location from the midline, then performed a formal inguinofemoral lymphadenectomy to examine the detection rate of the sentinel node procedure with consecutive standard inguinofemoral lympadenectomy, to determine the sensitivity and specificity of the method to predict the final lymph node status. The study evaluated the negative predictive value of the procedure and investigated a potential correlation between tumor location and accuracy of the procedure. Patients harboring negative sentinel lymph nodes received a step-sectioning and additional immunihistochemical staining by the pathologist to increase the detection rate of micrometastasis. The authors used both lymphoscintigraphy and blue dye to detect sentinel lymph nodes. The overall detection rate of sentinel lymph nodes was 99.1% and the detection rate was 98.3% for solely technetium-labeled sentinels. The reported sensitivity was 92.3% and false negative rate was 7.7%. Based on their results, the authors issued some recommendations, which agreed with the recommendations of the 6th Biennial International Sentinel Node Society Meeting in Australia, February 2008 (personal communication), that gynecologic oncologists should perform at least 10 groin dissections with successful identification of sentinel lymph nodes and no false negative sentinel lymph nodes before performing lymph node biopsy on their own. They also recommended performing the sentinel lymph node identification only in patients with tumors smaller than 4 cm. In case of a midline tumor, sentinel lymph nodes should be identified in both groins. If sentinel lymph nodes are not identified or any doubt exists regarding the correlation between a preoperative lymphoscinti-gram and the operative findings, the sentinel procedure should be abandoned and a formal inguinofemoral lymphadenectomy should be performed. A suspicious non-sentinel node should always be resected. They finally recommended ultrastaging for all removed sentinel lymph nodes (Hampl *et al.*, 2008b).

The ultimate goal of oncologic surgery is to reach complete cure, represented by high overall survival and progression-free survival rates. Johann and coworkers compared retro-spectively long-term outcomes of the sentinel lymph node procedure to those of a formal inguinofemoral lymphadenectomy. In this study, they analyzed data from 114 operated groins, with a sentinel detection rate of 95%, and a false negative rate of 2.2%. The median follow-up for patients who received a sentinel lymph node procedure and for those who re-ceived a formal inguinofemoral lymphadenectomy was 24 months and 111 months, respec-tively. Figure 3 shows the rate of development of local morbidity in the group that received a sentinel lymph node procedure and the group that received a lymphadenectomy (Johann *et al.*, 2008). Figure 4 shows the recurrence rate in both groups.

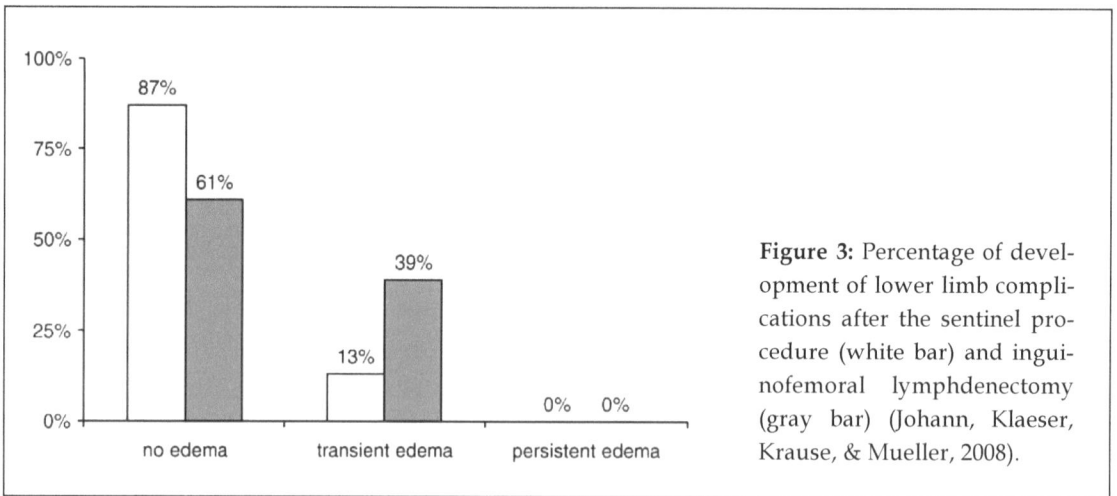

Figure 3: Percentage of devel-opment of lower limb compli-cations after the sentinel pro-cedure (white bar) and ingui-nofemoral lymphdenectomy (gray bar) (Johann, Klaeser, Krause, & Mueller, 2008).

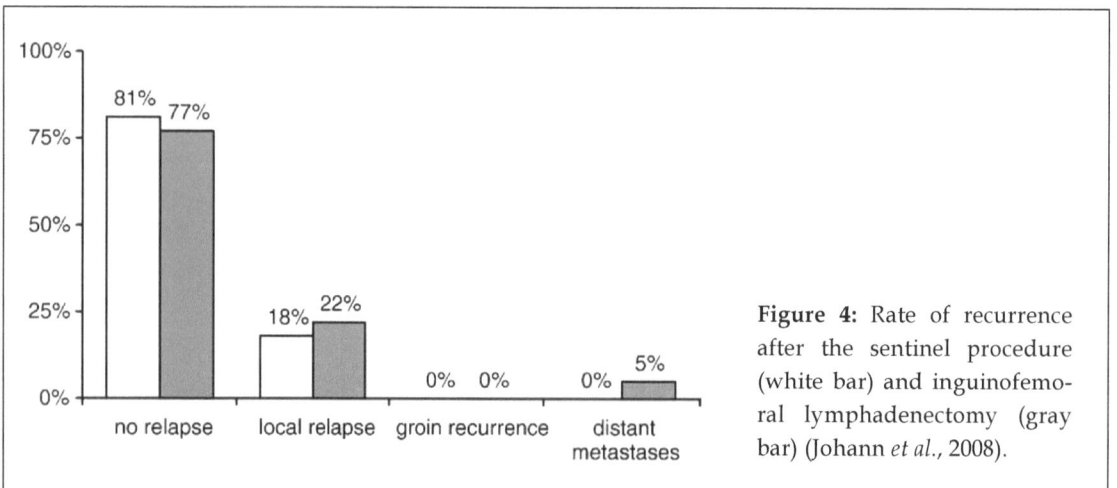

Figure 4: Rate of recurrence after the sentinel procedure (white bar) and inguinofemo-ral lymphadenectomy (gray bar) (Johann *et al.*, 2008).

Based on these results, the authors concluded that sentinel lymphadenectomy could be considered a feasible, accurate, and reliable method in a clinical routine setting for identifying nodal negative patients in vulvar cancer who will not benefit from a complete inguinofemoral lymphadenectomy (Johann *et al.*, 2008). They also concluded that the risk of groin relapse was not elevated after the sentinel procedure. Moreover, their results demonstrated that the risk of leg edema as a treatment-related morbidity after the sentinel lymph node procedure was considerably lower than that after inguinofemoral lymphadenectomy.

(Van der Zee *et al.*, 2008) conducted the largest prospective multicenter trial on the sentinel lymph node procedure, examining the accuracy, safety, local recurrence, and long-term outcome. A multicenter observational study on sentinel node detection using radioactive tracer and blue dye was performed in patients with T1/2 (< or = 4 cm) squamous cell cancer of the vulva. When the sentinel node was found to be negative at pathologic ultrastaging, inguinofemoral lymphadenectomy was omitted, and the patient was observed with a follow-up of 2 years every 2 months. Stopping rules were defined for the occurrence of groin recurrences. The sentinel node procedure was performed in 623 groins of 403 assessable patients. In 259 patients with unifocal vulvar disease and a negative sentinel node (median follow-up time, 35 months), six groin recurrences were diagnosed (2.3%), and 3-year survival rate was 97%. Short-term morbidity was decreased in patients after sentinel node dissection compared with patients with a positive sentinel node who underwent a subsequent inguinofemoral lymphadenectomy (wound breakdown in groin: 11.7% vs. 34.0%, respectively, p < 0.0001; and cellulitis: 4.5% vs. 21.3%, respectively, p < 0.0001). Long-term morbidity was also less frequently observed after removal of only the sentinel node compared with sentinel node removal and inguinofemoral lymphadenectomy (recurrent erysipelas: 0.4% vs. 16.2%, respectively, p < 0.0001; and lymphedema of the legs: 1.9% vs. 25.2%, respectively, p < 0.0001). This data is summarized in table 7.

	Sentinel	Inguinofemoral systematic lymphadenectomy	p-value
Wound breakdown	11.7%	34%	p < 0.0001
Cellulitis	4.5%	21.3%	p < 0.0001
Recurrent erysipelas	0.4%	16.2%	p < 0.0001
Lymphedema	1.9%	25.2%	p < 0.0001

Table 7: Rate of complications compared between sentinel and systematic inguinofemoral lymphadenectomy. p < 0.05 is statistically significant(Van der Zee *et al.*, 2008).

Based on these results, the authors concluded that in early stage vulvar cancer patients with a negative sentinel node, the groin recurrence rate was low, survival was excellent, and treatment-related morbidity was minimal. They even suggested that sentinel node dissection, performed by a quality-controlled multidisciplinary team, should be part of the standard treatment in selected patients with early stage vulvar cancer. In a subsequent analysis of a subset of the patients recruited to the study by (Van der Zee *et al.*, 2008), (Oonk *et al.*, 2009) performed a questionnaire on the quality of life after a sentinel procedure in comparison with that after a sentinel procedure followed by inguinofemoral lymphadenectomy due to positive lymph nodes. They found that patients who underwent a sentinel procedure alone reported less treatment-related morbidity compared with patients who underwent inguinofemoral lymphadenectomy, but this did not influence the overall quality of life. Patients who underwent the sentinel procedure without inguinofemoral lymphadenectomy were more content with the procedure they underwent and were more likely to recommend this new treatment option to relatives, probably because they themselves experienced the benefits of the new procedure. On the other hand, the patients who received an inguinofemoral lymophadenectomy after a sentinel procedure due to a positive lymph node were probably not going to recommend the new procedure to their relatives, for fear of false negative results.

Although pathological ultrastaging of the retrieved inguinofemoral lymph nodes using the sentinel technique is recommended from some authors (Sutton *et al.*, 2013; Van der Zee *et al.*, 2008), the role of HPV genetic material testing during frozen section and its role in adding more accuracy in detecting metastasis in inguinofemoral lymph nodes can be investigated as it proved useful in the field of cervical cancer as reported by some authors(Noventa, Ancona, Cosmi, *et al.*, 2014; Noventa, Ancona, Saccardi, *et al.*, 2014)

As discussed in this text, the treatment of vulvar cancer has evolved from a more radical procedure to a less radical one through the years, aimed at decreasing morbidity without compromising survival outcomes. It seems that the sentinel lymph node procedure, with its remarkable accuracy, low morbidity, and survival outcomes that are comparable to those of the tripe incision technique, may slowly become the standard surgical option in early stage vulvar cancer and replace the current standard of the triple incision technique. This can be achieved after gaining enough experience with the technique, accurately detecting sentinel lymph nodes, accurately ultrastaging them pathologically, and minimizing the false negative rate to almost nil.

References

Ansink, A., Sie-Go, D. M., van der Velden, J., Sijmons, E. A., de Barros Lopes, A., Monaghan, J. M., . . . Heintz, A. P. (1999). Identification of sentinel lymph nodes in vulvar carcinoma patients with the aid of a patent blue V injection: a multicenter study. Cancer, 86(4), 652-656.

Ansink, A., & van der Velden, J. (2000). Surgical interventions for early squamous cell carcinoma of the vulva. Cochrane Database of Systematic Reviews, 2.

Bell, J. G., Lea, J. S., & Reid, G. C. (2000). Complete groin lymphadenectomy with preservation of the fascia lata in the treatment of vulvar carcinoma. Gynecol Oncol, 77(2), 314-318. doi: 10.1006/gyno.2000.5790

Berman, M., Soper, J., Creasman, W., Olt, G., & Disaia, P. (1989). Conservative Surgical Management of Superficially Invasive Stage I Vulvar Carcinoma. Gynecol Oncol, 35, 352-359.

Burrell, M., Franklin, E., Campion, M., Crozier, M., & Stacy, D. (1988). The modified radical vulvectomy with groin dissection: an eight-year experience. Am J Obstet Gynecol, 159(3), 712-719.

Byron RL, L. E., Yonemoto RH. (1962). Radical inguinal node dissection in the treatment of cancer. Surg Gynecol Obstet, 114, 7.

Carlson, J. W., Kauderer, J., Walker, J. L., Gold, M. A., O'Malley, D., Tuller, E., & Clarke-Pearson, D. L. (2008). A randomized phase III trial of VH fibrin sealant to reduce lymphedema after inguinal lymph node dissection: a Gynecologic Oncology Group study. Gynecol Oncol, 110(1), 76-82. doi: 10.1016/j.ygyno.2008.03.005

Curry, S., Wharton, J., & Rutledge, F. (1980). Positive lymph nodes in vulvar squamous carcinoma. Gynecol Oncol, 9(1), 63-67.

De Cicco, C., Sideri, M., Bartolomei, M., Grana, C., Cremonesi, M., Fiorenza, M., . . . Paganelli, G. (2000). Sentinel node biopsy in early vulvar cancer. Br J Cancer, 82(2), 295-299.

de Hullu, J. A., Oonk, M. H., Ansink, A. C., Hollema, H., Jager, P. L., & van der Zee, A. G. (2004). Pitfalls in the sentinel lymph node procedure in vulvar cancer. Gynecol Oncol, 94(1), 10-15. doi: 10.1016/j.ygyno.2004.02.031

DiSaia, P., Creasman, W., & Rich, W. (1979). An alternate approach to early cancer of the vulva. Am J Obstet Gynecol, 133(7), 825-832.

Gaarenstroom, K., Kenter, G., Trimbos, J., Agous, I., Amant, F., Peters, A., & Vergote, I. (2003). Postoperative complications after vulvectomy and inguinofemoral lymphadenectomy using separate groin incisions. Int J Gynecol Cancer, 13, 522-527.

Gizzo, S., Noventa, M., & Nardelli, G. B. (2013). Gardasil administration to hr-HPV-positive women and their partners. Trends Pharmacol Sci, 34(9), 479-480. doi: 10.1016/j.tips.2013.07.001

Gould, N., Kamelle, S., Tillmanns, T., Scribner, D., Gold, M., Walker, J., & Mannel, R. (2001). Predictors of complications after inguinal lymphadenectomy. Gynecol Oncol, 82(2), 329-332. doi: 10.1006/gyno.2001.6266

Griffiths, C., Silverstone, A., Tobias, J., & Benjamin, E. (1997). Carcinoma of the vulva. In C. Griffiths, A. Silverstone, J. Tobias, & E. Benjamin (Eds.), Gynecol Oncol (pp. 79-94). Barcelona: Mosby-Wolfe

Hacker, N., Berek, J., Lagasse, L., Leuchter, R., & Moore, J. (1983). Management of regional lymph nodes and their prognostic influence in vulvar cancer. Obstet Gynecol, 61(4), 408-412.

Hacker, N., Leuchter, R., Berek, J., Castaldo, T., & Lagasse, L. (1981). Raidcal vulvectomy and bilateral inguinal lymphadenectomy through separate groin incisions. Obstet Gynecol, 58(4), 574-579.

Hampl, M., Deckers-Figiel, S., Hampl, J. A., Rein, D., & Bender, H. G. (2008). New aspects of vulvar cancer: changes in localization and age of onset. Gynecol Oncol, 109(3), 340-345. doi: 10.1016/j.ygyno.2008.01.041

Heaps, J., Fu, Y., Montz, F., Hacker, N., & Berek, J. (1990). Surgical-pathologic variables predictive of local recurrence in squamous cell carcinoma of the vulva. Gynecol Oncol, 38(3), 309-314.

Helm, C. W., Hatch, K., Austin, J. M., Partridge, E. E., Soong, S. J., Elder, J. E., & Shingleton, H. M. (1992). A matched comparison of single and triple incision techniques for the surgical treatment of carcinoma of the vulva. Gynecol Oncol, 46(2), 150-156.

Insinga, R. P., Liaw, K. L., Johnson, L. G., & Madeleine, M. M. (2008). A systematic review of the prevalence and attribution of human papillomavirus types among cervical, vaginal, and vulvar precancers and cancers in the United States. Cancer Epidemiol Biomarkers Prev, 17(7), 1611-1622. doi: 10.1158/1055-9965.EPI-07-2922

Johann, S., Klaeser, B., Krause, T., & Mueller, M. D. (2008). Comparison of outcome and recurrence-free survival after sentinel lymph node biopsy and lymphadenectomy in vulvar cancer. Gynecol Oncol, 110(3), 324-328. doi: 10.1016/j.ygyno.2008.04.004

Jones, R., Baranyai, J., & Stables, S. (1997). Trends in squamous cell carcinoma of the vulva: the influence of vulvar intraepithelial neoplasia. Obstet Gynecol., 90(3), 448-452.

Judson, P. L., Jonson, A. L., Paley, P. J., Bliss, R. L., Murray, K. P., Downs, L. S., Jr., . . . Carson, L. F. (2004). A prospective, randomized study analyzing sartorius transposition following inguinal-femoral lymphadenectomy. Gynecol Oncol, 95(1), 226-230. doi: 10.1016/j.ygyno.2004.07.022

Kaatsch, P., Spix, C., Hentschel, S., Katalinic, A., Luttmann, S., Stegmaier, C., . . . Wolf, U. (2013). Krebs in Deutschland 2009/2010. (9 ed.). Berlin: Robert Koch-Institut und die Gesellschaft der epidemiologischen Krebsregister in Deutschland e.V.

Leminen, A., Forss, M., & Paavonen, J. (2000). Wound complications in patients with carcinoma of the vulva. Comparison between radical and modified vulvectomies. Eur J Obstet Gynecol Reprod Biol, 93(2), 193-197.

Levenback, C., Burke, T., Gershenson, D., Morris, M., Malpica, A., & Ross, M. (1994). Intraoperative lymphatic mapping for vulvar cancer. Obstet Gynecol, 84(2), 163-168.

Levenback, C., Coleman, R. L., Burke, T. W., Bodurka-Bevers, D., Wolf, J. K., & Gershenson, D. M. (2001). Intraoperative lymphatic mapping and sentinel node identification with blue dye in patients with vulvar cancer. Gynecol Oncol, 83(2), 276-281. doi: 10.1006/gyno.2001.6374

Lin, J., DuBeshter, B., Angel, C., & Dvoretsky, P. (1992). Morbidity and recurrence with modifications of radical vulvectomy and groin dissection. Gynecol Oncol, 47(1), 80-86.

Lucci, A., McCall, L. M., Beitsch, P. D., Whitworth, P. W., Reintgen, D. S., Blumencranz, P. W., . . . American College of Surgeons Oncology, G. (2007). Surgical complications associated with sentinel lymph node dissection (SLND) plus *axillary lymph node dissection compared with SLND alone in the American College of Surgeons Oncology Group Trial Z0011. J Clin Oncol, 25(24), 3657-3663. doi: 10.1200/JCO.2006.07.4062*

Madhuri, T. K., Tailor, A., & Butler-Manuel, S. (2011). *Use of neutral plasma coagulation in groin node dissection for vulvar malignancy: a novel technique. Cancer Manag Res, 3, 253-255. doi: 10.2147/CMR.S19467*

Magrina, J., Gonzalez-Bosquet, J., Weaver, A., Gaffey, T., Webb, M., Podratz, K., & Cornella, J. (1998). *Primary Squamous Cell Cancer of the Vulva: Radical versus Modified Radical Vulvar Surgery. Gynecol Oncol, 71(1), 116-121.*

Manci, N., Marchetti, C., Esposito, F., De Falco, C., Bellati, F., Giorgini, M., . . . Panici, P. B. (2009). *Inguinofemoral lymphadenectomy: randomized trial comparing inguinal skin access above or below the inguinal ligament. Ann Surg Oncol, 16(3), 721-728. doi: 10.1245/s10434-008-0216-4*

Mansel, R. E., Fallowfield, L., Kissin, M., Goyal, A., Newcombe, R. G., Dixon, J. M., . . . Ell, P. J. (2006). *Randomized multicenter trial of sentinel node biopsy versus standard axillary treatment in operable breast cancer: the ALMANAC Trial. J Natl Cancer Inst, 98(9), 599-609. doi: 10.1093/jnci/djj158*

Morrow, C., & Townsend, D. F. (1987). *Malignant tumors of the vulva. In C. T. Morrow, DF. (Ed.), Synopsis of Gynecologic Oncology (3 ed., pp. 60-86). New York: John Wiley & Sons*

Morrow, M., Rademaker, A. W., Bethke, K. P., Talamonti, M., Dawes, L. G., Clauson, J., & Hansen, N. (1999). *Learning sentinel node biopsy: results of a prospective randomized trial of two techniques. Surgery, 126(4), 714-720.*

Noventa, M., Ancona, E., Cosmi, E., Saccardi, C., Litta, P., D'Antona, D., . . . Gizzo, S. (2014). *Usefulness, methods and rationale of lymph nodes HPV-DNA investigation in estimating risk of early stage cervical cancer recurrence: a systematic literature review. Clin Exp Metastasis, 31(7), 853-867. doi: 10.1007/s10585-014-9670-5*

Noventa, M., Ancona, E., Saccardi, C., Litta, P., D'Antona, D., Nardelli, G. B., & Gizzo, S. (2014). *Could HPV-DNA test solve the dilemma about sentinel node frozen section accuracy in early stage cervical cancer? Hypothesis and rationale. Cancer Invest, 32(5), 206-207. doi: 10.3109/07357907.2014.889707*

Oonk, M. H., van Os, M. A., de Bock, G. H., de Hullu, J. A., Ansink, A. C., & van der Zee, A. G. (2009). *A comparison of quality of life between vulvar cancer patients after sentinel lymph node procedure only and inguinofemoral lymphadenectomy. Gynecol Oncol, 113(3), 301-305. doi: 10.1016/j.ygyno.2008.12.006*

Patrelli, T. S., Gizzo, S., Peri, F., Franchi, L., Volpi, L., Esposito, F., . . . Modena, A. B. (2013). *Impact of Highly Active Antiretroviral Therapy on the Natural History of Cervical Precancerous Lesions: A 17-Year Institutional Longitudinal Cohort Study. Reprod Sci, 21(7), 837-845. doi: 10.1177/1933719113512531*

Podratz, K., Symmonds, R., Taylor, W., & Williams, T. (1983). *Carcinoma of the vulva: analysis of treatment and survival. Obstet Gynecol, 61(1), 63-72.*

Pompeo, A., Tobias-Machado, M., Molina, W. R., Lucio, J., 2nd, Sehrt, D., Pompeo, A. C., & Kim, F. J. (2013). *Extending boundaries in minimally invasive procedures with simultaneous bilateral video endoscopic inguinal lymphadenectomy (veil) for penile cancer: initial Denver health medical center and ABC school of medicine experience and surgical considerations. Int Braz J Urol, 39(4), 587-592. doi: 10.1590/S1677-5538.IBJU.2013.04.18*

Purushotham, A. D., Upponi, S., Klevesath, M. B., Bobrow, L., Millar, K., Myles, J. P., & Duffy, S. W. (2005). *Morbidity after sentinel lymph node biopsy in primary breast cancer: results from a randomized controlled trial. J Clin Oncol, 23(19), 4312-4321. doi: 10.1200/JCO.2005.03.228*

Rouzier, R., Haddad, B., Dubernard, G., Dubois, P., & Paniel, B.-J. (2003). *Inguinofemoral dissection for carcinoma of the vulva: effect of modifications of extent and technique on morbidity and survival. Journal of the American College of Surgeons, 196(3), 442-450. doi: 10.1016/s1072-7515(02)01895-1*

Saccardi, C., Gizzo, S., Noventa, M., Anis, O., Di Gangi, S., Patrelli, T. S., . . . Nardelli, G. B. (2014). *High-risk human papillomavirus DNA test: could it be useful in low-grade cervical lesion triage? Five-year follow-up. Reprod Sci, 21(2), 198-203. doi: 10.1177/1933719113492214*

Siegel, R., Ma, J., Zou, Z., & Jemal, A. (2014). *Cancer statistics, 2014. CA Cancer J Clin, 64(1), 9-29. doi: 10.3322/caac.21208*

Siller, B., Alvarez, R., Conner, W., McCullough, C., Kilgore, L., Partridge, E., & Austin, J. (1995). *T2/3 Vulva Cancer: A case-control study of triple incision versus en bloc radical vulvectomy and inguinal lymphadenectomy. Gynecol Oncol, 57, 335-339.*

Soliman, A., Heubner, M., Kimmig, R., & Wimberger, P. (2012). *Morbidity of inguinofemoral lymphadenectomy in vulval cancer. ScientificWorldJournal, 2012, 341253. doi: 10.1100/2012/341253*

Stehman, F. (2007). *Invasive cancer of the Vulva. In D. P. a. C. W (Ed.), Clinical Gynecologic Oncology (7th ed., pp. 235-264): Mosby*

Stehman, F., Bundy, B. N., Dvoretsky, P. M., & Creasman, W. T. (1992). *Early stage I carcinoma of the vulva treated with ipsilateral superficial inguinal lymphadenectomy and modified radical hemivulvectomy: a prospective study of the Gynecologic Oncology Group. Gynecol Oncol, 79(4), 490-497.*

Sultana, N., & Naz, S. (2007). *Radical vulvectomy by two different surgical incisions. J Pak Med Assoc, 52(2), 74-77.*

Sutton, A. J., Barton, P., Sundar, S., Meads, C., Rosenthal, A. N., Baldwin, P., . . . Roberts, T. E. (2013). *Cost-effectiveness of sentinel lymph node biopsy vs inguinofemoral lymphadenectomy in women with vulval cancer. Br J Cancer, 109(10), 2533-2547. doi: 10.1038/bjc.2013.631*

Taussig, F. (1940). *Cancer of the vulva: an analysis of 155 cases. . Am J Obstet Gynecol, 40, 764-779.*

Tobias-Machado, M., Tavares, A., Ornellas, A. A., Molina, W. R., Jr., Juliano, R. V., & Wroclawski, E. R. (2007). *Video endoscopic inguinal lymphadenectomy: a new minimally invasive procedure for radical management of inguinal nodes in patients with penile squamous cell carcinoma. J Urol, 177(3), 953-957; discussion 958. doi: 10.1016/j.juro.2006.10.075*

Van der Zee, A. G., Oonk, M. H., De Hullu, J. A., Ansink, A. C., Vergote, I., Verheijen, R. H., . . . Sluiter, W. J. (2008). *Sentinel node dissection is safe in the treatment of early-stage vulvar cancer. J Clin Oncol, 26(6), 884-889. doi: 10.1200/JCO.2007.14.0566*

Way, S. (1978). *The surgery of vulval carcinoma: an appraisal. Clin Obstet Gynaecol, 5(3), 623-628.*

Yuan, J. B., Chen, M. F., Qi, L., Li, Y., Li, Y. L., Chen, C., . . . Liu, L. F. (2014). *Preservation of the saphenous vein during laparoendoscopic single-site inguinal lymphadenectomy: comparison with the conventional laparoscopic technique. BJU Int. doi: 10.1111/bju.12838*

Zhang, X., Sheng, X., Niu, J., Li, H., Li, D., Tang, L., . . . Li, Q. (2007). *Sparing of saphenous vein during inguinal lymphadenectomy for vulval malignancies. Gynecol Oncol, 105(3), 722-726. doi: 10.1016/j.ygyno.2007.02.011*

Growths of the Cervix

Nirmala Duhan* and Mansi Juneja*

1 Benign Growths of the Cervix

1.1 Cervical Myomas

Cervical myomas are firm smooth muscle tumors that comprise about 3-8% of all myomas (Patel *et al.*, 2011). They are usually solitary and may arise from any part of the cervix. Majority of these actually arise from the uterine isthmus but the relative paucity of smooth muscle fibers in the cervical stroma may contribute to their apparent cervical origin. Most often the lesions are asymptomatic. When symptomatic, the presentation includes meno-metrorrhagia, blood tinged vaginal discharge and urinary symptoms like urgency, dysuria and frequency of micturition. At times, the myoma acquires a peduncle and is then termed cervical myomatous polyp. The condition is diagnosed by symptomatology and examination. Rarely, the polyp may extend outside the introitus (1 and 2) but is most often evident on a speculum examination which reveals a red, shaggy, rounded mass projecting out of the cervix. A larger cervical myoma may appear to be filling the upper vagina. Bimanual digital evaluation may reveal a large circular mass in upper vagina with the opposite cervical lip appearing stretched over the mass while a normal sized uterus may be felt sitting atop the large mass (Figure 3).

Microscopically, these tumors consist of circular smooth muscle bundles interspersed with thick, hyalinised blood vessels which are thought to be the source of origin of this tumor in the cervix (hence the term 'vascular leiomyoma').

The management depends on the symptoms, tumor size, patient's age and future reproductive plans. Very small and asymptomatic lesions qualify for expectant management while the larger ones may be treated surgically (myomectomy or hysterectomy). Medical treatment in the form of GnRH analogues may be used preoperatively to reduce the size and vascularity of the tumor though the cleavage planes may be obscured at surgery by these agents. Lateral growing myomas may invade between the leaves of the broad ligament and tend to push the ureters and uterine vessels posterolaterally thus posing a surgical challenge. For this reason, a preoperative intravenous pyelogram may be helpful in the presence of large cervical myomas. This anatomic proximity to important structures predisposes to increased risk of bladder, ureter or vascular injury. Rarely, urethrovaginal fistula may result due to a prolapsed cervical myoma (Lal *et al.*, 2006). Occasionally, a large cervical myoma may elongate and prolapse out of the uterus and even out of the introitus and present with retention of urine. Uterine artery embolization has also been tried as a conservative therapy and may predispose to degeneration and subsequent prolapse of the cervical tumor. A small pedunculated myomatous cervical polyp may be removed surgically by twisting the mass on its stalk while a large myoma with a thick stalk may be enucleated vaginally after clamping, cutting and

---

* Department of Obstetrics and Gynaecology, Pandit Bhagwat Dayal Sharma Post Graduate Institute of Medical Sciences, Rohtak, India

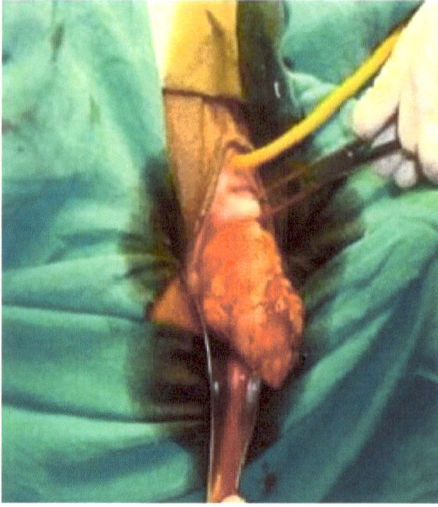

Figure 1: A small cervical polyp protruding at the external os.

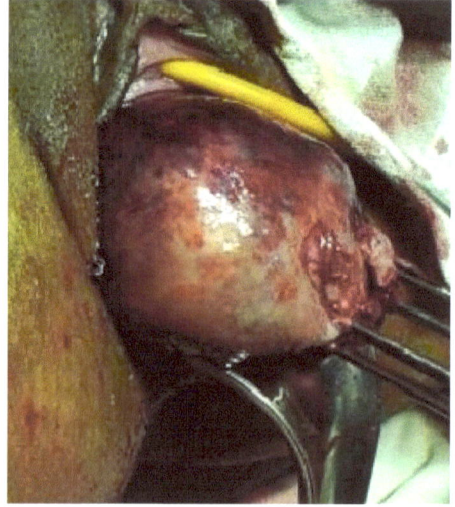

Figure 2: A large myomatous cervical polyp coming out of the introitus.

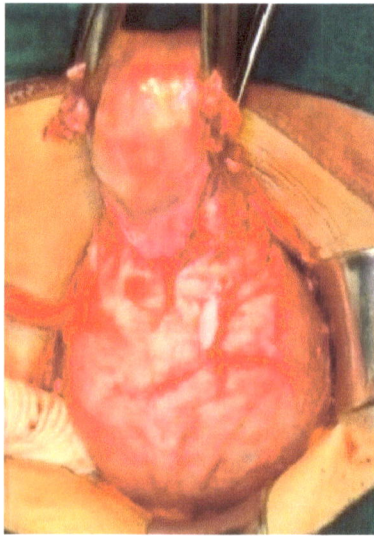

Figure3: An intraoperative picture showing a normal sized uterine body sitting atop a large cervical myoma.

ligating it. Large sessile cervical myomas are better approached abdominally and a myomectomy or hysterectomy may be carried out laparoscopically or by laparotomy, depending on the patient's age and desire for fertility preservation.

Microscopically, these tumors consist of circular smooth muscle bundles interspersed with thick, hyalinised blood vessels which are thought to be the source of origin of this tumor in the cervix (hence the term 'vascular leiomyoma').

The management depends on the symptoms, tumor size, patient's age and future re-productive plans. Very small and asymptomatic lesions qualify for expectant management while the larger ones may be treated surgically (myomectomy or hysterectomy). Medical treatment in the form of GnRH analogues may be used preoperatively to reduce the size and vascularity of the tumor though the cleavage planes may be obscured at surgery by these agents. Lateral growing myomas may invade between the leaves of the broad ligament and tend to push the ureters and uterine vessels posterolaterally thus posing a surgical challenge. For this reason, a preoperative intravenous pyelogram may be helpful in the presence of large cervical myomas. This anatomic proximity to important structures predisposes to increased risk of bladder, ureter or vascular injury. Rarely, urethrovaginal fistula may result due to a prolapsed cervical myoma (Lal *et al.*, 2006). Occasionally, a large cervical myoma may elon-gate and prolapse out of the uterus and even out of the introitus and present with retention of urine. Uterine artery embolization has also been tried as a conservative therapy and may pre-dispose to degeneration and subsequent prolapse of the cervical tumor. A small pedunculated myomatous cervical polyp may be removed surgically by twisting the mass on its stalk while a large myoma with a thick stalk may be enucleated vaginally after clamping, cutting and li-gating it. Large sessile cervical myomas are better approached abdominally and a myomec-tomy or hysterectomy may be carried out laparoscopically or by laparotomy, depending on the patient's age and desire for fertility preservation.

They are benign tumors projecting above the surface of the ectocervix and are found in 0.03- 1.4% of cervical biopsies (Simcock, 1994). Histologically, they consist of stratified squa-mous epithelium covering papillaryprocesses of connective tissue. The average age at presen-tation is 20 years in non-pregnant and 24 years in pregnant women.

1.2 Cervical Papillomas

Vaginal discharge is the commonest presenting symptom though the condition may be totally asymptomatic and may be detected incidentally at routine vaginal examination. Rarely, it may cause intermenstrual bleeding. A speculum examination may reveal multiple papillomas on the cervix which may also be present in the vagina. Cervical malignancy forms an im-portant differential diagnosis of this condition. Fluhmann in 1966 described two varieties of cervical papillomas.

1. Multiple papillomas on the cervix and similar lesions elsewhere in the genital tract (condyloma acuminata).

2. Solitary papilloma: This type was divided into two subtypes by Hertig and Gore (1960) on the basis of whether a co- existing pregnancy is present or not - papillomas of pregnancy and true papillomas.

The disease is caused by various strains of Human Papilloma Virus (HPV) and is most often self-limiting.

1.3 Cervical Endometriosis

The ovaries are the commonest sites affected by endometriosis, followed by uterosacral liga-ments and posterior uterine serosal surface. Rarely, the cervix, lungs, brain and eyes may also be involved. The condition is commonly asymptomatic and may be diagnosed on abnormal

Pap smear reports, at colposcopy or on histology of cervical biopsy or hysterectomy specimen. While endometriosis presents chiefly as dysmenorrhoea (in 60-80%women), infertility (in 30-40%) and pelvic pain (in 30-50%), cervical endometriosis may cause intermittent metrorrhagia and post coital bleeding in 12.5% cases (Veiga-Ferreira *et al.*, 1987). The lesions on the cervix are commonly flat, circular and cherry red or blue in colour. Rarely, they may be polypoid or may appear as a uterine like mass within the cervix (Kano &Kand, 2003; Fukunaga, 2001).

Cervical endometriosis, like endometriosis elsewhere, is affected by ovarian sex steroid variations during the menstrual cycle. As a result Pap smears of the affected women are likely to be misinterpreted as atypical glandular cells of undetermined significance (AGUS), high grade squamous intraepithelial lesion (HSIL) or adenocarcinoma in situ(Symonds *et al.*,1997; Lundeen *et al.*, 2002). FNAC has also been used to diagnose cervical endometriosis but is not the preferred modality (Veiga-Ferreira *et al.*, 1987).

Endometrioid adenocarcinoma and clear cell adenocarcinoma arising from cervical endometriosis have also been reported (Park *et al.*, 2009; Hiromura *et al.*, 2009). It has also been documented in a case of malignant pleural mesothelioma mimicking cervical cancer (Engel *et al.*, 2011).

Symptomatic cervical endometriosis responds to superficial electrocauterization, laser or cryotherapy. Sonography has also been used to localize and aspirate deep endometriotic cyst of the cervix (Coccia *et al.*, 2010).

1.4 Cervical Haemangioma

Vascular tumors, usually cavernous haemangiomas, are rare benign lesions arising from the cervix with less than 50 cases reported till date (Ozyer *et al.*, 2006). Most of these are asymptomatic and are detected incidentally on histology of hysterectomy specimens. Occasionally, they may present as menometrorrhagia and contact bleeding in women between 28 to 60 years of age (Bharti & Shah, 2012).Baxi in 2005 reported incidental detection of cavernous haemangioma in the cervix of a 61 years old lady who had undergone hysterectomy for uterine prolapse. Rarely the condition may cause intractable cervical bleeding requiring emergency hysterectomy (Riggs *et al.*, 2003). Attempts at biopsing the cervix in unsuspecting cases may result in torrential, life-threatening haemorrhage. Rapid growth in pregnancy is common and the condition is an important non placental cause of antepartum haemorrhage (Petry *et al.*, 1994).

Hemangioma of the cervix may occur in association with focal nodular hyperplasia of the liver and both these congenital vascular anomalies may exhibit increased growth under the influence of exogenous sex steroid administration (Padmanabhan *et al.*, 2001). The diagnosis can also be aided by sonography and magnetic resonance imaging though it is most often diagnosed on a speculum and vaginal examination (Haws, 1991). Cervical malignancy is an important differential diagnosis of the condition.

1.5 Cervical Tuberculosis

Cervical tuberculosis accounts for 0.1- 0.65% of all cases of tuberculosis and 5-24% cases of genital tract tuberculosis (Carter, 1990; Chowdhury, 1996). The condition commonly affects women of reproductive age group and is most often secondary to primary pulmonary affection. The fallopian tubes are invariably affected by genital tuberculosis through direct or lymphatic routes. Rarely, the cervix may be the primary site of infection from an infected partner (Richards & Angus, 1998).

The condition is usually asymptomatic or presents as vague abdominal or pelvic pain, menstrual irregularity (usually hypomenorrhoea) or infertility. Speculum examination of the cervix may reveal a vegetative or papillary growth accompanied at times by ulceration and may mimic a cervical malignancy (Shobin *et al.*, 1976).

Cervical cytology may occasionally reveal granulomata but the diagnosis is confirmed only if caseating granulomas are evident on histology of a cervical biopsy specimen. Conditions like sarcoidosis, schistosomiasis, brucellosis, amoebiasis and tularemia may cause a similar histological presentation and these conditions should also be excluded (Koller, 1975). The isolation of Mycobacterium tuberculosis from the lesion remains the gold standard for diagnosis even as one-third cases are culture negative. Polymerase Chain Reaction (PCR) for the causative organism is more sensitive but less specific than culture.

Pelvic ultrasound and magnetic resonance imaging have a limited role in the diagnosis. Pelvic lymphadenopathy and radiological appearance of the uterus mimicking that of Asherman's Syndrome may beevident due to extensive destruction of endometrium and intrauterine adhesions (Lamba *et al.*, 2002).

Multiagentantitubercular therapy for 6-9 months usually causes regression of the disease. Serial cervical biopsy specimens can confirm a therapeutic response though restoration of fertility may still be compromised due to healing by fibrosis (Lamba *et al.*, 2002; Sinha *et al.*, 1997).

2 Malignant Growths of the Cervix

Normally the ectocervix is lined by squamous epithelium, the endocervix and the glands have a tall columnar lining while the stroma is made of fibroblasts, muscle fibers, vessels and nerves. Usually the epithelial proliferation takes an upper hand as compared to the mesenchymal proliferation.

2.1 Carcinoma of the Cervix

Carcinoma of the uterine cervix is one of the leading causes of cancer death among women worldwide and it continues to be a significant health care problem especially in the third world countries. Cervical cancer is the third most common cancer in the world ranking after breast (1.38 million cases) and colorectal cancer (0.57 million cases) and the fourth mostcommon cause of cancer death ranking below breast (458,000 deaths), lung (427,000 deaths) and colorectal cancer (288,000 deaths). Eighty-five percent of all cervical cancers and 88% of all deaths caused by cervical cancer occur in developing countries (Ferlay *et al.*, 2010).

More than 80% of cases of carcinoma cervix are diagnosed at an advanced clinical stage and five-year survival in them is less than 40% (Siegel *et al.*, 2011). In many developed nations, a decline in the incidence and mortality caused by cervical cancer has been observed in the past 30 years as a result of screening by cytology. It is considered a preventable disease given its long pre- invasive state, availability of cervical cytology screening programmes and effective treatment of pre-invasive lesions. The mean age for cervical carcinoma is 47 years and the distribution of cases is bimodal, with peaks at 35 to 39 years and 60 to 64 years of age.

2.1.1 Risk Factors

Young age at first intercourse (less than 16 years), high parity, multiple sexual partners, chronic immune suppression, lower socio-economic status, race and consumption of tobacco are some of the risk factors for carcinoma cervix (International Collaboration of Epidemiological studies of Cervical Cancer, 2007). Oral contraceptive use has been proposed to increase cervical glandular abnormalities by causing cervical ectropion thus exposing the transformation zone to potential carcinogens. However, a definite role is debatable.

Infection with human papilloma virus (HPV) is believed to play a causal role in the development of cervical cancer, with herpes virus and Chlamydia trachomatis being cofactors. The role of HIV in causation of cervical cancer is believed to be mediated through immune suppression (Munger *et al.*, 1992).

2.1.2 Clinical Features

Vaginal bleeding is the most common symptom of carcinoma cervix. Most often, it presents as postcoital bleeding, but may occur as menorrhagia, metrorrhagia or post- menopausal bleeding. Many patients with advanced disease have a profuse and often malodorous discharge. Women with late stage disease may have obstructive uropathy, weight loss and obstructive bladder or bowel symptoms. Involvement of the lumbosacral and sciatic nerve roots by the disease may result in excruciating chronic pelvic bone pain radiating down the leg. Edema of the lower extremities may indicate obstruction of lymphatic or venous drainage by the malignant process.

In asymptomatic women, cervical cancer is most commonly identified through abnormal cytology screening evaluation. As the false negative rate for Pap smear in the presence of invasive cancer can be as high as upto 50%, a negative Pap test should not be relied upon in a symptomatic patient (Sasieni *et al.*, 2009).

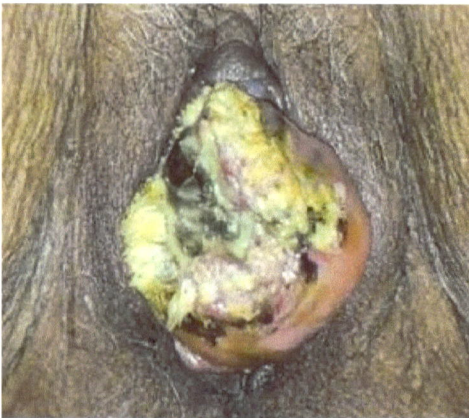

Figure 4: Fungating pale growth of the cervix coming out of the introitus.

2.1.3 Screening for Carcinoma Cervix

According to ACOG 2009, screening for cervical cancer should begin at the age of 21 years, regardless of the age of onset of sexual activity. It is recommended every 2 years for women aged 21-29 years with either conventional or liquid-based cytology.

More frequent screening is required in women who are infected with human immunodeficiency virus (HIV), are immunosuppressed (such as those who have undergone renal transplantation), exposed to diethylstilbestrol in utero or have been previously treated for CIN 2, CIN 3 or frankly invasive cancer.

Primary HPV testing is not FDA approved. However HPV co-test with cytology can be done for age >30 years, no more than every 3 years, if HPV negative and cytology normal, but not in women younger than 30 years. The screening should continue upto age 65-70 years with 3 consecutive normal cytology tests and no abnormal tests in the past 10 years; an older woman who is sexually active and has multiple partners should continue to have routinescreening (ACOG, 2009).

2.1.4 Evaluation

The supraclavicular, axillary and inguino-femoral lymph nodes should be examined to exclude the presence of metastatic disease in women with invasive cervical malignancy. On speculum examination vagina and cervix are inspected for suspicious areas. This may be aided by visual inspection after application of 3-5% acetic acid (VIA- Visual Inspection after Acetic acid) or Lugol's iodine (VILI- Visual Inspection after Lugol's Iodine) application can be done. The suspicious areas appear as noticeable opacity against normal pinkish hue of the cervix (Miller & Elkas, 2009). There may be a pale or cherry red, friable growth that bleeds to touch.

Digital examination may reveal a hard punched out or elevated growth on the cervix. It is important to establish cervical size and consistency and parametrial extension, particularly in women with endocervical malignancy. Rectal examination is important to help establish parametrial extension and involvement of rectal mucosa & is the only way to determine cervical size in women in whom the vaginal fornices have been obliterated by menopausal changes or by extension of the disease to parametrium (Miller & Elkas, 2009).

When obvious tumor growth is present, a cervical biopsy is sufficient for diagnosis. If gross disease is not present, a colposcopic examination with cervical biopsies and endocervical curettage is warranted. If the diagnosis cannot be established conclusively with colposcopy and directed biopsies, which may be the case with endocervical carcinoma, cervical conization may be necessary.

2.1.5 Spread of Carcinoma Cervix

Cervical carcinoma spreads by direct invasion (into the cervical stroma, corpus, vagina, and parametrium), through lymphatics (to pelvic and para-aortic lymph nodes), blood or by intraperitoneal implantation. Lesions that involve the cervix and vagina are designated as cervical primaries.

2.1.6 Staging of Cervical Carcinoma

Cervical cancer is a clinically staged disease. The FIGO staging system is applicable to all histologic types of cervical cancer. Table 1 depicts the FIGO staging system for carcinoma cervix.

The staging procedures recommended by FIGO are listed in Table 2. Investigations like lymphangiography, computed tomography (CT), magnetic resonance imaging (MRI), positron emission tomography (PET) suffer from poor sensitivity, high false-negative rates and variable availability. When there is doubt/ ambiguity about stage allocation, the earlier stage should be selected. After a clinical stage is assigned and treatment is initiated, the stage must not be changed because of subsequent findings by either extended clinical staging or surgical staging. The accuracy of clinical staging is limited as lymph node involvement, an important factor that affects prognosis, cannot be assessed, and thus surgical evaluation, although not practical and feasible in all patients, can more accurately identify metastatic disease (Miller & Elkas, 2009).

Stage I	The carcinoma is strictly confined to the cervix (extension to the corpus should be disregarded).
IA	Invasive carcinoma which can be diagnosed only by microscopy, with deepest invasion ≤ 5 mm and largest extension ≥ 7 mm
IA1	Measured stromal invasion of ≤ 3.0 mm in depth and extension of ≤ 7.0 mm
IA2	Measured stromal invasion of > 3.0 mm and not > 5.0 mm with an extension of not > 7.0 mm
IB	Clinically visible lesions limited to the cervix uteri or pre-clinical cancers greater than stage IAa
IB1	Clinically visible lesion ≤ 4.0 cm in greatest dimension
IB2	Clinically visible lesion > 4.0 cm in greatest dimension
Stage II	Cervical carcinoma invades beyond the uterus, but not to the pelvic wall or to the lower third of the vagina.
IIA	Without parametrial invasion
IIA1	Clinically visible lesion ≤4.0 cm in greatest dimension
IIA2	Clinically visible lesion >4 cm in greatest dimension
IIB	With obvious parametrial invasion (a). All macroscopically visible lesions — even with superficial invasion — are allotted to stage IB carcinomas. Invasion is limited to a measured stromal invasion with a maximal depth of 5.00 mm and a horizontal extension of not >7.00mm. Depth of invasion should not be >5.00mm taken from the base of the epithelium of the original tissue superficial or glandular. The depth of invasion should always be reported in mm, even in those cases with "early (minimal) stromal invasion" (~1 mm). The involvement of vascular/lymphatic spaces should not change the stage allotment. (b). On rectal examination, there is no cancer-free space between the tumor and the pelvic wall. All cases with hydronephrosis or non-functioning kidney are included, unless they are known to be due to another cause.
Stage III	The tumor extends to the pelvic wall and/or involves lower third of the vagina and/or causes hydronephrosis or non-functioning kidney.
IIIA	Tumor involves lower third of the vagina, with no extension to the pelvic wall
IIIB	Extension to the pelvic wall and/or hydronephrosis or non-functioning kidney
Stage IV	The carcinoma has extended beyond the true pelvis or has involved (biopsy proven) the mucosa of the bladder or rectum. A bullous edema does not permit a case to be allotted to Stage IV.
IVA	Spread of the growth to adjacent organs
IVB	Spread to distant organs

Table 1: FIGO Staging of Carcinoma of the cervix uteri (2009).

Physical examination	Palpate lymph nodes
	Examine vagina
	Bimanual rectovaginal examination anaesthesia
Radiologic studies	Intravenous pyelogram
	Barium enema
	Chest X-ray
	Skeletal X-ray
Procedures (a)	Biopsy
	Conization
	Hysteroscopy
	Colposcopy
	Endocervical curettage
	Cystoscopy
Optional studies (b)	Proctoscopy
	Computerized axial tomography
	Lymphangiography
	Ultrasonography
	Magnetic resonance imaging
	Positron emission tomography
	Radionucleotide scanning
	Laparoscopy

(a)   Allowed by the International Federation of Gynecology and Obstetrics (FIGO).

(b)   Information that is not allowed by FIGO to change the clinical stage preferably under.

Table 2: Staging Procedures.

2.1.7 Treatment Modalities

The therapeutic modalities for cervical carcinoma include surgery, radiation, chemotherapy and a combination of chemo-radiation. The modality chosen depends on the clinical stage and while radiation therapy can be used in all stages of the disease, surgery is limited to patients with stage I or IIa disease. Table 3 summarizes the stagewise management of the disease.

The 5-year survival rate for stage I cancer of the cervix is approximately 85% with either radiation therapy or radical hysterectomy (Brewster *et al.*, 2001). Surgical treatment may be preferred in the young as vaginal length is better preserved with surgery. Moreover, the ovaries may be left behind at surgery in these women without compromising results. Optimal therapy consists of either radiation or surgery so as to limit the increased morbidity of combination therapy.

Surgery

The surgical options for management of cervical cancer include conization, radical trachelectomy and radical hysterectomy.

Conization

Conization not only confirms the diagnosis but is also a treatment modality for stage IA1 disease when preservation of fertility is desired. For effective treatment, there must be no lymphvascular space invasion (LVSI) and both endocervical margins and curettings must be nega-

Stage	Extend	Therapeutic modality
IA1	≤3mm invasion, noLVSI	Conization or type I hysterectomy
	≤3mm invasion, w/LVSI	Radical trachelectomy or type II radical hysterectomy with pelvic lymphadenectomy
IA2	>3-5mm invasion	Radical trachelectomy or type II radical hysterectomy with pelvic lymphadenectomy
IB1	>5mm invasion, <2cm	Radical trachelectomy or type III radical hysterectomy with pelvic lymphadenectomy
	>5mm invasion, >2cm	Type III radical hysterectomy with pelvic lymphadenectomy
IB2		Type III radical hysterectomy with pelvic and para-aortic lymphadenectomy or primary chemoradiation
IIA1, A2		Type III radical hysterectomy with pelvic and para-aortic lymphadenectomy or primary chemoradiation
IIB, IIIA, IIIB		Primary chemoradiation
IVA		Primary chemoradiation or primary exenteration
IVB		Primary chemotherapy ±radiation

Table 3: Management of invasive cancer of the cervix (FIGO, 2009)

tive for dysplasia or anaplasia. If the endocervical margins or curettings are positive for dysplasia or malignancy, further treatment is necessary as there may be residual disease. In cases of adenocarcinoma in situ, the status of the cone margins is particularly important as there may be residual pre-invasive and invasive disease in upto 25% and 3% respectively, of cases with negative margins and upto 80% and 7% respectively in cases with positive margins (Wolf *et al.*, 1996).

Radical Trachelectomy

Radical trachelectomy is increasingly being used for women with stage IA2 and IB1 disease, who desire uterine preservation and fertility (Hopkins, 2000). The intent of the procedure is to resect the cervix, upper 1-2 cm of the vagina, parametrium and paracolpos similar to radical hysterectomy but sparing the uterine corpus. It is a fertility sparing surgery and is accompanied by cervical cerclage placement. Ideal candidates for this procedure are those with tumors less than 2 cm in diameter and negative lymphnodes. Lymph node dissection can be performed at the beginning of the procedure, and depending on the results, the procedure can be continued or abandoned further. Although radical trachelectomy is performed with curative intent, it must be remembered that if a recurrence develops, definitive therapy with surgery or radiation is necessary.

Type I Hysterectomy

Type I or simple extrafascial hysterectomy is an appropriate therapy for stage IA1 tumors without LVSI in women who are not desirous of future fertility.

Radical Hysterectomy

Primary radical surgery should be done if it is likely to result in complete removal of the central tumor with an adequate margin of tumor free tissue around it. This surgery should not be performed with the idea that radiotherapy with and/or chemotherapy can be used postoperatively to eliminate residual fragments of tumor tissue left behind after incomplete resection. Such women are better treated with concurrent pelvic radiation and chemotherapy from the outset. Various types of radical hysterectomy are Type II, III, IV and V (Piver *et al.*, 1974). Table 4 outlines the differences between type II and III procedures.

	Type II hysterectomy	Type III hysterectomy
Parametrium & paracolpos	Parametrium and paracolpos near the ureteral dissection	Divided near the sidewall lateral to ureter
Uterine vessels	Ligated at the level of ureter, preserving the ureteral branch to the ureter	Ligated at origin from hypogastric vessels
Anterior & posterior vesicouterine ligament	Anterior ligament is divided but posterior is conserved	Both ligaments are divided
Vaginal cuff	1-2cm removed	Upper one third removed

Table 4: Differences between type II & III Radical Hysterectomy (Boyce *et al.*, 1981)

In type IV extended radical hysterectomy, the periureteral tissue, superior vesicle artery, and as much as three fourths of the vagina is removed. In the type V operation, portions of the distal ureter and bladder are resected. However these procedures are rarely performed because radiotherapy can be used when extensive disease is encountered (Piver *et al.*, 1974).

Ovarian Conservation

Although the incidence of ovarian metastasis is slightly higher in women with adenocarcinoma of the cervix as compared to squamous cell carcinoma, ovarian conservation is recommended in young women (FIGO, 2009). Inpremenopausal patients, the ovaries may be surgically transposed to the paracolic gutters before initiation of radiotherapy (ovariopexy).

Pelvic Lymphadenectomy

The primary group of lymphnodes draining the cervix is parametrial, internal iliac, external iliac and obturator group of nodes. The lymphatics from primary group drain into common iliac and superior lumbar group. At the time of surgery lymphnodes that are suspicious for gross disease should be excised and evaluated by frozen section. If metastatic disease is identified, consideration should be given to abandoning radical surgery in favor of primary chemo-radiation therapy (Miller & Elkas, 2009). If the patient has no gross evidence of metastatic disease, the pelvic lymphadenectomy should be combined with the primary surgery.

Complications of Radical Hysterectomy

A variety of complications may result from radical surgery for carcinoma cervix. Hemorrhage (0.8%), pulmonary embolism (1-2%), small bowel obstruction (1%), ureterovaginal (1-2%) and vesicovaginal fistula (1%) formation and febrile morbidity (25- 50%) may complicate the acute phase of surgery (Hopkins, 2000).The subacute complications include bladder dysfunction, venous thrombosis and lymphocyst formation in upto 5% women. Adequate bladder drainage is an important preventive measure in the postoperative period. The pelvis should also be drained of all collected blood at the end of surgery. However, routine placement of pelvic drains at surgery is not recommended. Bladder denervation may cause chronic bladder hypotonia in 3% women (Boyce *et al.*, 1981). Nerve sparing radical hysterectomies have been described in an attempt to diminish the bladder dysfunction, sexual dysfunction andcolorectal motility disorders.

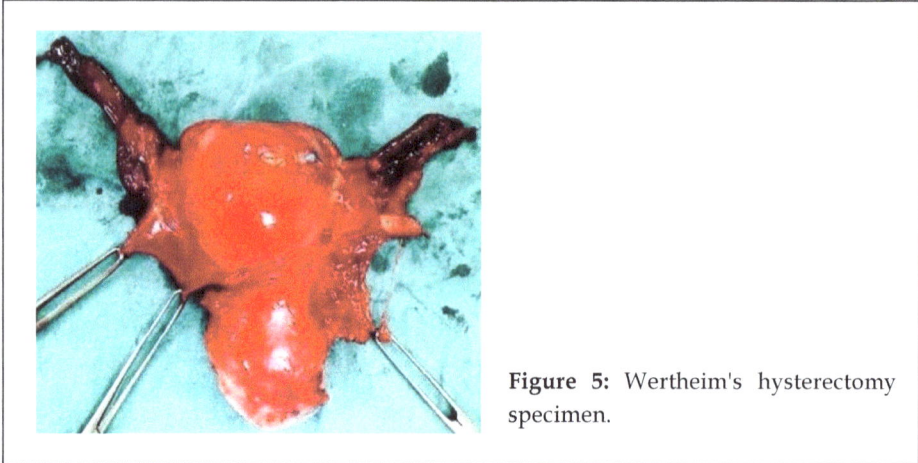

Figure 5: Wertheim's hysterectomy specimen.

Advantages of Surgery over Radiation Therapy for Early Stage Disease

The cure rates of primary radiation therapy and primary radical surgery are almost equal for early stage disease. Table 5 compares the surgical and radiation modalities of therapy for early cancer cervix.

Parameter	Surgery	Radiation
Survival	85%	85%
Serious complications	Urologic fistulas 1 – 2 %	Intestinal and urinary strictures and fistulas1.4% - 5.3%
Vagina	Initially shortened, but may leng then with regular intercourse	Fibrosis and stenosis, particularly in postmenopausal patients
Ovaries	May be conserved	Destroyed
Chronic effects	Bladder atonyin 3%	Radiation fibrosis of bowel and bladder in 6 – 8%
Applicability	Best candidates are those younger than 65years, weight<200lbs	All patients are eligible
Mortality	1% (surgical or anaesthetic complications)	1% (from pulmonary embolism during intracavitary therapy)

Table 5: Comparison of Surgery versus Radiation for Stage IB/IIA Cancer of the Cervix (Brewster *et al.*, 2001).

Athough neither surgery nor radiation is without complications, primary radical surgery offers several advantages for early stage disease (Hatch *et al.*, 1984). It helps in accurate evaluation of the extent of the disease and is helpful in determining prognosis by identifying those at greater risk of persistence or recurrence of disease necessitating additional therapy.

Ovariopexy also protects against premature loss of ovarian function following radiation therapy in young women. Marked fibrotic changes in the vagina and paravaginal tissues following radiation treatment may cause vaginal stenosis and dryness. The hypoestrogenism induced by radiation adds to this effect. The surgically shortened vagina on the other hand remains soft, pliant and moist and helps in better preservation of sexual function.

Late complications are less frequent with primary radical surgery while the progressive obliterative endarteritis may cause cystitis, proctitis, enteritis, pyelonephritis and colpocleisis several years after radiation treatment. Moreover, surgery offers psychologic benefits over radiation. Thus radical hysterectomy is preferred in women with early stage disease. However, women with lesions larger than 4 cm in diameter are better managed by primary radiation therapy. The complication rates can be minimized by careful selection of cases (Hatch *et al.*, 1984).

Conclusion

Carcinoma cervix continues to be a major gynecologic malignancy affecting Indian women. Various screening modalities have been devised for early diagnosis. Diagnosis is clinical and is confirmed by cervical histology. With recent advances in radiotherapy, the 5- year survival has improved in the last decade. However, given the large numbers affected by the disease, more needs to be done on the screening front so as to detect more and more cases in pre-invasive and early invasive stages.

2.2 Sarcomas of the Cervix

Primary cervical sarcomas are exceedingly rare neoplasms (<1% of all cervical malignancies) and are believed to be associated with poor prognosis (Rotmensch *et al.*, 1983). Most of the available data regarding these tumors is derived from case reports and small case series. Due to the rare occurrence of these tumors, treatment strategies are often derived from data for uterine and soft tissue sarcomas.

Rhabdomyosarcoma, most commonly of the embryonal subtype, represents the most commonly reported sarcoma at this location. Occuring most often in children and young adults, the tumor is composed of grapelike polypoid nodules commonly known as botryoid sarcoma. The diagnosis depends on the recognition of rhabdomyoblasts on histological examination (Rotmensch *et al.*, 1983).

Since cervical involvement by uterine corpus leiomyosarcomas (LMS) is not uncommon, the diagnosis of a primary cervical LMS requires the exclusion of origin of the tumor from uterine isthmus. Approximately 30 cervical LMS have been reported till date (Wright *et al.*, 2005). They generally occur in the perimenopausal and postmenopausal population in 4th to 6th decades of life. Women with these tumors most often present with abnormal vaginal bleeding and/or abdominopelvic pain and pressure symptoms (Abell & Ramirez, 1973). Grossly, the tumors are typically large, poorly circumscribed masses that either protrude from the cervical canal or widen andexpand it circumferentially (Figure 6 and 7). Kasamatsu *et al.* in 1998 reported the largest cervical LMS weighing 10.5 kg in a 47 year-old woman who had presented with hypermenorrhea and abdominal distention. The central least vascular area of a large leiomyoma may be the site of the sarcomatous change and hypoxia may have a role in its aetiology. The histologic findings for diagnosing cervical LMS should conform to

Norris and Taylor's criteria (1966) for LMS of the uterine corpus. Other criteria were proposed by Bell *et al.* in 1994. Microscopically, they display a spectrum of morphologic subtypes similar to those seen in their corpus counterparts, including the myxoid variant, epithelioid variant and cases with an abundance of xanthomatous cells apart from the conventional types. The epithelioid variety is an extremely rare variety with only 4 cases reported so far (Toyoshima *et al.*, 2005). The tumor is composed of bipolar fibroblasts with bizarre nuclei and light basophilic cytoplasm in myxoid stroma. There may be varying degree of cellular atypia, mitotic activity and coagulative tumor cell necrosis. In 2001 Gotoh *et al.* reported the first case of triple uterine cancer in which cervical epithelioid LMS was found coexisting with endometrial adenocarcinoma and cervical squamous cell carcinoma. Application of judicious immunohistochemical panel is useful. The prognostic indicators include tumor stage, grade and mitotic count. As the number of reported cases in the literature is exceedingly small, the optimum means of managing cervical leiomyosarcoma has yet to be established. Aggressive surgical treatment is the management of choice as these tumors have low metastatic potential.

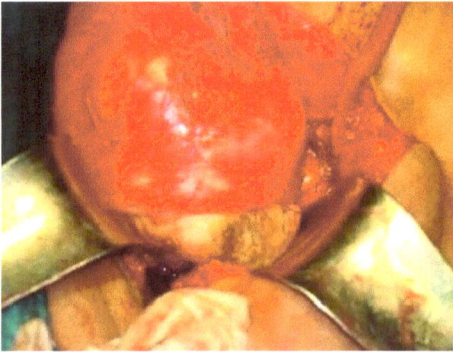

Figure 6: A large cervical leiomyosarcoma protruding out of the vaginal incision at hysterectomy.

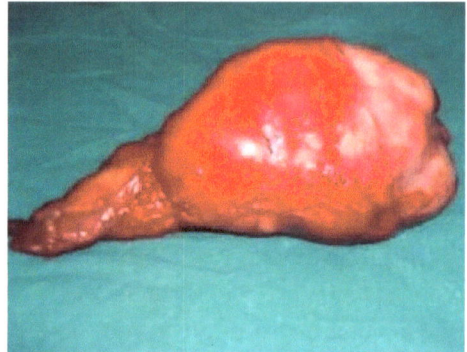

Figure7: Surgical specimen of the uterus with a large leiomyosarcoma of the cervix.

Complete surgical resection with a tumor free margin of 1cm is the treatment of choice. For disease confined to the cervix, total abdominal hysterectomy with bilateral salpingo-oopherectomy is usually sufficient. As these tumors are usually large, neoadjuvant chemotherapy may be given to reduce the size pre-operatively and ensure complete surgical resection (Bhaviskar & Angarkar, 2003).Given the low incidence of lymph node dissemination by eiomyosarcomas, the value of routine lymphadenectomy has been questioned. In the Gynecologic Oncology Group's surgicopathologic evaluation of uterine leiomyosarcomas, the incidence of nodal disease was only 3.5% (Major *et al.*, 1993). Likewise, in over 1200 soft tissue leiomyosarcomas, the incidence of lymph node involvement was found to be only 5.8% (Weingrad & Rosenberg, 1978). Accurate imaging and follow-up is essential for improving survival. There is no firm evidence from prospective studies as to whether adjuvant radiation therapy or chemotherapy is of benefit to women with uterine sarcomas. Several studies show a trend for improved local control in patients receiving pelvic radiation therapy; however, adjuvant radiation therapy does not appear to improve survival for patients with leiomyosarcoma of the uterus (Giuntoli *et al.*, 2003). Similarly, adjuvant chemotherapy has not significantly improved survival for patients with uterine leiomyosarcoma. Most patients with advanced disease are considered to be candidates for chemotherapy due to its tendency to metastasize haematogenously (Giuntoli *et al.*, 2003).

A number of other sarcomas like sarcomatoid carcinomas, adenosarcomas, endometrial stromal sarcomas (ESS), alveolar soft part sarcoma and neurofibrosarcoma have been reported to arise within the cervix (Brown *et al.*, 2003; Fukunaga *et al.*, 1998). Sarcomatoid carcinoma is a distinctive histologic variant of carcinomas typically characterized by a squamous cell component that merges with a spindle cell component. These tumors tend to be aggressive, and most patients with advanced stage disease are refractory to treatment (Brown *et al.*, 2003). Extrauterine endometrial stromal sarcomas (ESS) are rare tumors. Extrauterine ESS commonly arise within foci of endometriosis and histologically resemble ESS found in the uterus. The tumors have been reported in a varietyof locations including the peritoneum, omentum, and ovary. Extrauterine endometrial stromal sarcomas arising in the cervix are uncommon, with only two cases reported so far (Fukunaga *et al.*, 1998).

Based upon the data of sarcomas originating from other sites, it would appear logical to attemptsurgical extirpation in women with tumors confined to the cervix. Management usually consists of total abdominal hysterectomy with bilateral salpingo-oophorectomy followed by combination chemotherapy in the form of VADIC and Hydroxyurea, DTIC and Etoposide (Kasamatsu *et al.*, 1998). Further research into the natural history and optimal management of women with these rare neoplasms is warranted.

2.3 Metastatic Lesions on the Cervix

Metastatic lesions on the cervix from distant primary lesions are rare. Among the genital organs, breast carcinoma may metastasize to the ovaries, endometrium or cervix in that order of frequency. 56 Cervical involvements may be asymptomatic or manifest as intermenstural, postcoital or postmenopausal vaginal bleeding and dyspareunia. These lesions may be picked up on Pap smear or on colposcopy and cervical biopsy. Magnetic Resonance Imaging may detect the cervical mass and/or the parametrial involvement. Histologically, the lesion is identical to that at the primary site. Aggressive treatment of the isolated cervical metastasis is advocated where feasible (Bogoliolo *et al.*, 2010). In others, systemic chemotherapy with taxanes could be beneficial.

References

Abell, M.R., & Ramirez, J.A. (1973). *Sarcomas and carcinosarcomas of the uterine cervix*. Cancer, 31, 1176-1192.

American College of Obstetricians and Gynecologists. *Cervical cytology screening*. ACOG Practice Bulletin Number 109. Obstetrics & Gynecology, 149, 1409-1420.

Baxi, S. *Capillary haemangioma of the cervix- a case report*. (2005). Indian Journal of Pathology & Microbiology, 48(3), 373-375.

Bell, S.W., Kempson, R.L., & Hendrickson, M.R. (1994). *Problematic uterine smooth muscle neoplasms. A clinicopatho logic study of 213 cases*. American Journal of Surgical Pathology, 18(6), 535-558.

Bharti, P., & Shah, S.N. *Cavernous haemangioma of cervix- a case report* (2012). Journal of Indian Medical Association, 110(4), 258.

Bhaviskar, B.P., & Angarkar, N.N. (2003). Leiomyosarcoma of the uterine cervix. International Journal of Scientific Research, 2(4), 257-258.

Bogliolo, S., Morotti, M., ValzanoMenanda, M., Fulcheri, E., Musizzano, Y., & Casabona, F. (2010). Breast cancer with synchronous massive metastasis in the uterine cervix: a case report and review of the literature. Archives of Gynecology and Obstetrics, 281(4), 769-773.

Boyce, J., Fruchter, R., & Nicastri, A. (1981). Prognostic factors in stage I carcinoma of the cervix. Gynecologic Oncology, 12, 154-165.

Brewster, W.R., Monk, B.J., Ziogas, A., Anton-Cluver, H., Yamada, S.D., & Berman, M.L. (2001). Intent- to-treat analysis of stage IB and IIA cervical cancer in the United States: radiotherapy or surgery 1988-1995. Obstetrics & Gynecology, 97(2), 248-254.

Brown, J., Broaddus, R., Koeller, M., Burke, T.W., Gershenson, D.M., & Bodurka, D.C. (2003). Sarcomatoid carcinoma of the cervix. Gynecologic Oncology, 90(1), 23-28.

Carter, J.R. (1990). Unusual presentations of genital tract tuberculosis. International Journal of Gynecology & Obstetrics, 33, 171-176.

Chowdhury, N.N.R. (1996). Overview of tuberculosis of the female genital tract. Journal of Indian Medical Association, 94, 345-361.

Coccia, M.E., Rizzello, F., Castellacci, E., & Cammilli, F. (2010). Sonographic diagnosis of a large and deep endometrioma of the uterine cervix. Journal of Clinical Ultrasound, 38(4), 209-211.

Engel, J.B., Heuer, S., Segerer, S., Rauthe, S., Dietl, J., & Honig, A. (2011). Cervical endometriosis associated with malignant pleural mesothelioma mimicking cervical cancer- Occam's razor or the "third man". Fertility Sterility, 95(5), 1787, e5-7.

Ferlay, J., Shin, H.R., Bray, F., Forman, D., Mathers, C., & Parkin, D.M. (2010). Estimates of worldwide burden of cancer in 2008: GLOBOCON 2008. International Journal of Cancer, 127(12), 2893-2917.

FIGO Committee on Gynecologic Oncology. (2009). Revised FIGO staging for carcinoma of the vulva, cervix, and endometrium. International Journal of Gynecology & Obstetrics, 105, 103-104.

Fluhmann, C.F. (1966). The cervix uteri and its diseases. Philadelphia, Pennyslevania: Saunders.

Fukunaga, M., Ishihara, A., & Ushigome, S. (1998). Extrauterine low-grade endometrial stromal sarcoma: report of three cases. Pathology International, 48(4), 297-302.

Fukunaga, M. (2001). Uterus- like mass in the uterine cervix: superficial cervical endometriosis with florid smooth muscle metaplasia? Virchows Archive, 438, 302-305.

Giuntoli, R.L., Metzinger, D.S., DiMarco, C.S., Cha, S.S., Sloan, J.A., Keeney, G.L., & Gostout, B.S. (2003). Retrospective review of 208 patients with leiomyosarcoma of the uterus: prognostic indicators, surgical management, and adjuvant therapy. Gynecologic Oncology, 89, 460-469.

Gotoh, T., Kikuchi, Y., Takano, M., Kita, T., Ogata, S., & Aida, S. (2001). Epithelioid leiomyosarcoma of the uterine cervix. Gynecologic Oncology, 82(2), 400-405.

Hatch, K.D., Parham, G., Shingleton, H.M., Orr, J.W. Jr, & Austin, J.M. Jr. (1984). Ureteral strictures and fistulae following radical hysterectomy. Gynecologic Oncology, 19, 17-23.

Haws, D.R., Hemann, L.S., Cornell, A.E., & Yuh, W.T. (1991). Hemangioma of the uterine cervix: sonographic and MR diagnosis. Journal of Computer Assisted Tomography, 15(1), 152-154.

Hiromura, T., Tanaka, Y.O., Nishioka, T., Satoh, M., & Tomita, K. (2009). Clear cell adenocarcinoma of the uterine cervix arising from a background of cervical endometriosis. British Journal of Radiology, 82(973), e20-2. DOI: 10.1259/bjr/75304693

Hopkins, M.P. (2000). Adenocarcinoma in situ of the cervix: the margins must be clear. Gynecologic Oncology, 79, 4-5.

International Collaboration of Epidemiological studies of Cervical Cancer. (2007). Comparison of risk factors for invasive squamous cell carcinoma and adenocarcinoma of the cervix: collaborative reanalysis of individual data on 8,097 women with squamous cell carcinoma and 1,374 women with adenocarcinoma from 12 epidemiological studies. International Journal of Cancer, 120, 885-891.

Kano, H., & Kanda, H. (2003). Cervical endometriosis presented as a polypoid mass of portio cervix uteri. Journal of Obstetrics & Gynecology, 23, 84-85.

Kasamatsu, T., Shiromizu, K., Takahashi, M., Kikuchi, A., & Uehara, T. (1998). Leiomyosarcoma of the uterine cervix. Gynecologic Oncology, 69(2), 169-171.

Koller, A.B. (1975). Granulomatous lesions of the cervix uteri in black patients. South African Medical Journal, 49, 1228-1232.

Lal, S., Sowmya, S., Kriplani, Bhatla, N., & Agarwal, N. (2006). Urethrovaginal Fistula due to Prolapsed Cervical Myoma: A Case Report. The Internet Journal of Gynecology and Obstetrics, 7(1).

Lamba, H., Byrne, M., Goldin, R., & Jenkins, C. (2002). Tuberculosis of the cervix: case presentation and the review of literature. Sexually Transmitted Infections, 78, 62-63.

Lundeen, S.J., Horwitz, C.A., Larson, C.J., & Stanley, M.W. (2002). Abnormal cervicovaginal smears due to endometriosis: A continuing problem. Diagnostic Cytopathology, 26, 36-40.

Major, F.J., Blessing, J.A., Silverberg, S.G., Morrow, C.P., Creasman, W.T., Currie J.L., … Brady, M.F. (1993). Prognostic factors in early-stage uterine sarcoma. A Gynecologic Oncology Group study. Cancer, 71(4 Suppl), 1702-1709.

Miller, C., & Elkas, J.C. (2009). Cervical and vaginal cancer. Berek and Novak's Gynaecology (15th ed., pp. 1304-1349). Philadelphia: Lippincott Williams and Wilkins.

Munger, K., Scheffner, M., Huibregtse, J.M., & Howley, P.M. (1992). Interactions of HPV E6 and E7 oncoproteins with tumor suppressor gene products. Cancer Survey, 12, 197-217.

Ozyer, S., Uzunlar, O., Gocmen, M., Bal, S., Srvan, L., & Mollamahmutglu, L. (2006). Cavernous hemangioma of the cervix: a rare cause of vaginal bleeding. Journal of Lower Genital Tract Disease, 10(2), 107-108.

Padmanabhan, V., Mount, S.L., & Eltabbakh, G.H. (2001). Cavernous hemangioma of the cervix in association with focal nodular hyperplasia of the liver. A case report. Journal of Reproductive Medicine, 46(12), 1067-1070.

Park, H.M., Lee, S.S., Eom, D.W., Kang, G.H., Yi, S.W., & Sohn W.S. (2009). Endometrioid adenocarcinoma arising from endometriosis of the uterine cervix: a case report. Journal of Korean Medical Science, 24(4), 767-771.

Patel, P., Banker, M., Munshi, S., & Bhalla, A. (2011). Handling cervical myomas. Journal of Gynecological Endoscopic Surgery, 2(1), 30-32. Doi:10.4103/0974-1216.85277

Petry, K.U., Bernhards, J., & Jagla, K. (1994). Cavernous hemangioma of the uterine cervix in pregnancy. GeburtshilfeFrauenheilkd, 54(1), 62-64.

Piver, M., Rutledge, F., & Smith, J. (1974). Five classes of extended hysterectomy for women with cervical cancer. Obstetrics & Gynecology, 44, 265-272.

Richards, M.J., & Angus, D. (1998). Possible sexual transmission of genitourinary tuberculosis. International Journal of Tuberculosis & Lung Disease, 2, 439.

Riggs, J., Bertoni, M., Schiavello, H., Weinstein, A., & Kazimir, M. (2003). Cavernous hemangioma of the cervix with intractable bleeding. A case report. Journal of Reproductive Medicine, 48(9), 741-743.

Rotmensch, J., Rosenshein, N.B., & Woodruff, J.D. (1983). Cervical sarcoma: a review. Obstetrical & Gynecological Survey, 38, 456-461.

Sasieni, P., Castanon, A., & Cuzick, J. (2009). Screening and adenocarcinoma of the cervix. International Journal of Cancer, 125, 525-529.

Shobin, D., Sall, S., & Pellman, C. (1976). Genitourinary tuberculosis simulating cervical carcinoma. Journal of Reproductive Medicine, 17, 305-308.

Siegel, R., Ward, E., Brawley, O., & Jemal, A. (2011). Cancer statistics, 2011: the impact of eliminating socioeconomic and racial disparities on premature cancer deaths. CA: A Cancer Journal for Clinicians, 61, 12-236.

Simcock, M.J. (1964). Papillomas of the uterine cervix. Australian & New Zealand Journal of Obstetrics & Gynecology, 4, 174.

Sinha, R., Gupta, D., & Tuli, N. (1997). Genital tract tuberculosis with myometrial involvement. International Journal of Gynaecology & Obstetrics, 557, 191-192.

Symonds, D.A., Reed, T.P., Didolkar, S.M., & Graham, R.R. (1997). AGUS in cervical endometriosis. Journal of Reproductive Medicine, 42, 39-43.

Taylor, H.B., & Norris, H.J. (1966). Mesenchymal tumors of the uterus. Archives of Pathology, 82, 40-44.

Toyoshima, M., Okamura, C., Niikura, H., Ito, K., & Yaegashi, N. (2005). *Epithelioid leiomyosarcoma of the uterine cervix: a case report and review of literature. Gynecologic Oncology, 97(3), 957-960.*

Veiga- Ferreira, M.M., Leiman, G., Dunbar, F., & Margolius, K.A. (1987). *Cervical endometriosis: facilitated diagnosis by fine needle aspiration cytologic testing. American Journal of Obstetrics & Gynecology, 157(4 pt1), 849-856.*

Weingrad, D.N., & Rosenberg, S.A. (1978). *Early lymphatic spread of osteogenic and soft-tissue sarcomas. Surgery, 84(2), 231-240.*

Wolf, J.K., Levenback, C., Maslpica, A., Morris, M., Burke, T., & Mitchell, M.F. (1996). *Adenocarcinoma in situ of the cervix: significance of cone biopsy margins. Obstetrics & Gynecology, 88, 82-86.*

Wright, J.D., Rosenblum, K., Huettner, P.C., Mutch, D.G., Rader, J.S., Powell, M.A., & Gibb R.K. (2005). *Cervical sarcomas: An analysis of incidence and outcome. Gynecologic Oncology, 99, 348-351.*